D1490293

Florence Nightingale,
Nursing, and
Health Care Today

Lynn McDonald, PhD, LLD (Hon), completed her doctorate at the London School of Economics and then went on to pursue an academic career, publishing in criminology, political sociology, women's studies, the environment, and classical social theory, with a focus on women theorists. She also served as the president of Canada's largest women's organization and represented it when Canadian women got their "equal rights amendment" in the Charter of Rights. She went on to pursue a parliamentary career, variously working on issues of justice, communications and culture, and the environment. Her Non-Smokers' Health Act, 1988, was the first legislation in the world to establish smoke-free work and public places and influenced similar legislation in many countries. Her main work in recent years has been as director of the 16-volume (peer-reviewed) *Collected Works of Florence Nightingale* (www.uoguelph.ca/~cwfn), available in print and as ebooks. A short book, with highlights from the series, is *Florence Nightingale at First Hand* (2010).

Dr. McDonald currently gives much time and energy to work on the climate crisis. She is a co-founder of JustEarth: A Coalition for Environmental Justice, a voluntary organization, and a former member of the Board of Directors of Climate Action Network, Canada. She is a member of the Order of Canada and has an honorary doctorate.

Florence Nightingale, Nursing, and Health Care Today

LYNN McDONALD, PhD, LLD (HON)

SPRINGER PUBLISHING COMPANY

Copyright © 2018 Springer Publishing Company, LLC

All rights reserved.

No part of this publication may be reproduced, stored in a retrieval system, or transmitted in any form or by any means, electronic, mechanical, photocopying, recording, or otherwise, without the prior permission of Springer Publishing Company, LLC, or authorization through payment of the appropriate fees to the Copyright Clearance Center, Inc., 222 Rosewood Drive, Danvers, MA 01923, 978-750-8400, fax 978-646-8600, info@copyright.com or on the Web at www.copyright.com.

Springer Publishing Company, LLC
11 West 42nd Street
New York, NY 10036
www.springerpub.com

Acquisitions Editor: Margaret Zuccarini
Senior Production Editor: Kris Parrish
Compositor: Newgen KnowledgeWorks

ISBN: 978-0-8261-5558-0
ebook ISBN: 978-0-8261-5559-7

17 18 19 20 / 5 4 3 2 1

The author and the publisher of this Work have made every effort to use sources believed to be reliable to provide information that is accurate and compatible with the standards generally accepted at the time of publication. The author and publisher shall not be liable for any special, consequential, or exemplary damages resulting, in whole or in part, from the readers' use of, or reliance on, the information contained in this book. The publisher has no responsibility for the persistence or accuracy of URLs for external or third-party Internet websites referred to in this publication and does not guarantee that any content on such websites is, or will remain, accurate or appropriate.

Library of Congress Cataloging-in-Publication Data
Names: McDonald, Lynn, 1940- author.
Title: Florence Nightingale, nursing, and health care today / Lynn McDonald.
Description: New York, NY : Springer Publishing Company, LLC, [2018] |
   Includes bibliographical references and index.
Identifiers: LCCN 2017040350 | ISBN 9780826155580 (paper back) |
   ISBN 9780826155597 (ebook)
Subjects: | MESH: Nightingale, Florence, 1820-1910. | Philosophy, Nursing |
   Nurse's Role | Social Responsibility | Moral Obligations | History of Nursing |
   History, 19th Century
Classification: LCC RT84.5 | NLM WY 86 | DDC 610.7301—dc23
LC record available at https://lccn.loc.gov/2017040350

Contact us to receive discount rates on bulk purchases.
We can also customize our books to meet your needs.
For more information please contact: sales@springerpub.com

Printed in the United States of America by McNaughton & Gunn.

Contents

Reviewers

Laurie N. Gottlieb, PhD, RN, LLD (Hon), Professor, Ingram School of Nursing, McGill University, Montreal, Canada

Edward J. Halloran, PhD, RN, FAAN, Professor Emeritus, School of Nursing, University of North Carolina at Chapel Hill, Chapel Hill, North Carolina

Charlene Harrington, PhD, RN, FAAN, Professor Emeritus, School of Nursing, University of California San Francisco, San Francisco, California

Dame Janet Elizabeth Murray "Betty" Kershaw, DBE, FRCN, CStJ, Dean Emeritus, School of Nursing and Midwifery, University of Sheffield, Sheffield, United Kingdom

Preface

So much has been written about Florence Nightingale, as a war heroine, role model, nursing founder, and public health reformer, that one might wonder why another book, now. This book is geared to telling a story that has often been missed or botched by the use of poor secondary sources.

The extent and originality of Nightingale's writing is not fully appreciated. Along with her well-known *Notes on Nursing*—the only one of her books many nurses have read—are two other full books, plus numerous scholarly journal articles; letters to the editor (several substantial); pamphlets; and thousands of letters, professional and personal.

Nightingale material is now available to the dedicated scholar in a 16-volume *Collected Works*, in print and as ebooks. Seven of these volumes have significant amounts of nursing material but busy nurses, administrators, and nursing academics, as well as other health care professionals, may not want to wade their way through so much detail.

Florence Nightingale, Nursing, and Health Care Today is addressed to them, to nursing students, and to the interested general reader. Nightingale was far ahead of her time in setting out the core principles of the new nursing profession, with demanding ethical standards and continuing education to keep up with best practice. She was a gifted political activist who saw enormous strides made in the provision of quality services, including access to care for the most disadvantaged. Yet some of what she advocated has yet to be implemented.

Part I of the book shows what she wrote and did in key areas of nursing and health care: patient care, health promotion, ethics, pediatric care, long-term and palliative care, administration, and research and policy advocacy. Each chapter in this part of the book concludes with a discussion of where we are today on each of these issues.

Part II of the book takes the reader into Nightingale's best writing itself. Much of this material is new, even to nursing academics, for it goes well beyond her *Notes on Nursing*. Indeed, the excerpts from that book are from a seldom-read edition, the one geared to more educated readers. Her late papers show how far nursing had progressed in the decades after *Notes on Nursing* of 1860. The technical demands made on nurses by then were much tougher, reflecting the progress made in medical science. Two of the papers were written specifically for Americans.

Florence Nightingale, Nursing, and Health Care Today also shows how Nightingale interacted with leading physicians and other health science experts. She could draw on the latest information in medicine, medical statistics, and hospital architecture and engineering. She mentored nurses around the world, who brought her new information—material that has received scant attention to date.

My acquaintance with Nightingale comes from her expertise in social science—I am a social scientist, not a nurse or physician. I have also been a successful public health advocate when, as a Canadian Member of Parliament, I authored the Non-Smokers' Health Act of 1988. Thus, I have great appreciation for her ability to use the political process. As nursing and other health care leaders confront today's challenges—access to quality care, the rising cost of services, climate change, and the complications of globalization—Nightingale's willingness to take on the big issues can give us courage. Her goal was always to save lives, and with an impressive team working with her, she used the latest science available. She, and they, did save lives and published the data to prove it!

Nightingale faced and met the greatest challenges of her day. Why should today's nursing and health care leaders not aim just as high?

Lynn McDonald

Acknowledgments

Many colleagues assisted in the preparation of the book, hundreds if the background material on which it drew is considered—the 16 volumes of *The Collected Works of Florence Nightingale*. For the book itself, thanks go to several academic nurses who read an earlier draft of the book (in alphabetical order): Marilyn Gendek, MA, RN; Laurie N. Gottlieb, PhD, RN, LLD (Hon); Charlene Harrington, PhD, RN, FAAN (ret); Edward J. Halloran, PhD, RN, FAAN (ret); Betty Kershaw, DBE, FRCN, CStJ; and Marie Dietrich Leurer, PhD, RN.

Thanks to Patricia Warwick for much assistance in fact checking and proofing. Thanks to Janice Hicks for technical support at the University of Guelph, to Ken Simons, who also acts as technician for the Nightingale Society website, for technical support. Thanks to Margaret Zuccarini, nursing publisher emeritus, at Springer Publishing Company, who was wisdom and practicality at many stages of bringing this book into existence.

Part I: Nightingale's Nursing:
Then and Now

Chapter 1: Florence Nightingale: The Challenge, the Impact

It is Nature that cures, not the physician or nurse.

—Nightingale (1883, p. 1043)

WHY A NEW BOOK NOW

Why a new book now on Florence Nightingale's nursing? Her active career ran roughly from 1850 to 1900, and the bicentenary of her birth is 2020. She is recognized worldwide as the major founder of nursing, and International Nurses' Day is celebrated on her birthday, May 12. She still arouses controversy and probably will continue to, the consequence of the power and originality of her ideas and the concerted campaigns she waged to see serious system changes effected. In any event, few nurses are interested in the history of their profession. Nursing history courses or modules, which previously were common in nursing education, have largely been dropped from the curriculum.

The contention here is that many of Nightingale's key principles are still valid and that not only nurses but also health care decision makers would benefit by paying attention to them. Her insistence on high ethical standards, the centrality of the patient's needs, cautions about innovations—she advocated starting small and evaluating before wider application—are all good advice today. Medical science, technology, and hospital buildings have changed greatly since her day, but the new challenges of antibiotic-resistant disease germs call for new thinking and possibly a revisiting of old techniques. Her pioneering "evidence-based" approach to nursing and health care still holds (McDonald, 2001).

Nursing is not as old as medicine—Nightingale's school opened in 1860, a convenient date to mark the birth of the new profession. Earlier,

there were nuns who gave devoted care, but no regular, trained professionals. Medicine, by contrast, dates back to the fifth century BCE in the West.
Nightingale and her influence, in other words, do not date back to time
immemorial, but to a period not all that different from the present.

The creation of the new profession was a key goal, but nursing itself was
always a means to an end: quality health care. Hospital reform and broader
social reforms thus must always be kept in mind in pursuing Nightingale's
vision and work.

She was exceptionally well educated for her time, able to produce professional level reports and articles in all these areas, some with pioneering
charts to present the data. She was an effective writer, good at one-liners and
the equivalent of sound bites. Some of her ideas have yet to be implemented.

Eight key components of Nightingale's work and vision, it is argued,
are still pertinent to nursing and health care today; however, much of the
details have changed.

1. The prime purpose of nursing is to give high-quality, compassionate,
   patient care, which can be ensured only with adequate training and
   administration.
2. Best practice must evolve with advances in medical science, surgery, and
   related health sciences. Nightingale herself saw great progress made in
   reducing death rates by bringing in improved sanitary measures in the
   Crimean War of 1854–1856. She practiced this precept for the rest of her
   life. Best practice gets lip service routinely now, but serious implementation is more problematic.
3. When changes are made in care, they must be carefully monitored
   for both positive and negative results. Nightingale was herself a pioneer of what came to be called "evidence-based health care." It is
   acknowledged as essential now, although there is much resistance in
   practice.
4. Her goal in health care was quality care for all, including those unable
   to pay. Such a goal assumes a strong component of public provision for
   services, or "universal health coverage." It has been legislated in many
   countries, notably those with a social democratic ethos. The Germans
   pioneered coverage early via social insurance. It was first legislated,
   as a direct service, in Britain in 1946, in the National Health Act, and
   came into force through the National Health Service in 1948. It is perhaps no coincidence that the first instance of universal health care should
   have occurred in the country where the goal was first articulated—by
   Nightingale.

Canada's national Medicare shares this commitment, but with
threats of privatization. The American Affordable Care Act, known as

"Obamacare," extended coverage to millions more uninsured Americans, but still without reaching Nightingale's objective of quality care for all. Abolition of this limited measure was a promise of Donald Trump in his successful presidential election campaign of 2016. However, even with a Republican Congress, he has failed so far to get his substitute American Health Care Act adopted, or to repeal Obamacare. Extensive privatization in the British National Health Service has turned its health care coverage into a two-tier (or more) system, depending on ability to pay. In short, Nightingale's goal of quality care for the poorest as well as the rich is still far from realization. The increased coverage achieved in the United States with Obamacare may be reversed

5. Health status is greatly affected by surrounding environmental conditions, which are themselves influenced by income, status, and other factors, now termed the "social determinants of health." To promote good health thus requires attention to the quality, or not, of housing, nutrition, air, and water. As the gap in income and wealth increases in many countries, people at the bottom are at increased risk of illness and premature death.

As nurses today increasingly take on health care policy issues, Nightingale's example becomes ever more germane.

6. Quality care requires teamwork from many professionals. Nightingale herself led a team of medical doctors, statisticians, engineers, and architects in implementing change post-Crimea. All these professional men deferred to her for her vision, research ability, and effectiveness in implementation. She deferred to them in their areas of expertise.

7. Adequate health and safety measures must be put in place to protect nurses' health. During the 19th century, most nurses lived in hospital or district residences, so this meant measures for comfortable living conditions as well as health and safety on the job itself. Since living accommodation is no longer an issue in most jurisdictions, and unions now attend to working conditions, Nightingale's principles serve here only as a guide for comparison.

8. Priorities for action on health care matters should be based on extent of need and feasibility of achievement. Nightingale took on the highest death rates and worst social conditions of her day, and, with her team, made progress on both. Applying this principle today, the priorities that appear are the threats of climate change, hospital-acquired infections, prescription errors and accidents, lack of access to health care, and the continuing toll of tobacco-related deaths: quite different matters each. Nurses in many jurisdictions are actively involved in variations of these challenges, as policy advocates and experts as well as clinicians.

How far ahead of her time Nightingale was is seen as the developments a century later began to catch up with her eight components of practice. The definition of health, as "a state of complete physical, mental, and social well-being and not merely the absence of disease," adopted by the World Health Organization (WHO, 2017) on its formation in 1948, is an example, discussed further in Chapter 3. The WHO's Alma Ata Declaration of 1978 goes yet further, making "the highest attainable standard of health" to be "a fundamental right of every human being," a statement unanimously agreed to by 113 countries (WHO, 1978). The declaration then specified primary health care to be the chief means to this end. Nightingale did not use rights language herself, but her espousal of access to quality care for the very poorest members of society was an early step toward this understanding.

WHO WAS NIGHTINGALE AND WHAT WAS HER NURSING?

Florence Nightingale (1820–1910) is recognized as the major founder of the modern profession of nursing. Her training school, which opened at St. Thomas' Hospital, London, in 1860, was the first secular nurse training school in the world. That is, while limited training was given to Roman Catholic nuns and Anglican sisters before Nightingale's time, her school accepted pupils (all women at that time) of any faith and no faith. It trained nurses for full-time paid work, with a hierarchy of positions of increasing responsibility and salary to top administration.

The women called "nurses" before her reforms, apart from those in religious orders, were low paid, disreputable, and often drunk. They were mainly used as hospital cleaners. Their "cardinal sin," according to Nightingale, was demanding bribes for their services. Nuns, she readily acknowledged, were an exception to this charge, but not their servants. To establish high ethical standards was a decided challenge for the time (Sellman, 1997), which explains why Nightingale so often said that a "good nurse" had to be a "good woman."

Nightingale chose St. Thomas' for her school as the process of reforming nursing had already started there, with the appointment of Sarah E. Wardroper (1813–1892) as "matron," or nursing director, early in 1854. Wardroper was an army doctor's widow who had never nursed, but she had to earn a living for herself and her children. She raised the standards at St. Thomas', improved the pay and working conditions, and attracted better applicants. Nightingale met her before she left for the Crimea.

When Nightingale began the task of establishing her school post-Crimea, the need for trained nurses had gained wide acceptance. The failings of the old-style "Sairey Gamps" Charles Dickens ridiculed in his novel

Martin Chuzzlewit were well understood. There were serious analyses of the inadequacies as well, which soberly point out that the medical attendant at a hospital had to go his rounds at night to see that the wine or beer ordered for the patients was "not abstracted by the nurses" ("Hospital nurses," 1848, p. 540). But there were still many doctors content with the status quo. An eminent doctor at St. Thomas', Dr. John Flint Snow, published a pamphlet opposing nurse training in 1857, although he did not oppose Nightingale when the school opened.

Medical science, when Nightingale set to work, was at a rudimentary level. Anesthetics were new and experimental. Nightingale promoted their use during the Crimean War, although the principal medical officer, her superior, opposed them. Antiseptic surgery was yet another decade in coming, with Joseph Lister's great breakthrough publication in 1867 (Lister, 1867). Bloodletting, blistering, and violent purging of the bowels were standard treatments. Doctors were frustrated by their inability to treat the great epidemic fevers (typhoid and typhus, cholera, smallpox, measles, dysentery, and diarrhea). They used toxic substances like lead, mercury, arsenic, bismuth, and turpentine. Articles in medical journals, "materia medica," and medical textbooks show how widely accepted use of these substances was. Nightingale preferred cautious doctors and urged caution, which is discussed in Chapter 2 in the section "Heroic Medicine," "Bad Medicine."

Nightingale's "restorative" approach entailed a firm rejection of the prevailing "humors" theory of Galen and other ancients that the world was made up of four elements: air, fire, water, and earth. Human beings and animals, similarly, were thought to be composed of four elements: yellow bile, blood, phlegm, and black bile. Disease was the result of an imbalance in the humors, and so treatment required applying the contrary to redress it. Bloodletting, which continued to be used into the 20th century, was the cure for diseases of the blood, sweating and expectoration for diseases of excessive phlegm (Arikha, 2008, p. 4).

Nightingale nurses had to act on medical orders, and accordingly were trained on the application of leeches, but it seems they never had to participate in the more dire forms of bloodletting, such as by the lancet (the medical journal, *The Lancet*, takes its name from this widely practiced "treatment").

Referencing Nightingale's Work

Great care has been taken in referencing Nightingale's multitudinous writing. For her correspondence and hard-to-find printed works, reference is made to their publication in the *Collected Works of Florence Nightingale*, a sixteen-volume work, in print and ebook (McDonald, 2001–2012), for which there is an associated website that gives transcribed sources, in a searchable database, with biographical data on her correspondents, visitors, and authors she cited (www.uoguelph.ca/~cwfn/archival/index.htm). Manuscript sources cited here, the great number at the British Library, are given only when the item was not published in the *Collected Works* or another printed source.

Nightingale's writings include scholarly journal articles, letters to the editor, pamphlets, and thousands of letters in addition to her well-known full books. Large numbers of letters to and from nurses serve to flesh out what is known of Nightingale from the limited amount of her nursing work available in print. Seven of the volumes in the *Collected Works* have significant amounts of material on nursing. A short book, *Florence Nightingale at First Hand*, gives highlights selected from the whole collection (McDonald, 2010).

Part II of this book provides selections of her most important writing from 1858 to 1893, thus facilitating the tracing of her ideas as they evolved. Quotations in Part I are cross-referenced to those selections.

Because the titles of nursing positions have changed so much over the years, this text uses current terms. Thus, *matrons* and *superintendents*, even *lady superintendents*, have become *directors of nursing* here, except in direct quotations.

THE NEW PROFESSION OF PATIENT CARE

Nightingale's goal was a new, distinctive, profession of patient care. Given the poor educational level of nurses, medical orders would necessarily be the province of the physician or surgeon to determine. However, Nightingale was insistent that all decisions on hiring, promotion, discipline, and dismissal be made by senior nurse administrators, not doctors. A doctor who was dissatisfied with a nurse's performance would take that complaint to the nursing director, who reported to the senior hospital manager, as did the medical director. This manager would desirably not be a doctor—doctors made poor administrators, Nightingale thought. She also thought that they might prefer to practice their profession. To her friend, Sidney Herbert, she joked that there "must be something in the smell of the medicines which induces absolute administrative incapacity" (letter, May 25, 1859, in McDonald, 2009b, p. 123).

There is great misunderstanding in the secondary literature on Nightingale's use of the terms *profession, calling, art*, and *science* in relation to nursing. When it was crucial to demarcate the new trained nurses from the old-style nurses who drank and demanded bribes, Nightingale emphasized "calling." She stressed that it was the training, not the payment, that made someone a nurse, as it did a doctor. However, the profession was always to be paid work, and well paid, with good working conditions and opportunities for career advancement. She particularly regretted the low pay of workhouse nurses when the workhouse infirmaries began to employ trained nurses.

Nightingale had herself experienced a "calling," if not by an audible voice, a clear message she understood to be from God. However, nursing was always to be open to people of any faith or no faith, a secular profession, not a religious order. Its standards included moral qualities as well as technical knowledge and, most importantly, bedside skills, which could be learned only through apprenticeship-type training. Science was always part of the mix, to be introduced gradually—a reasonable strategy at the time, given the lack of education of the first nursing students.

Nightingale also linked "calling" with "enthusiasm":

> What is it to feel a *calling* for anything? Is it not to do our work in it to satisfy the high idea of what is the *right*, the *best*...? This is the "enthusiasm" which everyone...must have in order to follow his "calling" properly. Now the nurse has to do...with living human beings. (Nightingale, 1893, p. 193, in McDonald, 2004, p. 213, in Part II, Chapter 12)

In her article on nursing practice in Quain's *Dictionary*, she described nursing as "an art, and an art requiring an organized practical and scientific training" (Nightingale, 1883, p. 1043, in McDonald, 2009b, p. 736). In places, Nightingale exaggerated the "calling" aspect over the paid professional aspect. However, she strongly opposed unpaid nursing by "ladies" whose families did not want the indignity of their accepting a salary. Most nurses had to earn their living—some were supporting children or an aged parent. Unpaid nursing would depress wages, a decided wrong. A lady who did not need the salary should take it and donate it, Nightingale advised. Agnes Jones (1832–1868), the first professional nursing director of the Liverpool Workhouse Infirmary, who came from a well-off family, did precisely that.

When combating the state registration scheme proposed by the British Nursing Association, Nightingale argued that written examinations could not ascertain moral qualities. An experienced manager seeing the student's work in the ward could. Correspondence with Dr. Henry Acland, regius professor of medicine at Oxford, shows her stressing "calling" and deemphasizing "book learning." Nurse training was more about building character than technical knowledge, and she even said that nursing was not "a profession, but a calling" (letter, April 28, 1893, in McDonald, 2009b, p. 554).

In her 1893 paper, the last discussed in this book, Nightingale conveniently brought together the elements of art, science, profession, and calling. She began by announcing the creation, in the last 40 years of her career, of "a new art and a new science." She referred to a "threefold interest" in a nurse's work: "an intellectual interest in the case, a (much higher) hearty interest in the patient, a technical (practical) interest in the patient's care and cure" (in McDonald, 2004, p. 215, in Part II, Chapter 12). In the 1894 revision to her Quain's *Dictionary* practice article, Nightingale brought calling and technical aspects together. Nursing was "above all, a progressive calling," so that year by year, nurses had to learn "new and improved methods, as medicine and surgery and hygiene improve." Yet "year by year, nursing needs to be more and more of a moral calling" (in McDonald, 2009b, p. 749). Clearly, calling and profession were not either/or for Nightingale but both/and.

As early as her *Notes on Nursing*, Nightingale expressed her appreciation of the increase in knowledge in the medical sciences. Pathology especially— she became interested in it during the Crimean War—had seen a "vast" increase in knowledge, but there was "scarce any in the art of observing the signs of the change while in progress" (Nightingale, 1860, Chapter 13). In a later paper, she deplored doctors behaving "as if the scientific end were the only one in view, or as if the sick body were but a reservoir for stowing medicines into, and the surgical disease only a curious case the sufferer has made for the attendant's special information" (Nightingale, 1860, Chapter 13).

"Calling" for Nightingale personally was religious, as it was for many nurses of her time. Angelique Lucille Pringle (1846–1920) was nursing director at the Edinburgh Royal Infirmary, then later at St. Thomas' Hospital, who shared this sense (she later converted to Roman Catholicism). A Nightingale letter to Pringle refers to God showing "His love in calling us to His work" (letter, August 30, 1873, in McDonald, 2009b, p. 288). In her tribute on the death of Sarah Wardroper, director of nursing at St. Thomas' Hospital, Nightingale credited her with upgrading nursing from its disreputable past, to become a "new calling" (Nightingale, 1894, in McDonald, 2009b, p. 392). The Archbishop of Canterbury, who unveiled the memorial to Wardroper in the chapel at St. Thomas', made it a "high and holy calling" (Archbishop of Canterbury, 1894). In a late letter to nurses in 1897, Nightingale prayed that they would all be "true to our calling" (in McDonald, 2009b, p. 879), all the while insisting that the profession be open to believers of any or no faith.

In her last "address" to nursing students and former students, in 1900, Nightingale affirmed that nursing had "become a profession." Trained nursing was no longer an object, but "a fact." She also urged her nurses to "always keep up the honor of this honorable profession" (in McDonald, 2009b, pp. 880–881).

Working and Living Conditions for Nurses

All the while, Nightingale was also active in promoting decent wages and salaries and working and living conditions for nurses, all essential for the recruitment of better qualified people to the profession, in place of the old-style drunken nurses. She accepted that hours would be long for nursing students and nurses, but was most insistent that, when they reached the "Home" at the end of the day, they would find comfortable and warm quarters, good food with adequate variety, and a glass of wine. Much correspondence went to this endeavor. The point had to be made forcefully and often to hospital architects and administrators that nurses' residences had to provide private rooms (the walls must go up to the ceiling), have a window (which must open to the outside), decent furniture (chair, bookcase), and adequate washing and toilet facilities (separate from those used by patients). These were the responsibility of the director of nursing to ensure.

Nursing was onerous work, A nurse who had to get her own food and cook it, "'dog tired' from her patients," could be only "half a nurse," Nightingale explained in a fund-raising letter for a residence for district nurses: "she cannot do real nursing, for nursing requires the most undivided attention of anything I know…all the health and strength, both of mind and body," She repeated the point at the end of her appeal, asserting that "district nurses have quite other things to do than to cook for and wait upon themselves. They are the servants, and the very hard-worked servants, of the poor sick" (Nightingale, 1876, in McDonald, 2009a, p. 756, in Part II, Chapter 11).

Nightingale stipulated a month's holiday for all nurses. Isabel Hampton Robb, an American nursing leader, was content to accept 2 weeks. She, however, was successful in instituting an 8-hour day and substantially reduced the drudgery.

GENDER ISSUES IN NURSING

The profession Nightingale founded was geared to women, for good, historic reasons. When her school opened in 1860, women were not permitted in any profession—not the civil service, armed forces, politics, or religion as priests, ministers, or rabbis. Her goal in founding the profession was to improve patient care, not to provide jobs for women, but such jobs, with good salaries and working conditions, were a serious secondary objective. Nightingale recognized that men could be good nurses, and she expected that army nursing would be done mainly by men. She accordingly paid great attention to the selection, training, administration, and working conditions of men providing nursing care. This also held for nursing in the navy, but she was only peripherally involved in this issue.

Nightingale did not believe that being a woman made one a nurse, although women were typically expected, as women, to take on those tasks.

She was complimentary about men who were good nurses. Men in nursing are a logical development as the health care professions opened up to women. Here Nightingale's references to nurses are put into the plural where possible, to avoid expressions such as "the nurse, she," often coupled with the "doctor, he," which of course were correct statements in her day, with the occasional exception, late in her life, of a female doctor.

Many nursing leaders seem not to have understood the gender differences in education and opportunities that shaped the founding of their profession. Given these realities, why would anyone accuse Nightingale of "gender bias" or discrimination (Burkhardt, Nathaniel, & Walton, 2010, p. 7)?

A paper on men in nursing was critical of Nightingale, citing many negative secondary sources on the point, but not one by Nightingale herself (Brown, Nolan, & Crawford, 2009). These authors, further, had Nightingale's (presumed) opposition to men in nursing to cause her to "denounce male asylum nurses," considering that their duties were more like those "of prison warders than to nurses in general hospitals." Given that mental asylums at that time lacked trained nurses, they probably were.

Treiber and Jones (2015) oversimplified considerably, and incorrectly dated *Notes on Nursing* to 1881, having it set the "foundations for nursing as women's work" and even that Nightingale believed that it was "by its very definition, 'women's work,'" when she herself stressed that *training* was essential.

Nightingale knew men with good nursing skills, as correspondence with and about them shows. Sir Harry Verney's butler, for example, was an able observer on his employer's and other family members' illnesses, trusted to report both to the doctor and to her, and to administer medicines and food. He was the "excellent" and "admirable" Morey in 1889 correspondence, when he sent telegrams with urgent specifics and kept an hourly diary on the patient. Captain, later Sir, Edmund Verney was another who merited the "admirable nurse" title, again not for professional nursing but in the care of a family member at home (letter, February 6, 1889, Wellcome Ms 9012/110).

General Charles Gordon (1833–1885) would become known as "Chinese Gordon" for his exploits in China, then "Gordon of Khartoum," when he was assassinated there, but Nightingale saw him as a fellow nurse and hospital reformer. She praised him after his death for making his "battlefield" the hospital, the workhouse, the slums, the streets, and ragged schools: "His love of the sick and his experience made him of the same profession as I am." She commended him also for his earlier work in England when he looked after "waifs and strays" with fever at his own home. She recounted later that he had told her that, if his country did not require him for other service, "he hoped to devote the remainder of his life to hospitals" (letter, August 30, 1886, in 5:508).

That Gordon's opinion of nurses was high can be seen in his statement that he had not suffered "1/20 the part" of what the hospital nurse suffers, who, "forgotten by the world, drudges on in obscurity" (Gordon letter, April 22, 1880, in 5:492). He looked after his men when they were sick, and won their loyalty.

NURSE–PHYSICIAN RELATIONS

The physician prescribes for supplying the vital force, but the nurse supplies it.
—Nightingale (1893, p. 186, in McDonald, 2004,
p. 208, in Part II, Chapter 12)

In Nightingale's conceptualization, the nurse would always work under the orders of a physician or surgeon who made the diagnosis, prescribed any drugs and stimulants, and directed the treatment. Given the low educational level of nurses in her time, this could not have been otherwise. Women were excluded from universities and even secondary schools. Yet this seems to have escaped the notice of more recent commentators, so that Nightingale is said to have "deprofessionalized" relations between nursing and medicine (Gamarnikow, 1978, p. 114), as if those relations had been professional before.

Nightingale's challenge was to raise the status of the old-style nurse from that of a domestic servant to a junior professional. To make persons short of a secondary school education the equals of those holding a university degree and professional qualifications would be unrealistic.

With the great improvement in education since then, greater independence of nurses is possible. Nurse practitioners are a logical development of Nightingale's nursing. She anticipated—and promoted—rising standards in the proficiency required. Nurses had to keep up with advances in medical science and practice.

Nightingale has been much criticized for her insistence that nurses work under medical orders. It should be noted, however, that obedience was always qualified, "*intelligent* obedience," as she often said, meaning with discretion. She was influenced on this point by her early experience at Kaiserswerth: "There were the young deaconesses with their intelligent, animated, countenances, no mere instruments yielding a blind and passive obedience, but voluntary and enlightened agents, obeying, on conviction, an inward principle" (cited by Robb, 1912, p. 27). A Christmas letter to the first trained nursing director and nurses at Addenbrooke's Hospital, Cambridge, remarked on the obedience expected in the past. Then a nurse "was simply told what had to be done, and ordered to go and do it. *Now*, the utmost pains are taken to show her *why* it has to be done and *how*" (Nightingale, 1877).

Nightingale continued to make the point, for example, in 1890, that a nurse was not an "automaton," but "an intelligent human being who has to do with matters of life and death" (Nightingale, 1890, in McDonald, 2012, pp. 829–830). In her Quain's *Dictionary of Medicine* article on hospital nursing of 1883, the qualification was that the nurse must act "intelligently, using discretion" (in McDonald, 2009b, p. 751). In the nurse training article, also, she described training as enabling "the nurse to act for the best in carrying out her orders, not as a machine but as a nurse." The nurse was not to be "servile, but loyal to medical orders and authorities" (in McDonald, 2009b, p. 735). She contrasted the obedience required of a nurse with that of a soldier, who had no discretion to disobey orders.

While the doctor determined the diagnosis and treatment, the nurse had the ongoing task of carrying out the plan, observing its effects, and reporting back. As Nightingale put it, "The physician prescribes for supplying the vital force, but the nurse supplies it" (Nightingale, 1893, in McDonald, 2004, p. 208, in Chapter 12). In serious cases, long before the availability of antibiotics, the nurse's role could be critical. Some early doctors called for the establishment of nurse training for nurses precisely because this role was so crucial. The point is pursued in Chapter 2.

Status Issues and Titles: "Doctor," "Nurse," and First Names

Finally, on the use of titles and honorifics, it should be noted that Nightingale always referred to both doctors and nurses by their titles and surnames, such as "Dr. Sutherland," "Miss Jones," "Mrs. Wardroper," "Sister Charity," that being the name of the ward in her charge, never by their first names. Doctors and nurses, then, spoke to each other as fellow professionals, although not on an equal basis. The practice began some decades ago of nurses using first names for themselves and patients (whether they like it or not), while deferring to doctors with title and surname: "Dr. Smith will see you now, Sally," whatever the respective ages of the doctor and patient. This practice also violates Nightingale's goal that nurses be the patient's "advocate," for doctor superiority is enforced even when the patient objects. Why should today's nurses be status enforcers for doctors?

Raising the status of nurses took concerted efforts over many years. Nightingale was ever the stickler for cleanliness, and nurses should clean when the cleaner failed to do the job (the nurse had to check on the result).

But trained nurses were not the hospital cleaners of the old system. It was the hospital's responsibility to hire adequate staff, an ongoing problem as hospitals trim their budgets by contracting out these essential services.

> *A nurse must not be a scrubber. And a scrubber cannot be a nurse.*
> —Nightingale (1863, p. 54)

Nightingale's use of surnames and honorifics for nurses and nursing students shows her insistence that they be treated as professionals, when domestic servants were called by their first name if they were young, or surname if older, but not an honorific and surname. She insisted that the nursing director and nurses sent to Australia travel first class, as medical doctors would.

NIGHTINGALE'S MENTORING OF NURSES

Nightingale became a long-term mentor for many nurses trained at her school, assisting them with applications for higher posts, writing and organizing letters of references, and helping with advice and moral support when problems arose, as they very often did with those who became nursing directors.

To ensure that they were well prepared for the post in question, she sought short-term placements to give the person relevant experience. This could be done by the nurse filling in for a nursing director on a summer break.

Many of the nurses who obtained administrative positions needed advice and assistance on occasion. Nightingale made time for periodic meetings and invited those with difficulties to let her know. A number of nursing administrators faced opposition from their hospital authorities. Several were subjected to protracted investigations. Nightingale was usually able to help considerably, always gave comfort, but could not get every hospital to reverse a decision against a nursing head.

To boost a new director's status, Nightingale often sent a gift, such as flowers, to be delivered on her starting day, signaling to the administration that the new head had Nightingale herself watching over her.

Much information is available on this mentoring process, since Nightingale kept both the letters these nursing heads and senior nurses sent her and the notes she took of meetings with them. Correspondence from them shows gratitude for the understanding and support they got (often, Nightingale's letter to the nurse is missing). Nightingale understood that these early nursing administrators were on the firing line. They were typically the first trained head the hospital had ever had, for the old-style "matron" was merely the housekeeper, in charge of the female servants and linen. Some doctors were content with the old-style nurses or even preferred them. Nightingale mentored the next two generations of nursing leaders, not only in the United Kingdom, but also in Europe and the United States.

Nightingale understood that nursing, as medicine, surgery, and public health, was a work in progress. Nurses would have to renew and upgrade their skills to keep up with the demands on them. That was one reason why she so adamantly opposed the state registration scheme as it was initially formulated: It certified nurses immediately after their training and could not reflect the person's competence even a few years later. The answer to that concern is now typically met, in nursing as in many other professions, with required upgrading courses.

In her article on nurse training for Quain's *Dictionary of Medicine*, Nightingale suggested that a nurse needed "every five or ten years...after leaving the hospital, a second training nowadays." This followed from the advances made by "medicine, surgery, pathology, and above all hygiene [public health]" (Nightingale, 1883, Vol. 2, p. 1043).

Nightingale's writing shows that she paid great attention herself to keeping up with developments. She continued to debrief knowledgeable people about their work, into late in life. Her papers show her tracking operating theater preparations in 1896 (notes, August 1896, in McDonald, 2009b). Nurses visiting from other countries told her of improvements made there. British nurses visiting Europe reported back on innovations in place. A plague nurse in India gave her the latest news on inoculation in 1898. Nightingale was a dedicated and effective networker, yet one more reason why her writing is of such great interest.

NIGHTINGALE'S REPUTATION: HIGHS, LOWS, AND MISCONCEPTIONS

Nightingale was revered as the founder of nursing for decades after her death. Her status as a national heroine in the Crimean War was only the start. Her own school and her decades-long mentoring of nursing leaders around the world ensured that she was held in high regard. Nightingale's principles still appear frequently in nursing textbooks, but the fact of their origin in her writing is often unacknowledged.

The image of the "lamp" and use of the Nightingale pledge, which she did not write, are tributes to her influence but convey nothing of her own considered views. She has not been taught seriously in nursing schools in the West for decades. She typically gets casual mention in classes or a few lines or a paragraph or two in nursing texts, but seldom more.

Some nursing textbooks give at least minimal recognition of her work (Burkhardt et al., 2010; Chaska, 2001; D'Antonio, 2010; Ellis, Nowlis, &

Bentz, 1992; Haynes, Boese, & Butcher, 2004; Hinchliff, Norman, & Schober, 1994; Kelly & Joel, 1996; Lindeman & McAthie, 1999; Meleis, 1991; Taylor, Lillis, & LeMone, 1993).

Gottlieb is a significant exception to the general trend in drawing inspiration from Nightingale in her "strengths-based" philosophy of nursing (Gottlieb, 2012, pp. 41–42). "Strengths-based care" placed the person and family at the center; encouraged people to take charge of their own health, recovery, and healing; and required collaboration between the person/family and the health care provider. Gottlieb saw Nightingale using "strengths" in formulating health care policy, entailing "knowledge of people, their environments, and the political and social structure." The approach, Gottlieb contended, would help nursing get back on to Nightingale's vision and would move both nursing and the health care system in a new and better direction (p. 41).

Environmentally oriented nurses are also exceptional in continuing to find favor in Nightingale, for her highlighting the importance of environmental conditions in disease causation and healing (Libster, 2008; Selanders, 1993). For example, "Nightingale's environmental theory provides a basis for further theoretical development in nursing" (Hegge, 2013, p. 219). Her "thirteen canons," on ventilation, and so forth, differ "in specifics of application today, but the underlying principles remain sound" (Lobo, 2002, p. 59). A school of "holistic nursing" draws considerably on Nightingale (Dossey & Keegan, 2013), with a journal that reports on her influence, *The Journal of Holistic Nursing*. She is given enormous credit by environmentalists who work on health issues (Davies, 2013).

Meleis concluded that "Nightingale's attempts to establish professional nursing based on nursing's unique concern with environment for promotion of health were pre-empted by an illness-oriented training," which made it dependent on medicine (Meleis, 1991, p. 35). He evidently regretted that her followers, who continued to accept her advice on education and apprenticeship, "failed to continue in her footsteps, to differentiate the focus and goals of nursing and medicine and failed to further her theorization of nursing. Somehow the medical paradigm, better developed and more powerful, replaced what was starting to become a nursing paradigm (that is, concept of health, hygiene, environment and care)." The environment, he judged, has continued to be a central concept in nursing, but it is not treated with the same depth and conviction that Nightingale gave it (Meleis, 1991, pp. 190–191).

A nursing textbook credited Nightingale with being "an environmentalist before the term was ever coined." Both her *Notes on Nursing* and *Notes on Hospitals* provided "guidelines for ensuring the optimal physical environment for health and healing," including, in the latter, "detailed instructions on unit design so that patients are in clean, safe, and attractive surround-ings" (Lindeman & McAthie, 1999, p. 895).

Otherwise, however, it seems that the occasional reprinting of her iconic *Notes on Nursing* has been deemed a sufficient memorial to Nightingale, but typically not the best edition is chosen, and the introductions, by busy nursing administrators and academics, have missed a lot. *Notes on Nursing* predates the founding of her school and was not intended for professional hospital nurses, much as it is useful for setting out the basic principles of her environmental theory. A major example of comments from a "commemora-tive" edition is given in Part II, Chapter 10. These include obvious factual errors and even snide remarks.

Nursing textbooks with lists of models or systems of nursing begin with Nightingale's, typically noting its environmental focus. A major example specified 24 models, in five categories, beginning with Nightingale, flag-ging her "conditions for reparative process" theme (Potter, Perry, Ross-Kerr, & Wood, 2009, Table 5.1, p. 95). Henderson and Nite in 1978 cited three med-ical doctors and eight nursing theorists who articulated theories of nursing after Nightingale (Chapter 1). A more recent source has more than 20 theo-rists from Nightingale's environmental theory in 1860 to 2001 (Johnson & Webber, 2010).

Numerous examples could be cited of textbooks that use core Nig-htingale points without mentioning her name once. In a chapter on infection prevention and control, for example, five specific practices were outlined as necessary for all health care workers: handwashing, safe disposal of clini-cal material, wearing protective clothing, aseptic technique, and personal hygiene (Peto, 2004). All of these were assiduously promoted by Nightingale in her various writings.

Nightingale's reputation, as Sellman put it mildly, has been "tarnished" with the distortion of her approach, notably "by the zeal in which obedience above all else came to be seen as the primary virtue in a nurse." He referred to the "backlash of opinion" on her, adding, in understatement: "It is not fashionable to hold Nightingale in high esteem." He thought that she was unduly blamed for much of what is wrong in contemporary nursing, the result of her followers developing "a narrow interpretation of much of her work" (Sellman, 1997). This, in turn, results in her not being read directly, in favor of reliance on inadequate secondary sources.

The decline of interest in Nightingale's nursing in the West was accel-erated by a series of attacks, beginning with one by an Australian medi-cal historian (Smith, 1982). The second major author to attack her, focusing on her Crimean War work, was a management consultant (Small, 1998). Nurses, in other words, were not the instigators, but neither did any leading nurse or nursing organization defend her against either book, both of which were based on gross neglect of key sources and incorrect citation of others. Two films of the British Broadcasting Corporation broadcast hostile views of Nightingale to large audiences (BBC1, 2001; BBC2, 2008), rebroadcasted often in other countries. Several detailed refutations of Smith's often preposterous claims (1982) have already been published, with references to primary sources that counter his points (McDonald, 2001, Appendix B, 2009a, 2010, Secondary sources on Nightingale and the Crimean War). Further material on the attack on her reputation is provided in the Appendix to this chapter.

Statisticians have consistently, from her day to the present, treated Nightingale as a major and valuable contributor to their discipline. The president of the American Statistical Association in 2016 focused on Nightingale in her "President's Corner" article (Utts, 2016). A Nobel Prize winner in economics, Sir Richard Stone, gave her a high place in the history of social statistics (Stone, 1997).

That Nightingale continues to be valued as a social scientist can be seen in her inclusion in the *Palgrave Handbook of Social Theory in Health, Illness, and Medicine* (McDonald, 2015). There are sections on her in three earlier books on social theorists (McDonald, 1993, 1994, 1998), with substantial excerpts from her writing in the last of these three.

Hospital architects continue to pay tribute to her great reforms in the late 19th century and see parallels in the more "environmental" approach of the 21st century (Hammond, 2005; Marcus & Barnes, 1999; M. Nightingale [no relation], 1982; Verderber, 2005). Her high reputation in these fields holds for Britain, the United States, and Canada.

Misconceptions about Nightingale include unwarranted praise. She has often been credited with achievements not due her, nor which she ever claimed. The prime example is that of attributing the dramatic decline in hospital death rates during the Crimean War to her and her nurses' work (Haynes et al., 2004; Hood & Leddy, 2006; Kelly & Joel, 1996). She has also been incorrectly credited with inventing the triage of wounded soldiers during the war (Munro, 2010). These, and other, errors occur from citing poor secondary sources, not using Nightingale's own work. She herself gave the credit for the great reductions in death rates to the Sanitary and Supply Commissions.

Misconceptions on Germ Theory

One old favorite misconception has Nightingale as a lifelong denier of germ theory, stated by American (Kelly & Joel, 1996; Lundy & Bender, in Lundy & Janes, 2009), British (Baly & Matthew, 2004), Australian (Godden, 2006), Dutch (van der Peet, 1995), and Canadian (Helmstadter, 1997) nursing academics. There are misinformed medical doctors (Ayliffe & English, 2003; Cope, 1963; Wolstenholme, 1971), a director of the Army Medical Department (Cantlie, 1974), medical, military, and political historians (Brighton, 2004; Cannadine, 1998; Hays, 1998), plus a historian of ideas (Reverby, 1987); one medical historian published this incorrect view three times (Rosenberg, 1979, 1989, unpaged introduction, 1992).

According to a social historian, Nightingale was such a staunch opponent of germ theory that she went to her grave "believing that disease was caused by a bad smell" (Halliday, 2007, p. 81). Yet, if so, why did she state that the nurse "must be taught the nature of contagion and infection, and the distinctions between deodorants, disinfectants, and antiseptics," and that lives might have been saved had precautions always been "scrupulously observed" (Nightingale, 1883, Vol. 2, p. 1047)? She warned, in a late note, that "the risk with 'disinfectants'" was "that people think, if the smell is destroyed, the danger is gone" (note, British Library, Add Mss[1] 47767 f212).

Hospital architects tend to be highly favorable to Nightingale, but several, nonetheless, fell for the denier-of-germ-theory line (Stevenson, 2000; Thompson & Goldin, 1975). Numerous other examples are available (McDonald, 2009b), but those cited here are exceptional in coming from highly reputable authors and publishers, indeed from authors who otherwise made excellent contributions on her work.

One would have to have a badly distorted understanding of history to expect to see germ theory in her books of 1858 to 1863, before there was any documentation of the theory. That she did accept it can be seen in a publication in an Indian journal, where she urged that lectures be organized for villagers, with slides to show "the noxious living organisms in foul air and water," and thus prompt them to examine their water supply and take precautions (Nightingale, 1892, in Vallée, 2007, p. 363).

This "elite" list of misinformed authors should serve as a caution: Misconceptions about Nightingale are all too available, and great care must be taken in using sources.

FROM NIGHTINGALE'S VISION TO NURSING TODAY

The prime purpose of this book is to bring Nightingale's ideas and work to the attention of nurses today, not as a historical figure but as a source of principles, vision, and sound practice in the here and now. It is directed especially to nurses who have heard almost nothing about her in their training, or heard only the "tarnished" version.

---

[1] Further references to Add Mss (Additional Manuscripts) are also to the British Library.

This is not the place to describe what Nightingale did to establish professional nursing in any particular country, as much material is available elsewhere (McDonald, 2009a). The point is that she is a particularly useful source for nursing in countries where educational requirements are high and the profession well developed. In the United States and Canada, nurse practitioner positions are increasingly available. Many nurses take degrees past the bachelor's level, increasingly of doctorates. "Centers of excellence" promote a high level of professional activity. Some professional associations speak out on health care policy generally, not only professional nursing concerns, in line with Nightingale's own example of political activism.

The situation is quite different in Asia. Nightingale is still taught both in the school system and in nursing faculties in major Asian countries. She is seen as a moral example, as well as a source of relevant principles on nursing. After the dropping of the atomic bomb at Hiroshima in August 1945, hospital nurses treating the victims were brought together twice a day to recite the Nightingale pledge. The solemn pledge and reminder of their duty helped them to endure appalling conditions—vast numbers of dying in a nearly collapsed hospital (Nelson, in Nelson & Rafferty, 2010).

In Japan, not only is Nightingale's *Notes on Nursing* taught to nursing students, but her later, more advanced, writings are also available in Japanese translation. Professional societies exist to apply her principles in practice, notably the Nightingale KomiCare Society, which holds conferences and publishes a journal. Nurses at professional conferences discuss how they apply Nightingale's principles in acute, community, and palliative care, with patients reporting great satisfaction. There is, to my knowledge, nothing equivalent to this in Western nursing. However, so far, nurses in Japan have not taken on policy tasks nor pointed out failings in the health care system.

Nightingale is a serious model and example for nurses in India and China. In the case of India, there are links through her own attempts (with limited success) to bring in professional nursing in the late 19th century. In China, as in Japan, she has been revered as an example of self-sacrifice for the greater good. Yet again, her example as a policy advocate and whistleblower is ignored.

In the mid and late 20th century, nurse training made the transition to university, the United States and Canada leading the way. Yet continuities in priorities (health promotion and prevention), and even definitions of nursing, continue to show their roots in Nightingale. A leading American 20th-century nurse, Virginia Henderson, updated the definition of nursing to include the wider roles of administration and education, and to make clear that the work was *paid*, points left implicit in Nightingale's formulation.

Henderson's lengthier definition also follows Nightingale in assuming medical jurisdiction in diagnosis and prescription:

> The practice of professional nursing means the performance for compensation of any act in the observation, care, and counsel of the ill, injured, or infirm, or in the maintenance of health or prevention of illness of others, or in the supervision and teaching of other personnel, or the administration of medications and treatment as prescribed by a licensed physician or dentist, requiring substantial specialized judgment and skill and based on knowledge and application of the principles of biological, physical, and social science. The foregoing shall not be deemed to include acts of diagnosis or prescription of therapeutic or corrective measures. (Henderson, 1967, p. 3)

Henderson next defined "practical nursing" and gave its relationship to professional nursing. This definition is very much in line with the demarcation common in Nightingale's day, of a trained or "head nurse" and an untrained "assistant nurse" (Henderson, 1967, p. 3).

NIGHTINGALE'S LINK TO AMERICAN NURSING

That the first nursing schools in the United States, dating to 1873, were based on Nightingale's principles is well known (see the Appendix at the end of this book for a timeline of Nightingale's influence). Less well known is Nightingale's role in the important advances made in nursing organization late in the century, notably at the International Congress of Charities held in Chicago in 1893, which featured a paper by Nightingale, excerpted in Part II, Chapter 12. The congress brought together nursing leaders from many places in the United States and the United Kingdom. Isabel Hampton, principal of the training school at Johns Hopkins University Hospital, and before that at Cook County, Chicago, took advantage of the occasion to foster the formation of an organization of directors of nursing schools. It later became the National League for Nursing (she was president in 1909). She had earlier been instrumental in forming an alumnae organization at Johns Hopkins University Hospital (D'Antonio, 2000). The next step was a national organization of all accredited nurses. This was the Nurses' Associated Alumnae of the United States (and Canada), which became the American Nurses Association. She was the first president, 1897–1901. Nightingale was made an honorary member in 1899. Hampton Robb (as she was subsequently known) was also, later, a major force in the creation of the International Council of Nurses.

Shortly before she married, Hampton visited Nightingale in London in 1894 (Nightingale sent her the bridal bouquet). Hampton had published a full and comprehensive textbook, *Nursing: Its Principles and Practice for Hospital and Private Use* (Robb, 1893), a copy of which she gave to Nightingale (letter, September 20, 1894, Add Mss 45812 f189). She had extended the Johns Hopkins program from 2 to 3 years.

She was a gifted, innovative teacher. At Johns Hopkins she, as well as the doctors, gave lectures. For her lectures, she used such visual aids as a skeleton, a manikin for "visceral anatomy," specimens, and pictures. She is said to have been excellent also in bedside instruction. Hampton Robb highlighted lessons from Nightingale, on thorough cleanliness in the wards, pure air, and a sympathetic attitude (Baer, *Enduring Issues in American Nursing*). She drew on her lecture material when writing her influential textbook, *Nursing: Principles and Practices*.

It is perhaps no coincidence that Hampton looked to Nightingale for guidance when they met, specifically for advice on the new organization of nursing directors. From Nightingale's notes of the meeting, they evidently discussed this, as well as British–American differences in nursing and expectations (notes, July 8, 1894, in McDonald, 2009a).

Hampton Robb's own books, again no coincidence, can be seen as important bridges from Nightingale's core principles to the development of nursing in the 20th century, with a great increase in academic content and reduction in drudgery (D'Antonio, 2000). Her *Nursing: Its Principles and Practice* nowhere mentions Nightingale, but the influence is evident throughout in the stress on the biophysical environment, relations with doctors, and ethical concerns. It notably gives copious details of what nurses must learn, which go far beyond *Notes on Nursing*. By then, a 3-year program was in place, in contrast with 1 year at the Nightingale School. Hampton Robb used the material she taught in her classes at Johns Hopkins.

Hampton Robb's *Nursing Ethics* (1903), cites Nightingale explicitly and deferentially, and, again, shows Nightingale's considerable influence. It, however, has much on hospital "etiquette," or procedures, as well as ethics as such. Her *Educational Standards for Nurses* (1907) reflects another shared concern, a rigorous academic program for nurse education.

While Nightingale grudgingly accepted germ theory, Hampton Robb saw its importance and argued for at least the "broad principles of bacteriology" to be included in the curriculum for nurses. "How hopeless and dull, not to say irritating, would be the many washings and the various aseptic precautions which are now required from the nurse by the physician unless she had learned from bacteriology to appreciate the fact that there exists a surgical, a microscopical, cleanliness" (Robb, 1907, p. 99). In her ethics book also, she said that "bacteriologically practical training" was needed, and that the operating room nurse was no less important than any other member of the surgeon's staff (Robb, 1912, p. 35).

Nightingale continued to make (occasional) disparaging remarks about germ theory, even after accepting it, for example, in her paper on rural health, "Not bacteriology, but looking into the drains is the thing needed" (Nightingale, 1894, in McDonald, 2004, p. 617). Yet the two need hardly be either/or, as Hampton Robb well understood. Both were, and are, needed.

Nightingale's writing from the mid-19th century continued to be taught to nursing students well into the mid-20th century. Hampton Robb published a second edition of her *Principles and Practice* in 1906; then, after her death, her doctor husband brought out a third edition, with slight revisions, in 1914. The text was, at least partially, translated into Chinese for use when professional nursing was introduced into China (Dock, 1912, Vol. 4). Harmer brought out her similarly titled *Textbook of the Principles and Practice of Nursing* in 1922.

Nursing with its health approach would continue to be complementary to medicine, as Nightingale saw it (Potter et al., 2009). Harmer and Henderson were used into the late 20th century. Roy's Adaptation Model, noted in Chapter 2, gained much acceptance. It was based on core Nightingale ideas.

American nursing's ascendancy in the 20th century must owe something to its large numbers, but doubtless much must be attributed to its early promotion of university training and research. Hampton Robb was central to this development.

How well established was hospital nursing in the United States and Canada before Nightingale set to work? Florence Lees, on an inspection tour in 1873 to 1874 for William Rathbone, found nothing satisfactory to report. She visited New York, Albany, Boston, Chicago, and Cincinnati in the United States and Hamilton, Toronto, Ottawa, and Montreal in Canada. She found "scores" of young women willing to take nurse training in both countries, if any training school were established, but she knew of none, nor any serious plans to start one (this would soon change in the United States).

Lees judged the schooling of girls in Canada to be "admirable," for all children there learned "at least the *elements* of anatomy, physiology, and chemistry." Her opinion of Canadian hospitals, however, was even lower than that of American hospitals. There was "*nothing* to learn" in them, but they were "alike miserable in construction and arrangement," as well as "in their defiance of all sanitary laws, and in their miserably insufficient *nurses* for the sick" (Lees letter, December 3, 1873, Add Mss 47756 f219).

Her opinion was confirmed a couple of months later from Boston. Lees wrote to Nightingale: "The nursing in Canadian hospitals and (so far as I have yet seen) in the States, is utterly unworthy of the name" (Lees letter, February 12, 1874, Add Mss 47756 f228).

AN OVERVIEW OF CHAPTERS

From the abundant material Nightingale herself wrote on nursing, health promotion, and hospital safety, the task is to make the best of it available to active professionals today. As is shown in Chapter 2, Nightingale is still a good source on patient care. Have patients changed so much? Her positive, holistic definition of health and her pioneering analysis of the social determinants of health status still apply (Chapter 3). So also do her ideas on ethics (in Chapter 4).

Nightingale's most famous work took place during the Crimean War, under terrible hospital conditions. The lessons she learned from that experience took her into what came to be called infection control (Chapter 5). Ironically, her earliest and simplest advice on frequent handwashing remains the single most important method of combating the spread of infection. Large numbers of lives are lost annually around the world from lapses.

Nightingale never did pediatric nursing herself, but she was frequently asked for advice on it and she liaised with experienced people to provide answers. One of the first hospital plans on which she worked was for a children's hospital in Lisbon, and she continued to pay particular care to the needs of children in hospital care (Chapter 6).

Nightingale's own example in providing palliative care is of interest (see Chapter 7). Conditions have changed, and the numbers only increased as people live longer, increasingly in long-term care agencies. That she went beyond the call of duty is evident in this chapter.

Chapter 8 takes up the thorny issue of administration, relating Nightingale's own experience of it, her teaching on what is needed, and issues that arose in her ongoing mentoring of senior nurses. A number of the early nursing directors faced serious opposition by their hospital administrations, and Nightingale devoted time and energy to defend them. A recent example of gross failures in nursing (and other) care, the Mid-Staffordshire NHS Hospital, is examined in relation to Nightingale's principles of administration.

Finally, Nightingale's insistence on good research and its application in policy is as needed now as ever (Chapter 9). Many nurses want to play a stronger role in health care policy. The growing numbers of nurses with graduate degrees are prime candidates for this more significant role, but they require adequate tools. Nightingale is a formidable inspiration and an ongoing source of sound ideas for these challenges. That she led an interdisciplinary team of doctors, engineers, statisticians, and architects is scarcely known by today's nurses. Nor that the leading public health expert of Britain, if not the world, Dr. John Sutherland, for decades acted as her (unpaid) research and editorial assistant. Are there any nurses today that have such a team or produce anything comparable to what she and her team produced?

Part II gives selections, in chronological order, of Nightingale's writing of most enduring value. Chapter 10 has her first papers on hospital reform (1858), followed by the book that nurses most know, her *Notes on Nursing* (1860). Chapter 11 is devoted to her work to provide quality care for the poorest. It begins with her landmark 1867 brief for a Parliamentary committee, which made the case for quality, trained nursing in those dreaded places (e.g., the workhouse infirmaries). Next comes her 1868 tribute on the death of the first trained nursing director of a workhouse infirmary, Agnes Jones—a spirited call to women to take on the challenge. Then there is her letter to *The Times* promoting "district nursing," or home visiting or community nursing, to provide quality care while keeping patients out of hospitals and workhouse infirmaries.

Chapter 12 covers her last years of work on nursing, hospitals, and public health. Two items from the 1880s show how much nursing and hospitals had evolved since the opening of her school in 1860: an unpublished paper of 1880, and her entries in Quain's *Dictionary of Medicine* in 1883. A letter from 1884 written for *The New York Herald* gave urgent advice on an impending cholera epidemic. Finally, there is her paper for a world congress in Chicago in 1893. A tour de force, the paper goes back to key Nightingale ideas from her earliest work, with insights added from her decades of guiding the development of the growing profession. That congress also marks a great step in the evolution of the profession, with many nurses themselves giving papers of high standard. Isabel Hampton, then director of nursing at Johns Hopkins University Hospital solicited the paper, and read it for Nightingale.

In each case of the selected writings, the focus is on what is still relevant in the work. Thus, the rationale for a 28-bed ward and the horsehair mattress are omitted as no longer germane. Rather, the purpose is to relate Nightingale's core principles and their value today. The evolution of her ideas can be traced as nursing, medicine, and the health sciences generally developed. From early to late, her great gift of succinct and often witty expression will impress.

The chapters in Part I, apart from this introductory chapter, conclude with "Questions for Discussion." Some of the questions (not those first listed) are tough, suitable for nursing students doing degrees beyond the baccalaureate.

WHAT THIS BOOK IS NOT ABOUT

This book is not a biography, of which so many already exist. The best is still the two-volume official biography, for it quotes fully from Nightingale's own writing, a considerable merit (Cook, 1913). The secondary literature on Nightingale is vast and continues to grow: full books, scholarly articles, children's books, the popular press, websites, radio, and television. However, as is pointed out from time to time, it is highly error prone. Nightingale's writing is the best source of her views, and it is readily available, now more than ever before. She gave her best to her writing and wanted to be known by it. She was seldom boring, often provocative, and sometimes inspiring. Even when she exaggerated, she had something worth saying, as, for example: "The fear of dirt is the beginning of good nursing" (Nightingale, 1883, p. 1046, in McDonald, 2009b, p. 745).

QUESTIONS FOR DISCUSSION

1. Is Nightingale's short definition of health adequate for use today? What definition do you/your nursing school prefer?
2. How do Nightingale's views on the purpose of nursing relate to broader issues of health care?
3. How do nurses, in practice, cover the components of health promotion/disease prevention and giving patient care? Must these be specialized occupations?

REFERENCES

Archbishop of Canterbury. (1894). Unveiling of the Memorial to the late Sarah Elizabeth Wardroper, St. Thomas' Chapel. London Metropolitan Archives H1/ST/NTS/Y27/5.

Arikha, N. (2008). *Passions and tempers: A history of the Humours*. New York, NY: Harper Perennial.

Ayliffe, G. A. J. & English, M. P. (2003). *Hospital infection from miasmas to MRSA*. Cambridge, UK: Cambridge University Press.

Baly, M. E. & Matthew, H. C. G. (2004). Nightingale, Florence (1820-1910). *Oxford Dictionary of National Biography, 40,* 904–912.

BBC1. (2001). *Florence Nightingale: Iron Maiden.*

BBC2. (2008). *Florence Nightingale.*

Brighton, T. (2004). *Hell riders: The truth about the charge of the light brigade*. London, UK: Viking. ISBN: 9780805077223.

Brown, R., Nolan, P. W., & Crawford, P. (2009, September). Men in nursing: Ambivalence in care, gender, and masculinity. *Contemporary Nurse: A Journal for the Australian Nursing Profession, 33*(2), 120–129.

Burkhardt, M. A., Nathaniel, A. K., & Walton, N. (2010). *Ethics and issues in contemporary nursing* (2nd Cdn ed.). Toronto, ON, Canada: Nelson. ISBN: 9780176504595.

Cannadine, D. (1998). *History in our time.* New Haven, CT: Yale University Press. ISBN: 9780300077025.

Cantlie, N. (1974). *A history of the army medical department.* 2 vols. Edinburgh, UK: Churchill Livingstone. ISBN: 9780443010668.

Chaska, L. (Ed.). (2001). *The nursing profession: Tomorrow and beyond.* London, UK: Sage. ISBN: 978061919438.

Cook, E. T. (1913). *The life of Florence Nightingale.* 2 vols. London, UK: Macmillan.

Cope, Z. (1963, January). Review, a bio-bibliography of Florence Nightingale. *Medical History, 7*(1), 91–93.

D'Antonio, P. (2010). *American nursing: A history of knowledge, authority, and the meaning of work.* Baltimore, MD: Johns Hopkins University Press. ISBN: 9780801895647.

Davies, K. (2013). *The rise of the U.S. environmental health movement.* Lanham, MD: Rowman & Littlefield. ISBN: 9781442221376.

Dock, L. L. (1912). *A history of nursing: The evolution of nursing systems from the earliest times to the foundation of the first English and American training schools for nurses.* New York, NY: G.P. Putnam's Sons. ISBN: 185506-638-6.

Dossey, B. M., & Keegan, L. (Eds.). (2013). *Holistic nursing: A handbook for practice.* Burlington, MA: Jones & Bartlett. ISBN: 9781449645632.

Ellis, J. R., Nowlis, E. A., & Bentz, P. M. (1992). *Basic nursing skills* (5th ed). New York, NY: J.B. Lippincott [1988]. ISBN: 0395240697.

Gamarnikow, E. (1978). Sexual division of labour: The case of nursing. In A. Kuhn & A. Wolpe (Eds.), *Feminism and materialism: Women and modes of production* (pp. 96–123). London, UK: Routledge & Kegan Paul. ISBN: 0710000723.

Godden, J. (2006). *Lucy Osburn: A lady displaced: Florence Nightingale's envoy to Australia.* Sydney, Australia: Sydney University Press. ISBN: 9781920898397.

Gottlieb, L. (2012). *Strengths-based nursing care—Health and healing for person and family.* New York, NY: Springer Publishing. ISBN: 9780826195869.

Halliday, S. (2007). *The great filth: Disease, death and the Victorian life.* Stroud, UK: Alan Sutton.

Hammond, C. (2005, July). Reforming architecture, defending empire: Florence Nightingale and the pavilion hospital. *Studies in the Social Sciences , 38,* 1–24.

Harmer, B. (1922). *Textbook of the principles and practice of nursing.* New York, NY: Macmillan.

Haynes, L., Boese, T., & Butcher, H. (Eds.). (2004). *Nursing in contemporary society: Issues, trends, and transition to practice.* Upper Saddle River, NJ: Pearson. ISBN: 9780130941541.

Hays, J. N. (1998). *The burdens of disease: Epidemics and human response in Western history.* New Brunswick, NJ: Rutgers University Press. ISBN: 978-0813546131.

Hegge, M. (2013, July). Nightingale's environmental theory. *Nursing Science Quarterly, 26*(3), 211–219. doi:10.1177/0894318413489255

Helmstadter, C. (1997). Doctors and nurses in the London teaching hospitals: Class, gender, religion, and professional expertise 1850-1890. *Nursing History Review, 5,* 161–197.

Henderson, V. (1967). *The nature of nursing: A definition and its implications for practice, research, and education.* New York, NY: Macmillan [1964]. ISBN: 0887374948.

Henderson, V., & Nite, G. (1978). *The principles and practice of nursing* (6th ed.). New York, NY: Macmillan. ISBN: 0023535806.

Hinchliff, S., Norman, S., & Schober, J. (Eds.). (1994). *Nursing practice and health care: A foundation text* (3rd ed.). London, UK: Arnold [1989]. ISBN: (5th ed) 978 0 340 928882.

Hood, L. J., & Leddy, S. K. (2006). *Leddy and Pepper's conceptual bases of professional nursing* (6th ed.). Philadelphia, PA: Lippincott Williams & Wilkins [2003]. ISBN: 9781451187922.

"Hospital nurses as they are and as they ought to be." (1848, May). *Fraser's Magazine*, 539–542.

Johnson, B. M., & Webber, P. B. (2010). *An introduction to theory and reasoning in nursing* (3rd. ed.). New York, NY: Lippincott Williams & Wilkins. ISBN: 9781451190359.

Kelly, L. Y. & Joel, L. A. (1996). *The nursing experience: Trends, challenges, and transitions* (3rd ed.). New York, NY: McGraw-Hill. ISBN: 0071054839.

Libster, M. M. (2008, May-June). Elements of care: Nursing environmental theory in historical context. *Holistic Nursing Practice, 22*(3), 160–170. doi:10.109701 .HNP.000318025.37904.6c

Lindeman, C. A., & McAthie, M. (Eds.). (1999). *Fundamentals of contemporary nursing practice*. Philadelphia, PA: W.B. Saunders. ISBN: 072163527X.

Lister, J. (1867, September 21). On the antiseptic principle in the practice of surgery. *The Lancet, 90*(2299), 353–356. doi:10.1016/S0140-6736(02)51827-4

Lobo, M. E. (2002). Environmental model: Florence Nightingale. In J. B. George (Ed.), *Nursing theories: The base for professional nursing practice* (5th ed., pp. 43–60). Upper Saddle River, NJ: Prentice-Hall.

Lundy, K. S., & Bender, K. M. (2009). History of community health and public health nursing. In K. S. Lundy & S. Janes (Eds.). *Community health nursing: Caring for the public's health* (pp. 43–60). Burlington, MA: Jones & Bartlett. ISBN: 9781449691493.

Lynaugh, J. (2000). Isabel Hampton and the professionalization of nursing. In E. D. Baer, P. D'Antonio, S. Rinker, & J. E. Lynaugh (Eds.), *Enduring issues in American nursing* (pp. 42–84). New York, NY: Springer Publishing.

Marcus, C. C., & Barnes, M. (Eds.). (1999). *Healing gardens: Therapeutic benefits and design recommendations*. New York, NY: John Wiley. ISBN: 0471192031.

McDonald, L. (1993). *The early origins of the social sciences*. Montréal, Canada: McGill-Queen's University Press. ISBN: 0-7735-1124-5; soft 0-7735-1408-2.

McDonald, L. (1994). *The women founders of the social sciences*. Montréal, Canada: McGill-Queen's University Press. ISBN: 0886-29218-2; 0886-29219-0; 0-7735-2349-9.

McDonald, L. (Ed.). (1998). *Women theorists on society and politics*. Waterloo, Canada: Wilfrid Laurier University Press. ISBN: 0-88920-290-7.

McDonald, L. (2001–2012). *Collected works of Florence Nightingale*. Waterloo, Canada: Wilfrid Laurier University Press.

McDonald, L. (2001, July). Florence Nightingale and the early origins of evidence-based nursing. *Evidence-Based Nursing, 43*, 68–69. doi:10.1136/ebn.4.3.68

McDonald, L. (Ed.). (2004). *Florence Nightingale on public health care*. Waterloo, Canada: Wilfrid Laurier University Press. ISBN: 0-88920-446-2.

McDonald, L. (Ed.). (2009a). *Florence Nightingale: Extending nursing.* Waterloo, Canada: Wilfrid Laurier University Press. ISBN: 978-1-55458-170-2.

McDonald, L. (Ed.). (2009b). *Florence Nightingale: The Nightingale School.* Waterloo, Canada: Wilfrid Laurier University Press. ISBN: 978-1-55458-169-6.

McDonald, L. (2010). *Florence Nightingale at first hand.* London, UK: Continuum and Waterloo, ON, Canada: Wilfrid Laurier University Press. ISBN: 978-155458-191-7.

McDonald, L. (2015). Florence Nightingale: A research-based approach to health, health care, and hospital safety. In F. Collyer (Ed.), *The Palgrave handbook of social theory in health, illness, and medicine* (pp. 59–74). London, UK: Palgrave Macmillan.

Meleis, A. I. (1991). *Theoretical nursing: Development and progress* (2nd ed.). Philadelphia, PA: Lippincott. ISBN: 978-1-60547-211-9.

Munro, C. L. (2010, July). The "lady with the lamp" illuminates critical care today. *American Journal of Critical Care, 19*(4), 315–317. doi:10.4037/ajcc2010228

Nelson, S. (2010). The Nightingale imperative. In S. Nelson & A. M. Rafferty (Eds.), *Notes on Nightingale: The influence of a nursing icon* (pp. 9–27). Ithaca, NY: Cornell University Press. ISBN: 9780801449062.

Nightingale, F. (1860). *Notes on nursing: What it is, and what it is not.* London, UK: Harrison.

Nightingale, F. (1863). *Notes on hospitals* (3rd ed.). London, UK: Longman, Green.

Nightingale, F. (1876, April 14). Trained nurses for the sick poor. *The Times,* 6CD.

Nightingale, F. (1877). Letter to Miss Fisher. Retrieved from http://www .nursingworld.org/FunctionalMenuCategories/AboutANA/History/Florence -Nightingale-Letter-Transcription.pdf

Nightingale, F. (1880). Hospitals and patients. *The Nineteenth Century* (unpublished paper).

Nightingale, F. (1883). Nurses, training of and nursing the sick. In R. Quain (Ed.), *A dictionary of medicine* (Vol. 2, pp. 1043–1049). London, UK: Longmans, Green.

Nightingale, F. (1890). *Hospitals. Chambers's encyclopaedia: A dictionary of universal knowledge* (Vol. 5, pp. 805–807). Edinburgh, Scotland: W. & R. Chambers.

Nightingale, F. (1892). Letter to the Poona Sarvajanik Sabha. *The Quarterly Journal of the Poona Sarvajanik Sabha, 15*(1), 13–17.

Nightingale, F. (1893). Sick nursing and health nursing. In A. Burdett-Coutts (Ed.), *Woman's mission: A series of congress papers on the philanthropic work of women* (pp. 184–205). London, UK: Sampson, Low, Marston.

Nightingale, F. (1894). Nurses, training of and nursing the sick. In R. Quain (Ed.), *A dictionary of medicine* (Vol. 2, pp. 231–244). London, UK: Longmans, Green.

Nightingale, M. (1982, July 28). Buildings update: Part 2: Evolving wards. *Architecture Journal,* 47–50.

Nightingale Society. (2017, February 10). Letter to Sir David Cannadine, director, Oxford Dictionary of National Biography. Retrieved from http://nightingalesociety .com/to-Sir-David-Cannadine.director-oxford-dictionary-of-national-biography

Peto, R. (2004). Infection prevention and control. In M. Mallik, C. Hall, & D. Howard (Eds.), *Nursing knowledge & practice: A decision-making approach.* London, UK: Baillière Tindall.

Potter, P. A., Perry, A. G., Ross-Kerr, J. C., & Wood, M. J. (2009). *Canadian fundamentals of nursing* (2nd ed.). Toronto, ON, Canada: Mosby. ISBN: 9780779699933.

Reverby, S. M. (1987). *Ordered to care: The dilemma of American nursing, 1850-1945.* Cambridge, UK: Cambridge University Press.

Robb, I. H. (1893). *Nursing: Its principles and practice for hospital and private use.* Philadelphia, PA: W. B. Saunders.

Robb, I. H. (1907). *Educational standards for nurses: With other addresses on nursing subjects.* Cleveland, OH: E. C. Koeckert. ISBN: 0824065220.

Robb, I. H. (1912). *Nursing ethics: For hospital and private use.* Cleveland, OH: E. C. Koeckert [1900].

Rosenberg, C. E. (1979). Florence Nightingale on contagion: The hospital as moral universe. In C. E. Rosenberg (Ed.), *Healing and history: Essays for George Rosen* (pp. 116–136). New York, NY: Science History.

Rosenberg, C. E. (Ed., Intro.). (1989). *Florence Nightingale on hospital reform.* New York, NY: Garland.

Rosenberg, C. E. (1992). *Explaining epidemics and other studies in the history of medicine* (90–108). Cambridge, UK: Cambridge University Press.

Selanders, L. C. (1993). *Florence Nightingale: An environmental adaptation theory.* Newbury Park, CA: Sage. ISBN: 0803948603.

Sellman, D. (1997). The virtues in the moral education of nurses: Florence Nightingale revisited. *Nursing Ethics, 4*(1), 3–11. doi:10.1177/096973309700400102

Small, H. (1998). *Florence Nightingale: Avenging angel.* London, UK: Constable.

Smith, F. B. (1982). *Florence Nightingale: Reputation and power.* London, UK: Croom Helm.

Snow, J. F. (1857). *Facts relating to hospital nurses, also observations on training establishments for hospitals.* London, UK: Richardson Bros.

Stevenson, C. (2000). *Medicine and magnificence: British Hospital and asylum architecture, 1660-1815.* New Haven, CT: Yale University Press. ISBN: 030008562.

Stone, R. (1997). *Some British Empiricists in the Social Sciences 1650-1900* (pp. 303–337). Cambridge, UK: Cambridge University Press/Raffaele Mattioli Foundation. ISBN: 9780521128452.

Taylor, C., Lillis, C., & LeMone, P. (1993). *Fundamentals of nursing: The art and science of nursing care* (2nd ed.). Philadelphia, PA: Lippincott-Raven.

Thompson, J. D. & Goldin, G. (1975). *The hospital: A social and architectural history.* New Haven, CT: Yale University Press. ISBN: 0300018290.

Treiber, L., & Jones, J. H. (2015). The care/cure dichotomy: Nursing's struggle with dualism. *Health Sociology Review, 2,* 152–162. doi:10:1080/14461242.2014.999404.

Vallée, G. (Ed.) (2007). *Florence Nightingale on social change in India.* Waterloo, Canada: Wilfrid Laurier University Press. ISBN: 978-0-88920-495-9.

Verderber, S. (2005). *Compassion in architecture: Evidence-based design for health in Louisiana.* Lafayette, LA: Center for Louisiana Studies. ISBN: 9781887366632.

Wolstenholme, G. E. W. (1971). *All heal: A medical and social miscellany.* London, UK: Heinemann. ISBN: 0433285001.

World Health Organization. (1978). Declaration of Alma-Ata. Retrieved from http://www.who.int/publications/almaata_declaration_en.pdf

World Health Organization. (2017). Constitution of WHO: Principles. Retrieved from http://www.who.int/about/mission/en/

APPENDIX: THE ATTACK ON NIGHTINGALE'S REPUTATION

From examining misconceptions as to Nightingale's influence and reputation, in both directions, the focus here moves to two particularly influential negative sources. Both are British, for indeed American and other sources tend to be far more positive. Given their weight, however, and the tendency for bad news to travel, it seemed advisable to report on them here, so that readers, especially nursing leaders, can be forewarned.

David Cannadine's History of Our Time

The first source is David Cannadine, fellow of too many scholarly organizations and recipient of too many awards to mention, knighted for his "services to scholarship" in 2009. His *History of Our Time*, nonetheless, has numerous errors of fact, and, interspersed with many favorable comments on Nightingale's work, slurs on her character and achievements.

Cannadine depicted Nightingale as enormously selfish and demanding in personal relationships. For example, when her great collaborator Sidney Herbert became ill, according to him she "scarcely noticed" that he "was collapsing under the strain" (Cannadine, 1998, p. 203). But Herbert wanted to keep working as long as possible, and continued to write her with ideas for new projects; see his letters to her (Add Mss 43395); Nightingale thought that he was a bad patient—he went to a Belgian spa for treatment when he was dying of kidney disease. Her letters to him, as those to his wife (Add Mss 43396), do not suggest callousness, and Cannadine gave not one concrete example.

He had Nightingale "imperiously" telling newly qualified nurses "where to take employment, shamelessly promoting her proteges" (Cannadine, 1998, p. 202). Yet a massive number of letters by nurses to her is on record asking for her help in getting posts. She wrote numerous letters of reference, usually after meeting with the person herself to explore options (she kept the notes). Nightingale tried numerous times to get such leading nurses as Mary Jones and Florence Lees to take on workhouse infirmary work, yet continued to support them when they did not (Jones ran a convalescent home, Craven led in district nursing).

Cannadine blamed Nightingale for not acknowledging "those nurses who were not directly under her control" (Cannadine, 1998, p. 202), a matter belied by correspondence to her by nurses at many hospitals. Eva Luckes, nursing director at the London Hospital, is a good example, a nursing leader who sought her advice and help; yet she did not train at Nightingale's school and was never under her authority (Add Mss 47746). Alfhild Ehrenborg, first principal of the nursing school established by Queen Sophia in Sweden in 1883, is another example, as is Linda Richards, the first U.S.-trained nurse, who took Nightingale standards and methods to many American hospitals and, later, to Japan. Three Canadian-born American nurses were never under Nightingale's control but sought her advice and help—and got it; all ran their nursing services according to their own views, moving beyond her ideas: Isabel Hampton Robb, Louise Robinson Scovil, and Charlotte Macleod. Much surviving correspondence shows nurses reporting valuable material to her on best practice in their own and other hospitals. This was networking, and Nightingale benefited from material they brought her.

Another character flaw, according to Cannadine, Nightingale felt "personally affronted" if nurses under her "dared to get married" (1998, p. 203). Yet she sent greetings and good wishes on the wedding to some, sometimes the bridal bouquet, for example, Isabel Hampton, noted earlier in this chapter, and Emily Mansel Cheadle (Cheadle letter, August 6, 1892, Add Mss 45811 f124). Florence Lees was given both a wedding gift, one she would "treasure always," and a "beautiful" bouquet (Lees Craven letters, September 21 and November 23, 1879, Add Mss 47756 ff344 and 348). Nightingale took on such tasks as looking for help for Mrs. Craven and was godmother to a son. She sent a "nosegay" to a nurse of Adelaide ward on her wedding day (Haydon letter, September 13, 1897, Add Mss 45815 f9) and good wishes in 1901 to another on her wedding (Carpenter Davis letter, January 19, 1901, Add Mss 45815 f158).

On the development of nursing, Cannadine had Nightingale opposed "to the professionalization of nursing, to public examinations, and to state registration" (Cannadine, 1998, p. 204). Not quite: She opposed the scheme of state registration proposed by the Royal British Nursing Association for its giving too much power to doctors and for emphasizing written examinations, which would have excluded able working-class nurses from the profession (McDonald, "State registration of nurses," in McDonald, 2009b); she strongly supported high and increasing professional standards, but did not believe that written examinations sufficed to judge competence.

Yet another unfounded judgment has Nightingale not interested "in women's issues and women's rights" and no "feminist role model" (Cannadine, 1998, p. 206). Why then did she sign numerous petitions for the right to vote, support married women's property rights and higher education for women, mentor the first woman to win a senior civil service post, and vigorously oppose the discriminatory "Contagious Diseases Acts" that targeted female prostitutes? Suffrage leaders appreciated her support, as did John Stuart Mill, who led the struggle for the vote in Parliament.

The Oxford Dictionary of National Biography on Nightingale

The other highly prestigious negative source (again with positives interspersed) is the entry on Nightingale in *The Oxford Dictionary of National*

Biography (Baly & Mathew, 2004). Baly, who wrote the initial text, was the leading nursing historian at the time it was commissioned. Mathew, then the editor of the *Dictionary*, added much material from Smith (1982), a cool 15 additional citations, although Smith was known to be both inaccurate and derogatory.

In February 2017, the Nightingale Society protested the inadequate and hostile coverage to the then editor of the *Dictionary*, the same Sir David Cannadine, who succeeded to the editorship in 2014 (Nightingale Society, 2017). Disproportionate space went to Nightingale's family background, the complaint stated, leaving little for discussion of her work. There was no discussion of her influential *Notes on Hospitals* or her analysis of high death and illness rates in aboriginal schools and hospitals, none of her Franco-Prussian War work or her later nursing papers, and only scant coverage of her *Introductory Notes on Lying-in Institutions* and work on district nursing, which it dated incorrectly.

A heading in the entry has Nightingale "out of office" as early as 1870, a time when she was highly productive. The expression "out of office" was one she used, casually, in private correspondence, when a viceroy leaving for India did not come to see her (nor did the next one). However, the next three viceroys after them did call on her, and two became close collaborators on public health and broader social reforms (Lords Ripon and Dufferin). Far from being "out of office," she found new allies in Indian nationals, and wrote much for their public health journals.

The *ODNB* is grossly misleading as well in relegating Nightingale to "old age" in 1880, when she had 20 more years of useful work, including some of her best publications, which are simply ignored (they are excerpted in Part II, Chapter 12 of this book). These late works include new initiatives, a development entirely missed in the entry. And, while Nightingale continued to be sought out by leading medical and public health experts, the *ODNB* has her "out of touch" on those issues. The school itself is judged to have failed at providing good nursing training, although it gave not one example of a better school.

That these two examples are of sources normally considered reliable must suggest great caution to researchers in using sources. Primary sources, and biographies that rely heavily on them, such as Cook (1913), are recommended.

Chapter 2: Nursing: The New Profession of Patient Care

It may be said that you must fit your nursing arrangements to your sick, and not your sick to your nursing arrangements.

—Nightingale (1867, p. 74)

Providing the patient with good care was the original purpose of the new profession of nursing. Nurses would also play important roles in health promotion and disease prevention, but the initial impetus came from the need for ongoing care of the patient when the doctor left the sick room or ward. The doctor made the diagnosis and determined the treatment, including prescribing any drugs (few in Nightingale's time) and ordering special foods (the nurse's responsibility to cook, if necessary) and alcoholic drinks or "stimulants," frequently called on in lieu of drugs (wine or port were often prescribed, occasionally champagne).

Without antibiotics to kill the bacilli that cause the great fevers, the nurse at the bedside was often key to a patient's recovery. Before the invention of intravenous drips, nurses sat up with the patient, wiping a brow and spooning small quantities of liquids into the patient's mouth.

This chapter begins with the case for having a distinct occupation of patient care, a creation of the 19th century, at the instigation of doctors. Nightingale's view of disease as a "restorative" process is fundamental for understanding her purpose for nursing. It would be the duty of the bedside nurse to aid the body's natural "restorative" faculties, by ensuring the right biophysical conditions. Her *Notes on Nursing* (1860) laid out these essentials, chapter by chapter, which are briefly reviewed here. A special section notes the importance of nutrition.

Nightingale's "restorative" approach emerged at a time when the science of medicine had little to offer by way of known effective treatments.

"Heroic" or frankly "bad" medicine was widely practiced, including blood-letting, purging, and recourse to toxic substances, ostensibly to destroy the disease, but too often they weakened or even killed the patient.

The chapter then goes on to the particular field of midwifery, when obstetrics as a medical specialty was just emerging. Nightingale's own pioneering study of maternal mortality postchildbirth is briefly described.

Army nursing is the next subject, including Nightingale's own work to establish it with the same quality of professional care as could be had in civil nursing, against proposals for more amateur care.

District nursing or nursing by home visitors rounds out the chapter. This includes her work in the 1870s as the first British district nursing organization was established, to more ambitious measures late in the century in honor of Queen Victoria's jubilee. One last example is given of "health missioners" to rural mothers to teach health promotion, but without giving patient care. Again, we learn that disease prevention, for Nightingale, is always to be preferred to treating it later.

THE CASE FOR A PROFESSION OF NURSING

Some early doctors saw the need for ongoing bedside nursing, especially for fever patients. For example, a Dublin doctor, Robert James Graves, stated that he would not undertake a fever case without the assistance of a "regular fever nurse" to keep up the patient's strength, for family members and friends often counteracted the doctor's best efforts (Graves, 1843, p. 60). This advice was repeated more than half a century later by another leading doctor, that

> The most important element in the treatment is the conservation of the patient's strength with the preservation of his morale, and this can be best accomplished when the patient is constantly under the care of an experienced nurse, noting every symptom and averting every possible source of worry and every form of exhaustion of energy. (Walsh, 1907, p. 172)

Sometimes a doctor might take a "nurse" under his wing and give her some informal training; she would then look after his patients. Nightingale herself sought such experience at the Salisbury Hospital, where Dr. Richard Fowler, a family friend, was willing to train her, but her family would not allow it. She later learned how to dress wounds from a retired nurse, Eliza Roberts, who had been informally trained at St. Thomas' Hospital.

Given the limitations of medicine in her time, it is not surprising that Nightingale believed that neither medicine nor surgery, nor the nurse, cured the patient:

> Surgery removes the bullet out of the limb, which is an obstruction to cure, but Nature heals the wound. So it is with medicine. The function of an organ becomes obstructed; medicine, so far as we know, assists Nature to remove the obstruction, but does nothing more. (Nightingale, 1860, in Part II, Chapter 10)

The nurse's role, as the doctor's, was to assist Nature to effect the cure. Here, the nurse's role was no less important than the doctor's: "The physician prescribes for supplying the vital force—but the nurse supplies it" (Nightingale, 1883, in McDonald, 2009b, p. 734, in Part II, Chapter 12). Nature's "restorative processes" are fresh air, light, warmth, quiet, cleanliness, and care in diet (Nightingale, 1883, in McDonald, 2009b, p. 736–737, in Part II, Chapter 12).

Nightingale considered that the sick, at home or in a hospital, often suffered from defects in care as much as the disease itself. Nursing, she said, in *Notes on Nursing*, should mean more than the administration of medicines and poultices.

DISEASE AS A "RESTORATIVE" PROCESS

Disease for Nightingale was "a restorative process," its necessary suffering unknown. The nurse's task was to ensure that these restorative processes came into full play. Disease was, as she worded it later:

> Nature's way of getting rid of the effects of conditions which have interfered with health. It is Nature's attempt to cure—we have to help her. Partly, perhaps mainly, upon nursing must depend whether Nature succeeds or fails in her attempt to cure by sickness. Nursing is therefore to help the patient to live. (Nightingale, 1883, in McDonald, 2009b, p. 736 and Part II, Chapter 12)

Nursing today is just as committed to prioritizing health over chemicals. The definition is clear in Roy's "adaptation model" of nursing, that nursing is "a *profession* that uses specialized knowledge to contribute to the needs of society for health and well-being." Roy's reference to the "natural reparative processes" echoes Nightingale's words, down to the specifics of fresh air, light, warmth, cleanliness, quiet, and diet (Roy & Andrews, 1999).

THE BIOPHYSICAL ENVIRONMENT NEEDED TO RESTORE HEALTH

Nightingale's *Notes on Nursing* sets out the nurse's responsibility, chapter by chapter, to ensure adequate ventilation, warming, light, quiet, nutrition, and "petty management," or ensuring continuity of care when the nurse is not there.

Good ventilation topped Nightingale's priority list. The "first essential" was to keep the patient's air as pure as external air. Accordingly, ventilation and warming are the subjects of Chapter 1 of *Notes on Nursing*. However, with adequate central heating in most hospitals and homes today, and great improvements in mechanical ventilation, the insistence on open windows may now be irrelevant. In some countries, hospital windows are made not to open, and artificial ventilation is entirely relied on, a practice Nightingale strenuously opposed.

The amount of cubic space per patient in a ward was a major concern in hospitals of Nightingale's day. She herself gave the question considerable attention, although she thought that, for efficient nursing, superficial space around the patient's bed was even more important. Again, changes in hospital design make this less of a consideration. Large wards, of around thirty beds, still called "Nightingale wards," are now rare.

There is no point in belaboring this issue, for a nurse cannot open a window in a hospital where they were built not to open. The question for hospitals remains an empirical one, to be solved by comparing mortality rates and other indicators across buildings with differing modes of ventilation, including open windows with good cross ventilation, and different forms of air-conditioning. Given the high rate of hospital-acquired infections and resulting deaths, it is remarkable that firm data making these comparisons are not available. As well, data would be interesting on the simpler point of patient comfort. However, patient stays in hospital are now much shorter than in Nightingale's time, which reduces the importance of the mode of ventilation.

Opinion on this point, however, may change again, as microbiologists explore the "microbiome" and caution about excessive sterility, or killing the good germs with the bad. Nightingale's advocacy of opening windows to let fresh air in "can drastically change the microbes around us in the air," for the benefit of our health (Arnold, 2014).

Concern about effluvia from excretions is another matter largely solved in modern hospitals, thanks to great improvements in plumbing. Well-functioning toilets are close to patients in hospitals today, so that the routine use of bedpans is not necessary. The technology for cleaning and disinfection has improved vastly, as has the availability of disposable equipment and products.

The term "stress" was not used in Nightingale's day, but much of what she advocated under petty management was to reduce stress, both to the patient and to the nurse caregiver. "Petty management" entailed taking care of details, including time off for the nurse with suitable arrangements for care. Petty management evolved into the formulation and updating of a care plan.

How much difference does light make to a patient? Does the question even get asked? A Japanese nurse deliberately applying Nightingale's principles in palliative care reported on a patient being taken outside to enjoy the sunlight; the patient felt so much better as a result that he asked to be taken home for his last days, where he could enjoy a more natural setting.

Light got a whole chapter (Chapter 9) in *Notes on Nursing* and considerable attention in Nightingale's writing on hospitals. Second only to patients' need of fresh air was their need of light, specifically direct sunlight, Nightingale thought. It was not merely the patients' spirits that were affected, but the body. A sick person desirably would have two windows to look out of. Morning sun, when the patient was likely still to be in bed, was especially important.

A psychiatrist interested in "rewiring the brain" picked up on Nightingale's seeing the healing power of sunlight. He acknowledged that the ancient Greeks recognized the connection, with Apollo being both sun god and god of healing. Nightingale, however, not only advised exposure to sunlight for health and healing, but also promoted the pavilion model for hospital design because it maximized sunlight in wards: a north–south axis ensured sunlight coming in east–west windows from morning to night (Doidge, 2015, pp. 118–121).

Nightingale, of course, knew nothing of neurotransmitters, but did know, from observation, that people did better with sunlight. As she stated in *Notes on Nursing*, "People think the effect is upon the spirits only. This is by no means the case. The sun is not only a painter but a sculptor" (Chapter 9). Psychiatrist Doidge liked the "sculptor" metaphor, for suggesting that sunlight could "sculpt the circuitry of the brain" (Doidge, 2015, p. 121).

Noise got a chapter (Chapter 4) in *Notes on Nursing* and there is no reason to believe that hospitals have become quieter since. "Unnecessary noise" hurt the patient, Nightingale asserted. It was not the noise level necessarily, but noise that disturbed by creating an "expectation." Whispering, too, could cause anxiety, notably by the physician and patient's family or friends within earshot.

"Variety" got a short chapter (Chapter 5) in *Notes on Nursing*. The sick, especially the chronically ill, needed to see "beautiful objects." People were affected, body and soul, by "form, colour, and light." Variety and brilliance were "actual means of recovery" for the ill. Nightingale was firm that patients should be able, without raising themselves, to see "sky and sunlight at least," if nothing else.

The sick suffer from "mental as well as bodily pain," she said. It was, indeed, "one of the main sufferings of sickness." After a good diet, the state of the patient's nerves could be best relieved by "a pleasant view, a judicious variety as to flowers and pretty things." Light, "by itself, often relieved it." Any visitor to a typical hospital today, let alone a staff member, might wonder if anyone paid any attention to such concerns as beauty, form, and light.

Bed and bedding was given a full chapter (Chapter 8) in *Notes on Nursing*. Much of Nightingale's advice is now obsolete, for better beds are now commonly available, and good bedding is both inexpensive and easily laundered. The director of nursing is not tasked with their care.

The basics of Nightingale's advice on beds, however, still apply in the avoidance of any type that traps dust and dirt. The preference for a mattress in her day was horsehair, for its quality of not absorbing disease-laden humidity. The bed must be placed for convenient nursing, that is, with space on both sides, and for adequate light and ventilation, which would depend on the windows. "A patient's bed should always be in the lightest spot in the room, and he should be able to see out of window" (Chapter 8).

Cleanliness got two chapters in *Notes on Nursing*: Chapter 10 on cleanliness of rooms and walls, and Chapter 11 on personal cleanliness. As well, "the greater part of nursing consists in preserving cleanliness." Here she stated that the best ventilation would not suffice "where the most scrupulous cleanliness is not observed." Clearly both were needed and they reinforced each other: "Without cleanliness, you cannot have all the effect of ventilation; without ventilation, you can have no thorough cleanliness."

In her Chapter 11 on patient cleanliness, Nightingale stressed the "comfort and relief" the patient felt when carefully washed and dried. As good ventilation renewed the air around the patient, so good skin washing removed "noxious matter" and kept the pores free from "obstructing excretions." She articulated—when few others did—the need for frequent handwashing on the part of the nurse. She even compared the results of dirt removed from different procedures for washing, from hot water and soap to colder water. Use of a "rough towel" got better results than a light sponging. Nightingale also believed that washing with a large quantity of water, if soft, made the skin softer and more perspirable.

Nutrition

Notes on Nursing had two chapters on food, "Taking Food" (Chapter 6) and "What Food" (Chapter 7), on the nutritional value of various foods and common misconceptions about them. Chapter 6 stipulated care in the timing of meals. Weak patients often could not take food before 11 a.m., Nightingale reported. Such patients would become even weaker from fasting, after possibly a feverish night.

> A spoonful of beef tea, of arrowroot, and wine, of egg-flip, every hour, will give them the requisite nourishment and prevent them from being too much exhausted to take at a later hour the solid food which is necessary for their recovery. (Nightingale, 1860, Chapter 6, in Part II, Chapter 10)

If a patient could not take a teacupful of some food every 3 hours, the nurse should try a tablespoonful every hour, or a teaspoonful every quarter hour (Nightingale, 1860, Chapter 6, in Part II, Chapter 10). Exhaustion from "half starvation," as Nightingale put it, was a frequent cause of lack of sleep. Intravenous feeding, of course, was not available at the time.

Leaving untasted food at the patient's bedside might make the patient unable to eat at all later, Nightingale warned. She advised that the food be delivered at the expected time, and taken away, eaten or uneaten, soon after, "or you may disgust the patient of all food." A patient desirably should not have to see or smell the food of other patients or the nurses (Chapter 6 in Nightingale, 1860).

A patient's failure to eat could be caused by any of four defects, as she explained in *Notes on Nursing*:

1. Defect in cooking
2. Defect in choice of diet
3. Defect in choice of hours for taking diet
4. Defect of appetite in patient (Chapter 13 in Nightingale, 1860)

Yet commonly, Nightingale said, the first three were blamed on the last: the patient has "no appetite." Yet the patient might be too weak to complain.

Care must be taken not to spill anything into the patient's saucer, or the patient had to take extra care to drink, or would soil the sheets, pillows, or bedclothes with the slopped liquid. Such a small matter of patient comfort was important, as it affected some patients' willingness to eat at all. She advised on feeding patients with delirium or stupor.

"What Food?" has practical advice on getting nutrients into patients, from the frequent reliance on beef tea—getting enough beef in it—to the distaste for eggs by many patients, preference for cream and butter, and inability, for many, to digest cheese, although it was a good nutrient and craved by others. Nightingale said that some patients became "scorbutic" from the excessive reliance of meat in their diets, referring to the disease caused by lack of vitamin C. Milk must be provided with the utmost care to avoid any sourness. Buttermilk was good, especially for feverish patients. Scorbutic patients often liked sweet jams, but other patients, she found, did not like sweets.

Nightingale warned against reliance on arrowroot, which was not very nutritious, while easy to fix, and jelly (she seems to be writing about the ubiquitous hospital gelatins).

Nightingale's fundamental point about nutrition was that the patient's stomach had to be the judge, and there was great variation in what the patient could take:

> The main question is what the patient's stomach can derive nourishment from, and of this the patient's stomach is the sole judge. Chemistry cannot tell this. The patient's stomach must be its own chemist. The diet which will keep the healthy man healthy will kill the sick one. (Chapter 7, "Taking Food")

Nightingale was a great believer in the restorative power of coffee and tea (Chapter 7, in Part II, Chapter 10). Coffee was the better restorative, but a greater impairer of digestion: "Let the patient's taste decide." For people coming out of a fatiguing activity, or about to start one, tea was best, a finding from the experience of many people. She approved of "real tealeaf tea," although it was expensive and considered a luxury, because it alone had the restorative power needed (Chapter 7). Cocoa was not a good substitute, for it added fat, but not nutrients. When brandy was ordered for the patient, it should not be overly diluted, as often the patient could not take the bulk, and thus missed the brandy.

Chapter 12 in *Notes on Nursing* is the source also on the usefulness of companion animals for the sick. "A small pet animal," even a bird in a cage, was recommended, especially for a chronic patient (Part II, Chapter 10). "Pet therapy," or "animal-assisted therapy," is now a recognized service some hospitals provide, with trained visiting animals. Its importance has even been recognized in a critical care journal (Halm, 2008).

CLEANLINESS AND DISINFECTANTS

Nightingale continued to write on the fundamental points laid out in *Notes on Nursing* over the next decades. Her advice grew increasingly more specific as medical science evolved, especially antiseptic surgery and the use of aseptic procedures. Her Quain's *Dictionary* entry on nursing practice gives detailed quantities and solutions of disinfectants to use. Procedures for preventing "blood poisoning" or septicemia were developed, which again reflect increased knowledge from her first admonitions on soap and water and handwashing.

Student nurses at her school were taught about disinfectants and antiseptics in the program of lectures taught by the medical instructor. Beginning in 1873, they were acquainted with a rudimentary version of germ theory (Croft, 1873, Lesson XIX).

The routine failure of caregivers to wash adequately is known to cause millions of unnecessary hospital deaths worldwide. Good handwashing has been found to be the most effective way of avoiding hospital-acquired infections (Angus et al., 2001). The subject, accordingly, is pursued further in the discussion on infection control.

Nightingale advised on the best ways of washing dysenteric patients while "maintaining their dignity." These patients needed "perpetual washing ... to prevent abrasion of the skin." Yet it could not be done at a lavatory table. Cases confined to bed should be washed by the nurse. For convalescents, there ought to "a convenience in the lavatory," providing privacy, a kind of bidet (Nightingale, 1861).

Issues of patient dignity and autonomy will be dealt with more in the chapter on ethics, but a note should be made here that these were basic to good patient care. This occurs in such mundane matters as making it possible for patients to open their windows, except for delirious patients. Food should be served so as to avoid spills and cause embarrassment. Nightingale urged that nurses sit down when the patient was speaking to them, to "show no signs of hurry" and give "complete attention."

Ease of management was an important consideration in hospital design. Whatever the form of hospital construction, provision was needed for inspections at "unexpected times." As hospital scandals come to light, a subject pursued in later in this text (Chapter 8, on administration), the merit of this requirement only becomes more obvious.

Nightingale's consistent view was that hospitals should be avoided whenever possible, and patients moved out as soon as the necessary medical or surgical interventions were completed. Convalescent care, in healthy surroundings, desirably the seaside, would then follow.

Her extensive work for nursing at home, or "district nursing" as it was called in the United Kingdom, shows this basic preference. She remarked to the philanthropist William Rathbone who funded the first project, in Liverpool, that "Hospitals are but an intermediate stage of civilization," and repeated the point in her letter to the editor appealing for money to fund district nursing (letter, August 13, 1860, in McDonald, 2009a, p. 255; Nightingale, 1867, in Part II, Chapter 11).

"HEROIC MEDICINE," "BAD MEDICINE"

In Nightingale's days, treatments such as bloodletting and blistering were widely practiced. Doctors, frustrated by the lack of effective remedies, turned to extreme measures, even metals now known to be poisonous at any dose. Lead, mercury, and arsenic were commonly used, as can be seen in articles in professional medical journals and books on "materia medica."

Recent commentators have noted the verdict of medical historians, that, in the 1850s, and for some time before, "patients that received no medical care would probably have fared better than those who received the conventional medications given at the time." This occurred because "the 1850s still belonged to the era of so-called 'heroic medicine,' when doctors probably did more harm than good." Further, the "richest patients were the most heroic, because they endured the most severe treatments" (Singh & Ernst, 2008, p. 108). American medicine also relied on bleeding, purging, and blistering, so that "many patients lost their lives" thanks to the use of "these drastic methods" (Mottus, 1981, p. 1).

The use of such extreme measures has been more simply named "bad medicine" (Wootton, 2006). With the benefit of hindsight, it is easy to see that many of these "remedies" harmed the patient. They were questioned at the time, but the continued use of ineffective and even harmful treatments is a well-known, unhappy fact of medical practice.

Nightingale, however, was on the side of cautious medicine. She had learned from the cholera patients treated at Middlesex Hospital, London, and then at the Scutari Barrack Hospital, during the Crimean War, that the "heroic medicine of the day, which was based on infusions of arsenic, mercury, opiates, and bleeding, hastened the death of many more patients than it saved." She came to believe that, "by keeping patients well-fed, warm, comfortable, and above all clean, nursing could solve many problems that 19th century medicine could not" (Gill & Gill, 2005, endnote 12). The kind of patient care she advocated kept the patient warm, nourished, and comfortable, and reduced stress to the minimum possible, with minimal cost to the "vital powers" as Nightingale put it.

How revolutionary this was is still not fully realized, as "heroic," drastic, medicine was the norm. Such "treatments" are now so unthinkable that the effort it took to move on is not evident. The breakthroughs in medical science that led to more effective treatments were late in coming. Nightingale's articulation of a restorative process, in which nurses could play a central role, was a valid, important contribution. She continued to make the case from *Notes on Nursing* on.

However, her statements that neither medicine nor surgery cures no longer holds, for there are many medicines that do cure, notably antibiotics, and many effective surgical treatments and vaccines, plus radiation, chemotherapy, stem cell therapy, and alteration of DNA itself. Nightingale's words, in short, need modification: Support is required to aid Nature in effecting a cure, that is, the best medical and surgical treatments available, and the work of doctors, surgeons, and nurses.

The emergence of effective medical and pharmaceutical advances, however, is not problem free. Medicines may have harmful side effects, and some are addictive. Thalidomide is an example of the former, prescribed for morning sickness for pregnant women, but the cause of serious effects on the fetus. Opioid prescriptions for acute pain are an example of the latter, as large numbers of patients prescribed opioids turn to unsafe street drugs after addiction.

All the precautions Nightingale urged on unintended consequences should come into play: New treatments must be monitored for unintended consequences. They should be tested in smaller numbers before being generalized.

MIDWIFERY NURSING

Nightingale never herself did midwifery nursing. She attended the delivery of a child by her friend Elizabeth Herbert, but there is no reference to her attending any others. Yet she thought midwifery nursing to be so important that, in 1861, only a year after her school at St. Thomas' Hospital opened, she got a midwifery ward and training program opened at King's College Hospital. It made sense at the time, that better training of midwifery nurses would save lives. Women then died more from "accidents" of childbirth, such as breech births, than from the great disease of childbirth, puerperal fever or childbed fever, not identified as a staphylococcal infection until 1902. Better training of midwives could be expected to reduce deaths.

The midwifery program was run by Mary Jones (1812–1887), the nurse Nightingale most respected in the world. The experienced Jones sought no help and did not inform Nightingale of the problems as they emerged. There were no deaths in their first year, but three in the next year, rising to nine in 1867. The medical authorities then notified Nightingale that the ward was to be closed. No newborns died at King's College Hospital, although infant deaths were also common from puerperal fever. Jones was preoccupied all the while by a dispute with the governing authorities of her religious order and seems to have been unaware of the increasing number of deaths.

After the closing of the ward, Nightingale, with the help of her closest collaborator, Dr. John Sutherland, sought to ascertain the cause of the high death rate and to consider changes to be made to permit another attempt. The result, published in 1871, was *Introductory Notes on Lying-in Institutions*, a powerful, pioneering study of maternal mortality post-childbirth (Nightingale, 1871, in McDonald, 2005, pp. 249–329). Its lessons, which required concerted, difficult data collection, are, however, not relevant to current issues of maternal mortality in prosperous, industrial countries. Death rates of birthing mothers are now measured per million. Puerperal fever still occurs, but can usually be treated successfully with antibiotics.

What is relevant from Nightingale's struggle with the issue is the basic question of where women can most safely give birth. She affirmed unequivocally: "Unless from causes unconnected with the puerperal state," no woman ought to die in giving birth, and there ought to be, in a maternity establishment, "no death rate at all" (Nightingale, 1871, "Influence of the time spent in a lying-in ward on the death rate," in McDonald, 2005, p. 299). More realistically, she pursued the question: "what is the real normal death rate" of birthing women? Then, "having ascertained this to the extent which existing data may enable us to do, we must compare this death rate with the rates occurring in establishments into which parturition cases are received in numbers" (Nightingale, 1871, in McDonald, 2005, p. 253).

The data analysis led to her substantial rethinking on maternity care. She greatly admired the French system, where the midwives were the best trained in the world, a full 2-year program. Yet the French death rates were the highest in the world. Semmelweis's Vienna experience explains why, a subject pursued in Chapter 5, "Infection Control."

Nightingale also discovered that the rates of death were lower in workhouse infirmaries, even though birthing mothers in them were less healthy than women in regular, fee-paying hospitals. Autopsies were not conducted in workhouse infirmaries because they had no pathologists on staff and only minimal medical attendance. Here, then, is a great dilemma. Superior education and experience is associated with higher death rates. Women in higher income families were the exception to the normal pattern of death rates declining with rising income, despite their enjoyment of better housing and nutrition.

Thus, although the precise questions will be different today, Nightingale's approach is still useful: Is it safer for a woman to give birth with a midwife or doctor, at home or in a hospital? These questions, of course, come with further specifications as needed for the mother and the professional.

As women began to move into medicine, albeit in small numbers, Nightingale wanted them to practice midwifery. She also wanted doctors and midwifery nurses to teach infant care to new mothers, especially cleanliness and nutrition.

In Nightingale's time, women with resources hired a "monthly nurse" to help them in the first month after giving birth. Desirably these "monthly nurses," who were not trained nurses, would be trained not only in their duties to the new mother, but to give the mother basic health care lessons for the infant. She recognized that poor women had at least as great a need for this assistance, yet seldom got it.

Postpartum depression is not a subject that comes up at all in Nightingale's writing. Her concern for good care of the mother postchildbirth, however, makes one wonder if she had some knowledge of the problem. Japanese birthing practices stress rest for the mother, the baby to be kept in a nursery and brought in for feeding, but kept away enough for the mother to rest. Stays of a week after birth are standard in Japan. Empirical data on postpartum depression and the length of hospital stay and adequacy of maternal rest would be of interest.

Nightingale considered that a good rest after giving birth was needed. Birthing mothers should not leave the ward in less than 3 weeks: "The parts are not replaced in less time and the woman suffers afterwards from prolapsus uterus." However, she acknowledged that that was better than puerperal fever (Nightingale note, 1868, British Library Add Mss[1] 45753 f156).

ARMY NURSING

Army nurses needed the same basic training as civil nurses, Nightingale believed, and for that they had to be trained at regular, civil hospitals. Army hospitals in peacetime lacked the array of serious cases needed for training. In wartime, they would be too busy dealing with large numbers of sick and wounded to be able to train. Note that Nightingale always said "sick and wounded" in that order, since there were far more sick than wounded. During the Crimean War (1854–1856) the ratio was at least seven times as great, and the ratios continued to be high in later wars.

In the 1860s in the United Kingdom, professional nursing was established in the major army hospitals, the general hospitals, but not the small, more numerous "regimental hospitals." In those hospitals, in Nightingale's view—and no one seems to have challenged this—the men were not sick enough to require trained nurses. In the army, when a soldier became ill, he had to report to the regimental hospital, whereas an ordinary person—a civilian—with a minor illness would simply stay home and go to bed. Home, for army men, meant a barracks, with no family support.

---

[1] Further references to Add Mss (Additional Manuscripts) are also to the British Library.

The same sorts of problems had to be solved in army nursing as in civil nursing, notably adequacy of recruits and administration. Progress was slow. A considerable problem in army nursing is related in Chapter 8 on administration.

Where there were no professional (female) nurses, sick or wounded soldiers were looked after by an army buddy he chose or orderlies. Doctors attended. In time, the army developed an Army Hospital Corps of male orderlies. Improving the care they gave by having trained female nurses as managers was one strategy to improve care generally. Nightingale expected—and no one disagreed—that most army nursing (as most nursing in the Navy) would be done by men orderlies. She sought better training and working conditions for them. In short, there were important compromises in the development of professional (trained) nurses in the army.

Britain did not take part in the next European wars, the wars of Italian independence, the Austro-Prussian War, the Franco-Prussian War, or the Balkan wars. For the Franco-Prussian War of 1870 to 1871, and the Balkan wars of the 1870s, British doctors and some nurses served as volunteers. Nightingale was much involved in aid for the Franco-Prussian War, but little of this involved nursing (McDonald, 2011, pp. 603–829).

Nightingale always wanted the same caliber of trained nursing for army sick and wounded as for civilians, hardly a matter that would be contested now. She had considerable support for this among army doctors, but a scheme was proposed to accept a lower level of training. The instigator was Viscountess Strangford, a dedicated and well-organized activist. She had initially tried to persuade hospital boards to accept ladies for a shorter period of training and a much lower workload (Strangford, 1874). It seems that this did not happen.

In 1876, Strangford took on raising money, doctors, and nurses for war in Bulgaria. She was an able fundraiser and organizer, as can be seen in the considerable coverage she got in *The Times*. Nightingale was not persuaded: "I think these private undertakings, without any rules or organization, a great and useless expense doing little good in proportion" (letter, April 29, 1878, in McDonald, 2011, pp. 837–839). A Miss Jackson, who had served for 2 months at Strangford's hospital in Adrianople, later reported to Nightingale that the hospital was "swarming with vermin" and the mortality rate high, although there was an "abundance of stores." She complained that the nurses had to "leave the patients and dress and come to dinner at 6 p.m. (in the hall of the open house, all the patients groaning) *with everybody*...and then go into the garden and smoke a cigarette—*such* confusion, such nonsense, and then sit up all night" with the patients (Notes from a meeting, April 29, 1879, in McDonald, 2011, p. 838).

Strangford's next scheme was to give some short training to soldiers' wives to become nurses, which was supported by the secretary for war and the commander-in-chief. It began in 1880, facilitated by the St. John Ambulance Association (*The Times*, 1880).

Nightingale strongly disapproved of both schemes. "Lady Strangford has done infinite harm in lowering the standard," she told Douglas Galton (letter, May 27, 1881, in McDonald, 2009a, pp. 669–670). A draft note Nightingale wrote is more pointed, with a description of Strangford as "a quack who promises a short cut to health" (undated draft note, Add Mss 47720 f146).

Nightingale was closely involved in the selection and sending of nurses when the British Army was itself belligerent, but not for these other efforts. By the time of the Anglo-Zulu War, in 1879, and the Transvaal War, of 1881, there was a reasonable supply of trained army nurses ready to serve. Nightingale kept in touch with them (McDonald, 2011, The Anglo-Zulu and Transvaal Wars, in McDonald, 2011, pp. 882–964).

How much nursing had developed can be seen in the emergence both of army nurses who could provide Nightingale with detailed assessments of how the work was going and of other women acting in a voluntary capacity, fully capable of sending back detailed reports. Amy Hawthorn, wife of a colonel, visited hospitals and made observations while posted with her husband. She first made contact with Nightingale through her cousin, the famous General Gordon.

By the Egyptian campaigns of 1882 and 1885, when Nightingale was also much involved in selecting the nurses and mentoring them, further evolution can be seen. Army nurse Sybil Airy, who nursed at the cholera hospital in Cairo in 1883, was an excellent informant on the work. Her reports back to Nightingale also show a decided change in relations with doctors. "Young Dr. Acland," as she called Thomas Dyke Acland, son of Henry Dyke Acland of Oxford, a friend of Nightingale's, invited Airy to visit his hospital. He wanted her to show the doctors there the correct way to pad splints. He also asked her for a recipe for beef tea, which their Arab cooks did not know how to make. She delivered on both (Airy letter, October 30, 1883, Add Mss 45775 f140). The visit shows unusually easy, collegial relations—both were St. Thomas' trained—rather than those of superior to subordinate.

A great increase in confidence in their ability on the part of nursing leaders can be seen in the example of a nurse on a hospital ship off the African coast later in the century. "Sister Gray," the nursing director on the Coromandel, reported to a colleague, who passed it on to Nightingale, that they had had, in fact, no casualties to look after, but a naval officer, Prince Henry of Battenberg, died of disease. His death could have been averted, she said, if he had been sent to them, "if only for a week," to have a proper rest, but was in fact sent off with a temperature of 105°F (Joan A. Gray letter, April 20, [1896], Add Mss 47751 f260).

While professional nursing spread successfully throughout army hospitals in Britain and most of the world, this did not apply to army hospitals in India. Not only did Nightingale's early efforts to bring in professional nursing in them fail, there were few efforts later, and none that succeeded in her lifetime. Army hospitals in India routinely had well-qualified doctors on their staffs, but not nurses.

In 1881, with a new, sympathetic viceroy, Lord Ripon, Nightingale tried again. She sent him a lengthy description of the appalling care in the army hospitals in India, "*the worst nursing in any existing army.*" She gave grim details: the complete lack of trained nurses, the (ongoing) use of an army buddy to assist a sick soldier, and reliance on low-caste "ward coolies," also untrained, for most of the work. However, she thought that these Indian men were better than the British soldiers who gave care—good material, "invariably sober," physically strong, kind, and tender. She wanted them trained and supervised, but this never happened. Patients were routinely left entirely unattended at night, and some with seizures were neglected for hours (letter, April 14, 1881, Add Mss 43546 ff158-75). These Indian employees were not enlisted men, so that when trouble occurred, they simply ran away.

In 1886, Lady Roberts, wife of the commander-in-chief in India, frustrated by the (unchanged) lack of nursing in the hospitals, undertook the promotion of *voluntary nurses*, not a scheme Nightingale would have wanted (she always wanted nurses to be paid well). Lady Roberts explained her rationale that only the best qualified "ladies" would be useful in India, yet they would not come for the amount of money that could be raised by donations to pay them. She issued a printed appeal arguing that having qualified hospital nurses would save lives, and that the doctors themselves deplored the loss of lives that nursing could have saved. An initial financial appeal was geared to providing "homes in the hills" for these (yet-to-arrive) nurses during the summer (Roberts, 1886, 1887).

Nightingale seems to have limited her remarks to pointing out that it was a very bad time for soliciting donations, as people had been giving into the Queen's jubilee fund, which was also to support nursing (letter, August 6, 1887, in Vallée, 2007, pp. 785–786).

The next stage in getting (professional) nursing care for the soldiers in India occurred in 1888, when the Army Medical Department sent several nurses to Rawalpindi (now in Pakistan). However, the doctors at the hospital would not let them attend the dangerous cholera cases. The nurse Nightingale mentored, Catherine G. Loch, reported back to her:

> I do not know why, but all the medical men were set against our
> having anything to do with the cholera cases, and for some time

we were absolutely refused permission to see them. They argued that it was a dreadful sight, which we said was not the point.

The principal medical officer finally relented and let them look after a small number of cholera patients. The local medical officer was very pleased with their work, to conclude that "several lives were due entirely to their close assiduous nursing." He sent in a report to that effect. (Loch letter, September 18, 1888, Add Mss 45808 f237)

A breakthrough was made in 1897 when British nurses were sent to India to nurse victims of plague. Nightingale met with the departing nurses (Vallée, 2006, pp. 791–795), and kept in close touch with one of them, Georgina Franklin, who published their correspondence later, under a pseudonym (Lamorna, 1910).

AFTERCARE–CONVALESCENCE

Convalescent hospitals must be as like a home and as unlike a hospital as possible.

—Nightingale (1890, p. 807)

In large hospitals now, aftercare referrals are normally the province of a department of medical social work. In Nightingale's time, arrangements for aftercare were haphazard, shared among nurses, doctors, and the family. The head of the ward or the nursing director might arrange a referral to a convalescent home or hospital.

At that time, before the availability of antibiotics, hospital stays were longer and the patient who survived a severe fever did so with depleted resources. An adequate, sometimes lengthy, period of convalescence was needed. Nightingale considered that convalescent care could have the important result of preventing a family becoming paupers for generations. She saw this occur too often, when "a little timely good nursing, good food (and a change of air for the convalescent)" could save the father or mother from "incurable infirmity—children from consequent pauperism" (letter, April 27, 1867, in McDonald, 2009a, pp. 718–719). Families went into the workhouse when either the breadwinner, the father, could not earn or when the homemaker, the mother, could not look after the family.

Nightingale always wanted convalescent institutions to be in the countryside. Convalescents needed good air, rest, food, and, past the acute phase, did not need proximity to a great medical school for treatment.

She began making aftercare arrangements at her Harley Street Hospital in 1853 and was at it until her departure for the Crimean War. Her quarterly reports and some correspondence give some interesting details:

1. Two days after a patient had a severe epileptic seizure, the chaplain brought in an "insane governess"; this patient who escaped, raised a mob, but was recaptured. On Dr. Bence Jones's advice, she was to be sent to St. Luke's Hospital. (letter, January 17, 1854, Wellcome Ms 8994/93)
2. A few weeks later the "insane governess" returned—she had been at the home of her sister, who could not keep her. Bence Jones and another doctor signed a certificate that she was of unsound mind and had to go to a lunatic asylum. A private asylum was found at Oxford and sufficient extra money provided by a friend. Nightingale advised this friend that a pauper asylum would, "in the opinion of her medical men, in all probability confirm her in insanity." (letter, February 24, 1854, Wellcome 8994/ unnumbered)
3. One patient left "somewhat improved" for the Brompton (Consumption) Hospital. (Nightingale, 1854/1970, 3rd. Quarter, in McDonald, 2009b, p. 108)

Nightingale took up organizing aftercare referrals again post-Crimea, particularly for patients she had had admitted to hospital.

She was pleased that a convalescent home would be built as a memorial on the death of her friend Sidney Herbert. The architect was one she esteemed, T. H. Wyatt, and she worked with him on the plans. The foundation stone for the Herbert Convalescent Home was duly laid in September 1865, with the public statement that "the plans for the new building received the approval of Miss Nightingale" (*The Times*, 1865).

When the Prudhoe Convalescent Home was opened in 1869, its "fine building" and commanding view of the coast were praised, its arrangement on the pavilion plan, "which has prevailed in Germany and France so many years, and which Miss Florence Nightingale and the Crimean Commissioners have so strongly recommended" (*The Times*, 1869).

To a doctor's wife who was organizing a convalescent institution later, she called "the benefits of convalescents homes" to rank

only second to those of hospitals, and indeed that no hospital is complete without its convalescent adjunct—so few patients leave hospital able to return at once to their work and their poor homes. And this dooms them sooner or later "to the parish" in too many cases, i.e., to be dependent on the poor rates, to a life of infirmity. (letter, June 24, 1880, Add Mss 45806 f40)

Nightingale regularly supported and sent cases to the Ascot Convalescent Home in Berkshire, run by an Anglican sisterhood. One referral she made was especially touching, and she followed the case for the next years. This was a little boy, a spinal case, from a family she knew in Derbyshire. She made arrangements for his admission to St. Thomas', then transfer to Ascot when St. Thomas' would not keep him on after 2 years, as incurable, and back and forth again.

The child made "great progress" at St. Thomas' Hospital, Nightingale reported, was growing and able to go back to the convalescent home (letter, January 2, 1879, Derbyshire County Record Office, in McDonald, 2009a, p. 285). She subsequently met with the Ascot mother superior, who had served with her in the Crimean War, who told her that the boy was "much stronger, happier, very intelligent, and a great pet, but she wished him to return for a time to St. Thomas', as she thought he must need surgical attendance. The surgeon who saw him reported that the child had a large abscess on the spine; the parents were told that chances of recovery were less than they had been" (letter, February 21, 1880, in McDonald, 2009b, pp. 328–329).

The Ascot home was exceptional in not being *for* incurables, but for convalescents, but they did not require a patient found to be incurable to leave, "unlike all other institutions of the kind," Nightingale told Sir Harry Verney. They would continue to nurse them until they died. Her example, "little Harry Lee of Lea," was there for 4 years (letter, January 14, 1882, Wellcome 9009/3). A note on the matter later recounted that he lived at Ascot "two years very happily and died there after two years more," presumably not happily (letter, February 27, 1897, Wellcome Ms 5476/94).

An advertisement for the "London and Ascot Convalescent Hospital," which mainly served the poor in the East End of London, used Nightingale's support in its fund-raising: "Eminent physicians approve of the working of the hospital. Miss Nightingale gives her name as a referee." Features of the hospital included 43 acres of pines, heath, and recovered heath, so that "the fragrance of the pines adds much to the salubrity of the dry and exhilarating air. Chronic bronchitis has been healed there" (*The Times*, 1882).

When Amelia de Laney, a nurse Nightingale mentored, took on the matronship of an epileptic institution, Nightingale took careful notes on what she told her. The care of epileptics could be improved by good nursing care. For "wet and dirty patients," she explained, this required "inculcating and practising cleanliness, keeping up their minds with a little cheerful talk." They had "very few such inveterate cases," de Laney told her, after this care (notes, May 7, 1894, Add Mss 47764 f65).

DISTRICT NURSING, HOME VISITING, COMMUNITY NURSING

Trained district nursing saves expense to the parish, makes it possible to nurse incurable cases at home, which otherwise go into the workhouse infirmary, while tiding cases over a temporary illness and setting them on foot so that they need not go either into hospital or infirmary at all.
   —(Nightingale, letter December 2, 1887, in McDonald 2009a, p. 802)

District nursing brings together two core Nightingale principles: a healthy fear of hospitals and belief that the poor deserve as high-quality care as the rich. Well-off people at the time avoided hospital typically by engaging a private nurse at home. For the poor, however, the options were a charity ward at a hospital or the workhouse infirmary, the latter supported by local taxes. Keeping the destitute sick out of workhouse infirmaries thus saved tax money, just as home visiting nurses today keep people out of costly hospitals and emergency departments.

Before Nightingale, a form of home visiting was provided by the Ranyard Mission, or the "Bible women," as they were known. Founded by Ellen Ranyard in 1857, the mission gave working-class women 3 months training in the Poor Law, hygiene, and scripture, with ongoing oversight by more educated "ladies." The visitors reputedly went out on their calls with the Bible under one arm and Nightingale's *Notes on Nursing* under the other. Nightingale respected the organization, but wanted improvements in their unhygienic practices. In 1875, she sent them a check for £20 with her gratitude to God, and prayer for the work's extension, plus a hint that the money be used to pay for "waterproof cloaks" or "washing gowns for summer and washing linen sleeves to take on and off, and washing aprons or washing money for two or three of the nurses in the very poorest district, where there is no local lady to look after these things for the nurses" (Bunford, 1948, pp. 10–11).

Much later, Nightingale wondered if the Bible women might be the means of teaching "*sanitary* monthly nursing for the sick poor" (letter, April 30, 1892, Add Mss 45776 f297). It seems, however, that the Ranyard nurses never met her goal of adequate training.

The Roman Catholic Sisters of Mercy also did home visiting of the sick, but their objects were much more the saving of the patient's soul than care to the body. They were not trained in nursing (Sullivan, 1995, Table 1, pp. 297–299).

William Rathbone, the Liverpool philanthropist who funded the first professional nursing care at a workhouse infirmary, was the benefactor also for the first district nursing project using trained nurses. He authored two books on their efforts, for which Nightingale wrote the introductions (Rathbone, 1865, 1890).

Training for district nurses, as Nightingale saw it, had to be more rigorous than for hospital nurses, for the simple reason that the nurse visiting at a patient's home had no doctor to refer to on the spot. As well, they had to be able to make referrals to social agencies and to advise municipal authorities of sanitary defects. Training started with the same hospital experience, for otherwise they would not see a sufficient range of difficult cases. Then they required supervised experience in the field. District nurses may be seen as an early version of nurse practitioners and medical social workers.

It took many years, and several different organizations, before any concerted system of district nursing was put in place. Nightingale continued to play a background role, drawing on the Nightingale Fund, money which had been raised in her honor during the Crimean War, to provide (limited) financial support (most of the Fund, however, went into regular nurse training). In the mid-1870s, Florence Lees (1840–1922) took over leadership of the work. At Rathbone's request, she conducted a study of what was available in England. This led to the organization of the major district nursing organization, the Metropolitan and National Nursing Association, housed in Bloomsbury Square, London (McDonald, 2009a, pp. 707–899). Lees also made a trip to the United States, with a brief foray into Canada, to see nursing there, but this did not lead to any advances in practice.

Nightingale assisted with the fundraising for district nursing by sending a lengthy letter to the editor of *The Times* in 1876 (see Chapter 11), in effect a justification for the whole project. She sent a further fundraising letter in 1878 to be read at the second annual meeting of the organization. She forcefully presented the great advantages to be gained with district nurses. The district nurse helped to "pull through" cases of life and death, cases that it would be an honor for the best hospitals, with all their appurtenances, to pull through. The district nurse would "show rich and poor what nursing is and what it is not," both "preventing disease and stopping infection and the causes of disease." The dual roles were always a good selling point. Again, Nightingale cited cost-effectiveness: The visiting nurse kept "whole families out of pauperism by preventing the home from being broken up and nursing the breadwinner back to health" (Nightingale, 1878).

A new initiative in district nursing occurred in 1887 on Queen Victoria's jubilee, or 50 years after her accession to the throne. The Queen decided that the fund raised in her honor would be used to establish a new organization, the Queen Victoria Jubilee Nurses. Again, Nightingale played a significant role in shaping its goals and standards.

Similar district nursing projects came into existence in the United States and other countries, somewhat later. There were numerous, sporadic projects that started district nursing earlier, but none of them lasted. American nursing leader Lillian Wald (1867–1940) is typically credited with its founding in 1893, with the opening of the Henry Street Settlement in New York City, which included home visiting nursing in its work. The settlement became the Visiting Nurse Service of New York and Wald herself became the first president of the National Organization for Public Health Nursing, and a reformer in such other causes as racial integration, women's suffrage, and pacifism. She coined the term "public health nursing."

District nursing was later still in coming to Canada. It was only finally established in Canada in 1898, in honor of the Queen's diamond jubilee. The organization, which is still in existence, took the name "Victorian Order of Nurses."

"Health Missioners" for Rural Mothers

Another late initiative of Nightingale's to promote health and prevent disease, without recourse to hospitals, was "health missioners," women trained to take health practices to rural mothers. The medical officer of health of Buckinghamshire organized classes for the missioners, who were not nurses, but specially trained for home visiting. A proper training organization was set up, with examinations and certification. There were obvious social-class challenges to overcome, as the "ladies" might cause offence to the poor, uneducated mothers they were to train. Nightingale considered that they passed the test when the rural mothers welcomed them into their homes.

Nightingale included an addendum, "Health-nurse training," with a syllabus for the lectures, in her paper for the Chicago World Congress of 1893 (Nightingale, 1893, p. 201). The lectures, not less than 15, would be given by the medical officer of health, to include elementary physiology and the science of hygiene, with supervised visits to the cottages. Examinations were conducted by an independent examiner.

As late as 1904, Nightingale was encouraging district nursing in other parts of the world, as a letter to the District Trained Nursing Society of South Australia shows (letter, November 7, 1904, in McDonald, 2009a, p. 899).

NIGHTINGALE AS "NURSE PRACTITIONER"

While Nightingale never worked in a hospital again post-Crimea, she continued until late in life to organize nursing care for many people: friends, relatives, employees, villagers at Lea Holloway (near the Nightingale home in Derbyshire) and Claydon House (her sister's home in Buckinghamshire), and sometimes for old soldiers. She wrote letters of referral to doctors, and kept in touch as treatment continued. She organized admission to hospitals and care facilities of various sorts, and often convalescent care after that. Correspondence on this ranges from before the Crimean War to 1902 (McDonald, 2004, pp. 623–672). A few examples here will have to suffice.

Nightingale paid the local doctor at Lea Hurst on a quarterly basis for his seeing what we would term her "caseload." On one occasion, she wrote to ask him, "Do you not think it very bad for the two sisters, one convalescent and one very ill of typhoid, to lie in the same bed, and both in the same room with the mother?" She had made arrangements specifically for a separate room at "Widow Brown's" (letter, September 7, 1879, Derbyshire County Record Office).

In 1880, she declined a meeting with Colonel Gordon as she was busy sending off a patient to the Dover Convalescent Home (note, February 11, 1880, in McDonald, 2003, p. 492). She had a subscription to Miss Marsh's Convalescent Home, Black Rock, Brighton, so that she could send patients there regularly (receipt, July 5, 1890, Add Mss 45810 f20). Indeed, she donated frequently to small convalescent institutions, partly to support care of a particular patient and partly because of the dangers of hospitals.

QUESTIONS FOR DISCUSSION

1. How important is convalescence as a stage of health care today? How do "rehabilitation" hospitals compare with "convalescent hospitals" of earlier times? Are separate convalescent institutions needed now? If so, why?

2. How are home visiting nurses organized in your area? What qualifications are required for appointment, beyond those of a registered nurse? To what extent does home care enable patients to avoid hospital stays? (Desirably, this could be ascertained by comparing hospitalization rates and lengths of stay by availability of home visiting nurses.)

3. Aftercare arrangements: To what extent are these the task of nurses (hospital or home visitor) to organize? In your area, are these handled by medical social workers instead? What are the comparative merits of arrangements by nurses and by social workers?

4. Nurse practitioners: what role do they play in your area? What additional qualifications are required? What more could nurse practitioners do (a) in giving care and (b) in preventing disease or relapse?

REFERENCES

Angus, D. C., Linde-Zwirble, W. T., Lidicker, J., Clermont, G., Carcillo, J., & Pinsky, M. R. (2001, July). Epidemiology of severe sepsis in the United States: Analysis of incidence, outcome, and associated costs of care. *Critical Care Medicine, 29*(7), 1303–1310.

Arnold, C. (2014, July). Rethinking sterile: Hospital microbiome. *Environmental Health Perspective, 122*(7). doi:10.1289/ehp.122-A182

Bunford, A. M. (1948). *Ninety years a mission 1857-1947.* London, UK: Ranyard Mission.

Croft, J. (1873). *Notes of lectures at St. Thomas' Hospital.* London, UK: St. Thomas/ Blades, East & Blades.

Doidge, N. (2015). *The brain's way of healing: Remarkable discoveries and recoveries from the frontiers of neuroplasticity.* Harmondsworth, UK: Penguin. ISBN: 9781925016374.

Gill, C. G. & Gill, G. (2005, June 16). Nightingale in Scutari: Her legacy re-examined. *Clinical Infectious Diseases, 40*(12), 1799–1805. doi:10.1086/430380

Graves, R. J. (1843). *A system of clinical medicine.* Dublin, Ireland: Fannin.

Halm, M. A. (2008, July). The healing power of the human-animal connection. *American Journal of Critical Care, 17*(4), 373–376.

Lamorna [Georgina Franklin]. (1910, September 3). Some personal reflections of Miss Florence Nightingale. *Nursing Mirror and Midwives' Journal,* 347–349.

McDonald, L. (Ed.). (2003). *Florence Nightingale on society and politics, philosophy, science, education, and literature.* Waterloo, Canada: Wilfrid Laurier University Press. ISBN: 0-88920-429-2.

McDonald, L. (Ed.). (2004). *Florence Nightingale on public health care.* Waterloo, Canada: Wilfrid Laurier University Press. ISBN: 0-88920-446-2.

McDonald, L. (Ed.). (2005). *Florence Nightingale on women, medicine, midwifery and prostitution.* Waterloo, Canada: Wilfrid Laurier University Press. ISBN: 0-88920-466-7.

McDonald, L. (Ed.). (2009a). *Florence Nightingale: Extending nursing.* Waterloo, Canada: Wilfrid Laurier University Press. ISBN: 978-1-55458-170-2.

McDonald, L. (Ed.). (2009b). *Florence Nightingale: The Nightingale School.* Waterloo, Canada: Wilfrid Laurier University Press. ISBN: 978-1-55458-169-6.

McDonald, L. (Ed.). (2011). *Florence Nightingale on wars and the war office.* Waterloo, Canada: Wilfrid Laurier University Press. ISBN: 978-1-55458-382-9.

Mottus, J. E. (1981). *New York Nightingales: The emergence of the nursing profession at Bellevue and New York Hospital, 1850-1920.* Ann Arbor, MI: UMI Research Press. ISBN: 97808375711678.

Nightingale, F. (1854/1970). *Florence Nightingale at Harley Street: Her reports to the governors of her nursing home, 1853-54.* London, UK: J.M. Dent & Sons.

Nightingale, F. (1860). *Notes on nursing: What it is, and what it is not.* London, UK: Harrison.

Nightingale. F. (1861, March 2). Letter to R. Rawlinson. Bonhams sale 29/311.

Nightingale. F. (1867). *Suggestions on the subject of providing training and organizing nurses for the sick poor in workhouse infirmaries* (pp. 67–76). London, UK: HMSO.

Nightingale, F. (1871). *Introductory notes on lying-in institutions.* London, UK: Longmans, Green.

Nightingale, F. (1876, April 14). Trained nurses for the sick poor, *The Times,* 6CD.

Nightingale, F. (1883). Nurses, training of, and nursing the sick. In R. Quain (Ed.), *A dictionary of medicine* (Vol. 2, pp. 1038–1049). London, UK: Longmans, Green.

Nightingale, F. (1890). Hospitals. In *Chambers's encyclopaedia: A dictionary of universal knowledge* (Vol. 5, pp. 805–807). Edinburgh, Scotland: W. & R. Chambers.

Nightingale, F. (1893). Sick nursing and health nursing. In A. Burdett-Coutts (Ed.), *Woman's mission: A series of congress papers on the philanthropic work of women.* London, UK: Sampson, Low, Marston.

Rathbone, W. (1865). *The organization of nursing in a large town.* Liverpool, UK: Holden.

Rathbone, W. (1890). *Sketch of the history and progress of district nursing from its commencement in the year 1859 to the present date.* London, UK: Macmillan.

Roberts, N. (1886, July 29). Printed paper (untitled). British Library Add Mss 45807 ff267-268.

Roberts, N. (1887, July 8). Lady Roberts's "Homes in the Hills" for Nursing Sisters Employed in the British Military Hospitals in India. British Library Add Mss 45807 f269.

Roy, C., & Andrews, H. A. (1999). *The Roy adaptation model* (2nd ed.). Stamford, CT: Appleton & Lange. ISBN: 0838522718.

Singh, S., & Ernst, E. (2008). *Trick or treatment: Alternative medicine on trial.* London, UK: Bantam. ISBN: 9781409081791.

Strangford, Viscountess. (1874). *Hospital training for ladies: An appeal to the hospital boards in England.* London, UK: Harrison.

Sullivan M. C. (1995). *Catherine McAuley and the tradition of mercy.* Notre Dame, IN: University of Notre Dame Press. ISBN: 0168008116.

The Times. (1865, September 18). The Herbert Convalescent Home, 8F.

The Times. (1869, September 16). The Prudhoe Convalescent Home, 10C.

The Times. (1878, February 21). Trained nurses, 8A.

The Times. (1880, December 9). Instruction for Nurses, 11A.

The Times. (1882, June 30). London and Ascot Convalescent Hospital, 13B.

Vallée, G. (Ed.). (2006). *Florence Nightingale on health in India.* Waterloo, ON, Canada: Wilfird Laurier University Press. ISBN: 10-0-88920-468-3.

Vallée, G. (Ed.). (2007). *Florence Nightingale on social change in India.* Waterloo, Canada: Wilfrid Laurier University Press. ISBN: 978-0-88920-495-9.

Walsh, J. J. (1907). *Makers of modern medicine.* New York, NY: Fordham University Press; 1970. Freeport, NY: Books for Libraries. ISBN: 0836915380.

Wootton, D. (2006). *Bad medicine: Doctors doing harm since Hippocrates.* Oxford, UK: Oxford University Press. ISBN: 9780199212798.

Chapter 3: Health Promotion

It is much cheaper to promote health than to maintain people in sickness.
—Nightingale (1894)

Nightingale was consistent throughout her working life on the importance of health promotion and disease prevention, although the care of the sick would be the main task of nurses and the primary focus of their training. This chapter shows that Nightingale's definition of health would be widely accepted, and still is. The chapter goes on to the social and environmental determinants of health, the factors that have to be addressed to improve health status. Housing was a major factor for Nightingale and remains no less important today, as can be seen by numerous later documents on health promotion.

Nutrition, for improving health among troops and food in hospitals for patients and nurses, was an early and ongoing concern.

The chapter goes on to setting priorities, á la Nightingale, for disease prevention, by looking at the statistics. Today's greatest cause of preventable mortality is cigarette smoking, not an issue Nightingale dealt with. Several countries, Western and Asian, are considered in relation to their smoking and death rates, and control measures or lack of them. Obesity as an issue of disease prevention follows, again not an issue for Nightingale, but one that qualifies for inclusion according to her criteria of preferring to prevent disease rather than treat it, and the fact of its increase worldwide.

A section follows on occupational health and safety, an important matter from the beginning of professional nursing because of the high number of nurse deaths.

Finally, some context to Nightingale's approach is given by examining her broader concerns of environmentalism.

NIGHTINGALE'S DEFINITION OF HEALTH

Of the many definitions of health now available, Nightingale's short, positive one continues to please: "Health is not only to be well, but to be able to use well every power we have." It appeared first in her entry in Quain's *Dictionary of Medicine* (Nightingale, 1883), and she repeated it in her paper to the Chicago world congress in 1893 (Nightingale, 1893). The World Health Organization (WHO) definition, from 1948, is similar: "Health is a state of complete physical, mental, and social well-being and not merely the absence of disease or infirmity." Nursing textbooks since have typically offered lengthier definitions, but with the same core substance.

Health promotion was a major goal of Nightingale's throughout her life, shared with a small number of doctors. It would become increasingly the goal of major nursing organizations, notably the International Council of Nurses and the American and Canadian national organizations, and of national governments and the United Nations' WHO. The four components have to be linked: health promotion, disease prevention, cure, and the alleviation of suffering. Nursing has a role in all four.

Nightingale's approach can be seen in the National Health Service established in the United Kingdom after the Second World War. Its 1946 legislation aimed at no less than the "improvement in the physical and mental health of the people of England and Wales and the prevention, diagnosis, and treatment of illness."

INTERNATIONAL ENDEAVORS ON HEALTH PROMOTION

Numerous international efforts have been made to promote health and health care, from the WHO's definition of health in 1948 to the declaration at Alma Ata in 1978 that the highest attainable standard of health should be "a fundamental right of every human being." The declaration reflects the principles Nightingale formulated in her first work after the Crimean War of 1854 to 1856, making disease prevention and education the means of achieving those goals. Food supply, nutrition, safe water, basic sanitation, and maternal and child care were specified in the Alma Ata declaration, as was the need for the participation of other sectors, such as agriculture and public works (United Nations, 1978; WHO, 2015). This would be all familiar material to anyone who has read Nightingale.

Since the focus of this chapter is health promotion, which was only one of Alma Ata's concerns (which had a significant focus on primary health care), two other conferences are key. The WHO's 14th World Health Assembly, in 1977, set out the aim of "health for all" by the year 2000, through better measures at health promotion.

Its 1986 meetings in Ottawa, Canada, went on to adopt a charter, approved by delegates from 38 countries, aimed at an "economically productive" level of health, again for the year 2000. This charter specified five "action areas," all of which are consistent with Nightingale's views:

1. Building healthy public policy
2. Creating supportive environments
3. Strengthening community action
4. Developing personal skills
5. Reorienting health care services toward prevention of illness and promotion of health

The charter holds that these goals cannot be achieved by the health sector alone but require collaboration by all levels of government. The more of the "action areas" in operation, the better the chances of achieving health promotion. Public health nurses and other professionals see the Ottawa Charter of 1986 as a useful tool for advancing health promotion goals, and note that it is entirely consistent with Nightingale's approach.

The "Right" to Health

Nightingale herself did not use "rights" language, but she believed that quality care should be available to all, regardless of the ability to pay, as noted in Chapter 1. Rights, of course, do not effectively exist unless someone has the duty to provide what is needed. Nightingale did much to promote the idea of societal responsibility for health care and of societal benefit from having a healthy population.

Prominent nurses and nursing organizations have taken up universal access to care as a cause. Virginia Henderson, probably the most influential American nursing leader in the 20th century, in a guest editorial looked to health care needs being met by "universal health coverage" in the United States: "Certainly it is high time to recognize that meeting them is a *shared responsibility* of the recipients and providers of care." She looked to health care, like education, being recognized as a right of all members of society, as it was in "virtually every industrialized society except the United States." Henderson added arguments of cost-effectiveness for "some sort of universally available, affordable, effective, national health insurance that reduces the numbers of needlessly dependent individuals in a given society" (Henderson, 1990). That was 1990, and universal access has yet to be established in the United States.

When nursing organizations began to establish formal codes of ethics, a matter discussed in Chapter 4, the goals they set out included health promotion, understood in broad terms, not only care of the sick.

> Let us reform our hospitals now, and as we improve our cities and towns, they will be less required.

—Nightingale (1858, p. 643)

SOCIAL/ENVIRONMENTAL DETERMINANTS OF HEALTH

Nightingale had a keen sense that the conditions in which people live and work have a powerful impact on their health status, and these of course are greatly determined by social status. Air and water quality, nutritious food, and decent housing are frequent subjects in her writing from beginning to end. She was well aware that the poor were more vulnerable to illness than those better off, although there were scandalous cases of death from poor drainage even in the homes of the rich and in elite public (fee-paying) schools.

Housing was fundamental to health status, in Nightingale's understanding, as she told Dr. Sutherland in 1872: "To make the people's dwellings fit for sick, or rather such as will *not make* sickness . . . is of course our first duty" (letter, March 15, 1872, in McDonald, 2012, p. 769). This she contrasted with building hospitals to heal the sick.

Right in her *Notes on Nursing*, Chapter 2, she set out five "essential points" to secure the health of the house: pure air, pure water, efficient drainage, cleanliness, and light. Without them "no house can be healthy," and the house will be unhealthy in proportion to their lack. Bad housing was the norm in her day. More light was especially needed in the homes of the poor. An extra pane of glass or a skylight that opened could make a great difference, Nightingale thought.

The same principles applied when the "home" for ordinary soldiers was a barracks. Nightingale and her colleagues devoted considerable efforts post-Crimea to improving ventilation and other amenities in barracks (nutrition is discussed shortly below). She had discovered in the course of her Crimean War mortality research that death rates among soldiers living in barracks in London were twice that of the population at large, although the men had had to pass a physical examination to be accepted in the army (the British Army then was entirely voluntary).

The reformers were rewarded in their efforts by seeing substantial declines in death rates. The laws of health worked: Provide adequate ventilation, space, light, nutrition, exercise, and so forth, and health status improves and hospital stays and deaths decline. As a tribute to her great collaborator on army reforms, Sidney Herbert, after his death in 1861, Nightingale (1862) published those statistics, with charts, showing the decline in death rates. The work had to be well coordinated to be effective, another lesson she/they learned.

When the army's Royal Victoria Hospital was planned for Netley, on the south coast of England, its large size was based on the proportion of troops expected to be sick, 7 percent, before the reforms were made. By the time it opened in 1863, sickness rates and lengths of stay had declined to 3.5% to 4%. Nightingale then joked, "Really, it is not our *fault* if the number of sick has fallen so much that they can't fill their hospitals" (letter, March 14, 1865, in McDonald, 2012, p. 442). The hospital was not filled to capacity until the Boer War.

Nightingale's emphasis on fresh air has been taken up more recently by microbiologists who study the microbiome. A paper at the 2009 meeting of the American Association for the Advancement of Science cited her advocacy of fresh air in *Notes on Nursing*, comparing the community of bacteria in the air with that in the gut. Just as antibiotic use can wipe out the "good bacterial community," excessive disinfection can destroy bacteria that fight disease pathogens. Data from a University of Oregon study show that clinics that kept their windows open had a wider range of bacteria, "while those that were kept sealed had a higher proportion of potentially harmful germs" (Collins, 2012).

Measuring Health Status

When the U.K. national census was being planned in 1860, Nightingale sought to have questions added both on health status and housing, which she always saw as closely linked. The former would give an overall picture of the state of the nation's health, on "one spring day," as she told medical statistician William Farr. (The census was taken in April—not the coldest, nor the hottest time of the year.) Mortality data were then routinely collected, but Nightingale pointed out that these gave only "a very imperfect standard of health." The only real standard is *"how many people, are well, how many ill* and the *diseases."* Further,

> We have absolutely no information on the sanitary state of the people....how many sick there are in the population, and in what kind of houses the population live are fundamental points.... [They] would afford a better basis upon which to build up social progress than any information the census now gives. (letter, May 11, 1860, in McDonald, 2003, pp. 99–100)

The Toronto Charter for a Healthy Canada list of "social determinants of health" closely resembles Nightingale's concerns, however, adding terms not in use in her day, such as "social exclusion" and "social safety nets":

- Employment and working conditions
- Income and income distribution
- Food insecurity
- Housing
- Early childhood development
- Education
- Health care: primary, secondary, tertiary
- Social exclusion
- Social safety nets

The authors note that, in Canada, "poverty is the strongest determinant of health, and poverty rates have not improved over the last two decades" (Wilkinson & Marmot, 2003).

IMPROVING NUTRITION IN THE ARMY AND IN HOSPITALS

In addition to the two chapters on food in her *Notes on Nursing*, discussed in Chapter 2, Nightingale devoted much attention to adequate diet, especially for the army (both for soldiers on active duty and the sick) and nurses (both nursing students and employed hospital nurses).

During the Crimean War, given that the British Army did not provide anything close to a balanced diet for its soldiers, scurvy was frequent. "Scorbutic disease," meaning scurvy related, appears frequently in official reports of admissions and deaths. Furthermore, men weakened by poor diet and overwork were much more vulnerable to infectious disease. Improving the food became a major concern for Nightingale in the first year of her war work. That may account for nutrition getting two chapters in her *Notes on Nursing* (discussed in Part II, Chapter 10).

For the army, Nightingale succeeded in getting a cooking school established at the large army base at Aldershot. The volunteer chef, Alexis Soyer, had succeeded in improving the food for hospitals during the Crimean War. However, his giving a demonstration did not bring about any practical improvement. A program of cooking classes was needed, not a single example. It seems that the new regime instituted post-Crimea was successful, for the health status of ordinary soldiers improved.

There was no separate specialty of nutrition when her school opened and no occupation of nutritionist, and so nurses were responsible for cooking special meals when the regular menus were inadequate. Cooking classes were sometimes organized for the students.

The importance of nutrition has not declined since, but nurses now need only to learn the general principles, as others take charge of the cooking and meal planning.

Nightingale periodically looked over the "dietary," or menus, for St. Thomas' Hospital. She passed on complaints, especially of poor variety, lack of milk, and, for nurses having to come to meals late, sometimes not enough food at all, especially hot food. Nurses worked hard and needed decent food for their health. She insisted that there be a hot meal ready for student nurses on return to their residence, with nutritious food and good variety. They should be able to make themselves a hot cup of tea at any time, in a warm lounge. Beer or wine was provided as part of the meal. Specific complaints she sent in included lack of green vegetables and inedible carrots, greens, turnips, and potatoes; "meat inferior and ill cooked" (notes, January 15, 1876, in McDonald, 2009b, p. 305). Decent food for night nurses was an ongoing concern.

With the benefit of hindsight, Nightingale's "diets," as meal plans were then termed, can be seen to have met good nutritional standards. A study conducted of her army diet found it somewhat low on fiber, but good otherwise (Calkins, 1989). Nightingale worked hard on this subject, notably consulting the best expert on nutrition, Edinburgh Dr. Robert Christison.

Food issues of course have changed markedly since Nightingale's time. Fast food and obesity simply do not appear in her writing. Bad food then meant food that was rotten or otherwise dangerous from industrial production or poor storage when there was no state provision for food inspection. Obesity as a health issue is turned to shortly.

NIGHTINGALE'S OPTIMISM ON DISEASE PREVENTION

In later writing, Nightingale showed herself to be optimistic about disease preventive measures, improving public health through education and local organization. Partnership was required among local authorities, citizens volunteering their time, and people/women obtaining the necessary training to do the work. The county council could be "one of the strongest engines" in its favor, she thought. Enlightened public opinion was essential, "wise in principles, wise in details." These elements had to "contend against centuries of superstition and generations of indifference," but she nonetheless saw a "great impulse . . . for national health against national and local disease," all words chosen carefully (Nightingale, 1892).

The county council needed a "Sanitary Committee," which could gather information and support the work of the medical officer of health, instead of "quashing" his reports. In summing up the core message she, as she often did, included the practical advantage of cost:

> We will not have cholera, we will not have fever, nor infantile complaints, the true test of what is sanitary or insanitary— sickly children growing into sickly parents. We will have good water supply, good drainage, no overcrowding, pure air, pure water, pure earth, for disease is more expensive than sanitation. (Nightingale, 1892, in McDonald, 2004, p. 595)

DISEASE PREVENTION: SETTING PRIORITIES FOR TODAY

Nightingale's practice was to look at the big picture, to seek change where new policies could prevent deaths and promote health. Applying her principles to current conditions, we would ask what are the greatest threats to health, and set about to reduce them. Practically, this means deciding where taking action would save the most lives. Recommended actions themselves then have to be followed up to ascertain their actual results, for harmful unintended consequences are always possible.

Top of the list for its potential to kill in our age would be climate change, with the risk of full-scale species extinctions as well as massive illness and deaths, which have already begun to occur, a subject to be pursued in Chapter 9 on policy. For a lesser, but still major, cause of unnecessary deaths, cigarette smoking is the priority, the world's greatest cause of preventable mortality, estimated at 6,000,000 annually, which includes 600,000 deaths from second-hand smoke.

Other diseases for which substantial reductions in mortality could be achieved are malaria, tuberculosis, and HIV/AIDS. Deaths from hospital-acquired infections are considered in Chapter 5 on infection control.

Reducing Death Rates From Smoking

Tobacco use is the greatest cause of preventable mortality worldwide, with roughly 10% of adult deaths globally due to smoking. In low-income countries, not surprisingly, smoking-related deaths are exceeded by deaths from low birth weight, or malnutrition, and indoor smoke (from kitchen fires). Still, tobacco use is significant in low-income countries, ranking seventh (WHO, 2002).

An overview of the toll of smoking in the United States shows that it reduces life expectancy by more than 10 years among current smokers, compared with those who never smoked. More happily, the same study reported that adults who quit gained in life expectancy, although they did not reach that of nonsmokers (Jha et al., 2013, p. 341).

Many countries, notably Canada, parts of the United States (California leading the way), and many in the European Union, have taken strenuous measures to reduce smoking and to protect nonsmokers from second-hand smoke. Other countries have done little, enacted token measures only, or failed to enforce legislation they did enact. Here two contrasting American examples are given: Virginia, a tobacco-growing state with no statewide legislation, and California, the most effective state in reducing smoking prevalence and deaths.

Since smoking and death rates are particularly high in Asia, two examples, both countries with high rates, are examined: Japan, an advanced industrial country, and Vietnam, a rapidly industrializing country. Globally, 29% of people aged 15 years and older were regular smokers in 1995. For East Asia the rate was 38%. Males there constitute 80% of all smokers.

Desirably all these unhappy facts will become obsolete with reforms, but the trend is still going the other way. The decline in smoking rates and deaths in Western countries is more than made up for with the rise in smoking in Asia especially. Cigarette companies continue to make ample profits from selling this product.

American Examples: Virginia and California

Virginia, a tobacco-growing state, ranks 12th of the American states in the proportion of adults who smoke. There is no statewide law to protect people from second-hand smoke in public areas or workplaces, or any statewide ban on cigarette advertising or promotion. State law does not allow municipalities to enact smoke-free provisions, but only to regulate the promotion, sampling, and display of tobacco products.

The rate of cigarette taxation in Virginia is low, at $.30 per pack, making it 49th among the 50 states. Funding for tobacco control programs is well below the recommended level, giving Virginia a rank of 32nd among the states.

When municipalities in California began to bring in nonsmoking regulations, the state had a higher prevalence rate than the nation generally. The restaurant and bar smoking bans were well liked and led to much tougher, statewide measures.

A comprehensive program, the California Tobacco Control Program, was established by the Tobacco Tax and Health Promotion Act of 1988, which was approved by California voters. This program increased taxes and paid for a bold media campaign. In 1995, California became the first state to enact a statewide smoking ban. Other states have since followed.

An estimated 1 million Californian lives have been saved since the antitobacco program began. Health care costs have declined. In 2011, the adult smoking rate in California hit a record low of 12%, from 26% in 1984. Declines, as elsewhere, had begun earlier, probably from increased awareness of the risk of smoking.

Canadian Example

Canada became a world leader in tobacco control in 1988 with the passing of the Non-smokers' Health Act, which established smoke-free work and public places in areas under federal regulation, and named tobacco a hazardous product. Controls over packaging were brought in through separate legislation, and, some years later, a complete ban on advertising and sponsorship was introduced (Cunningham, 1996). Smoking remains the largest cause of preventable mortality, with an estimated 37,000 dying each year.

As in the United States, smoking rates had begun to decline in the 1970s with the growing awareness of the ill effects of smoking. In Canada, smoking rates declined from 49% in 1965, to 35% in 1985, 30% in 1991, and 20% in 2013 (Gilmore, 2000). Canada tops the list of (four) countries where declines of smoking of more than 50% for both men and women have been achieved (Taylor, 2014).

Asian Examples: Japan and Vietnam

About 130,000 people die each year in Japan of tobacco-related diseases, according to WHO. Smoking accounts for the largest number of premature deaths in Japan, triple the number of suicides and 10 times the number of traffic fatalities. The incidence of smoking there is decreasing, but the rates are still high. Japan Tobacco is the third largest cigarette producer in the world and the Japanese government is its largest owner. That tobacco is grown in Japan is thought to be partly responsible for government inaction on the problem, a point that holds also for the state of Virginia. The Japanese government, until recently, not only permitted smoking in its own offices, but also gave out free cigarettes to the elderly.

Each year 350 billion cigarettes are smoked in Japan, or 2,770 cigarettes per person, compared with 2,350 for the United States. Some 36.6% of men smoked in 2010, compared with 24% for the United States. The rate for Japanese men fell below 40% for the first time in 2005. The smoking rate for Japanese women is lower, 11.3% in 2005 (Hays, 2009).

Regulations have reduced the amount of smoking in public places, but there is still no effective ban, and large numbers of Japanese employees are routinely subjected to second-hand smoke at their places of work. The Health Promotion Law of 2003 prohibits smoking in public places, but lacks penalties and an enforcement agency. Indeed, WHO's monitoring survey published in 2014 reported that Japan had implemented none of the five top recommended measures to reduce smoking. Smoking is permitted in universities teaching nursing and health care! Many doctors and nurses smoke.

Cigarette taxes in Japan are low, and so the price of cigarettes is roughly half that in other industrialized countries. The budget for smoking cessation programs is a bad joke. Its health ministry did not add so much as one expert on smoking to its staff when the 2003 law was passed. Cigarette advertising is still permitted, as is "soft advertising," such as by showing attractive characters smoking in films and on television.

Warnings on cigarette packages in Japan are weak and even misleading. They advise people to "be careful," that smoking "too much" can harm one's health, when the evidence is unequivocal that smoking any amount is harmful, both to the smoker and others who breathe the second-hand smoke. There is no "safe" amount to smoke actively or passively. Fetuses, too, are affected by second-hand smoke.

Japan's legislation needs to be strengthened to be effective, notably by the institution of regulations prohibiting smoking in the workplace, with penalties and enforcement. The low budget for antismoking measures would appear to be a false economy. With increased taxes on cigarettes, significant increases in programs for smoking prevention and cessation would be feasible. Again, this is typical Nightingale strategy, that it is more effective to promote health and prevent disease than to treat it after the fact.

In Vietnam, as elsewhere, tobacco-related illnesses are the leading cause of death, accounting for 40,000 deaths each year, three times the number from traffic injuries. More than half of Vietnamese men smoke, 56.1%, while only 3.4% of women are active smokers. More than half of Vietnam's non-smokers report frequent exposure to second-hand smoke, not surprising when 65% of smokers report smoking in their offices and 90% at least sometimes at home.

WHO points out that a 20% increase in tobacco taxes in Vietnam would save 100,000 lives over the next 40 years (WHO, 2015). Taxes account for only 45% of the retail price, while the World Bank recommends that they be in the range of 66% to 80%.

The Government of Vietnam has issued a Resolution on National Tobacco Control Policy with the aim of reducing smoking prevalence. It was one of the first Asian countries to sign the WHO's Framework Convention for Tobacco Control in 2004. Smoking bans have been enacted, however, to date, they have not been enforced.

The Framework Convention of WHO, incidentally, was one of the most supported agreements ever. It had 168 signatory countries and was based on rigorous evidence. Yet its effects have been scattered, and countries with poor health care systems have rising cigarette use. The best international efforts, in other words, can be subverted by concerted advertising drives by cigarette companies, aided by lax enforcement by governments.

If Nightingale's principles are considered, large numbers of deaths, illness, and absences from work would be treated as problems to be addressed. Examples of successful reductions of tobacco-related mortality in other countries would be studied, for many countries have brought in measures that cut their smoking rates and reduce mortality.

WHO tracks both the prevalence of tobacco use by country and countries' implementation of reduction measures. Its "Tobacco-free Initiative" is exemplary in being evidence based (WHO, 2017). The good news is that those countries that adopt more (if not all) of the reduction measures see greater reductions in smoking than those that adopt fewer. The bad news is that most low-income countries have not implemented any such measures, or only very partially. The question remains then, for those countries that have seen reductions, is part of this success due to younger people especially taking up "vaping," or the use of e-cigarettes? In the United States, more young people "vape" than smoke regular cigarettes.

Vaping or E-cigarettes: The New Tobacco Epidemic?

The U.S. Surgeon General, who alerted the world to the high death toll of tobacco in 1964, has reported the serious threat of electronic cigarettes "e-cigarettes," or "vaping," from the use of an aerosol rather than burning tobacco. That the tobacco industry has invested heavily in e-cigarettes is cause for concern. So is the fact that it uses all the ploys of cigarette advertising and sponsorship for this new product—glamour, daring, risk. Just as it earlier argued "harm reduction" for new tobacco products, such as "light" cigarettes and filters, it now argues that e-cigarettes help smokers to quit (U.S. Centers for Disease Control and Prevention, 2016).

E-cigarettes have not been in use for long enough for any full assessment of their harm to have been made. Nicotine is addictive and known to be harmful to brain development, up to the age of 25. Yet Canadian legislators, to give one example, as this is written, are considering a minimum age of 18 for legal access to e-cigarettes. E-cigarettes are widely sold and advertised everywhere.

Generalizing the Lessons Learned on Tobacco Control

Three measures, when combined, have been successful in many Western countries in reducing smoking prevalence and ensuing disease and death: smoke-free workplaces, higher cigarette prices through taxes (especially a deterrent for the young), and a ban on all forms of advertising and sponsorship. A complete ban is essential, for cigarette companies are adept at finding loopholes. Smoking cessation aids such as nicotine patches and enhanced medical counseling on cessation may also assist, but are unlikely to be effective without these stronger measures.

None of these proposed measures requires new research. Policy makers need only consult the best research available (an abundance of sources), which all point in the same direction. Nightingale would surely call nurses and doctors to set an example and quit smoking themselves. Health care facilities should ensure a smoke-free environment for all their employees and patients.

Tobacco use has declined per capita in Western, industrialized countries in recent years, thanks to well-targeted campaigns. It is still high in Japan, China, and other Asian countries where regulations have been late in coming and their implementation half-hearted. East Timor has one of the world's highest rates of smoking, with more than two thirds of men smoking, an increasing rate among young people, and an as yet unseen impact on health care, given the lead time on disease and death. There are no bans on smoking anywhere; teachers and pupils smoke in the classroom; the infamous "Marlboro Man," who died of emphysema, still appears on billboards there (Taylor, 2014).

International studies show a reduction in the proportions of people smoking, but with population increases, the number of cigarettes smoked (and sold) worldwide increases steadily (Ng et al., 2014).

Smoking and vaping are prime subjects for health promotion today over treatment of disease later. Can nurses make a difference here? The means needed to reduce smoking mainly require political action: higher taxes, bans on smoking in work and public places, graphic warnings, and plain packaging. Clinical measures, such as quitting programs and tobacco patches, can play only a minor role. The "vaping" threat is a new challenge.

Tobacco use is not an issue Nightingale or anyone of her time addressed, as the harmful effect of smoking was not then known (or they were thought to pertain to character, not morbidity or mortality). But it is the kind of issue in which her approach could be useful: The data on harm and what works to reduce it are both abundant and persuasive. There is, in short, no lack of useful experience from countries that have led in reductions. A concerted, multisectoral approach is needed, with critical attention paid to the profit motive of cigarette corporations and advertisers, and the ability to counter their moves.

Obesity

In Nightingale's time, famine and malnutrition were great problems, and still are in some places. Now obesity is a present and growing health issue in most countries. Wealthy countries were the first to see rising obesity rates, but now there are increases as well in developing countries. Obesity appeared in the United States during the Depression, for sugar and starch were cheap foods. Obese persons suffer more illness than others, including heart disease and diabetes. Obese persons have a lower life expectancy than other people.

As predicted, life expectancy, after many years of increases, has begun to decline. In the United States, it declined for men from 2014 to 2015 from 76.5 to 76.3 years, and for women from 81.3 to 81.2 years (Xu, Murphy, Kochanek, & Arias, 2016).

The problem is complex and experts do not agree on the relative causal importance of genetic makeup, lack of exercise, and patterns of food consumption, especially of fats versus sugar. The case for sugar as the major cause now has considerable backing. Advocates for the sugar industry and related packaged food producers argue that there is no firm scientific evidence. They are correct, and there never can be, short of a draconian experiment with people variously assigned to diets with differing levels of sugar, fats, and so on, to be tested over a period of decades for diabetes, heart disease, cancers, and degenerative diseases like Alzheimer's.

The arguments are reminiscent of the tobacco wars of the 1970s, when cigarette companies argued that there was no proof that smoking caused lung cancer, or any other disease, or was addictive.

Using Nightingale's method, we would want to look at the numbers. The increase in per capita sugar consumption, worldwide, has been enormous over the last two centuries (it began earlier, but more gradually). In 1800, estimates of consumption were 1 to 2 kg per person on average worldwide. In 1900, estimates of average consumption were 5 kg, rising to a staggering 50 to 65 kg per person in 2010 (Gibson, 2012). There is no other remotely comparable change in consumption patterns. Charts show a close relationship between rising sugar consumption, obesity, and diabetes.

The extent to which sedentary lifestyles, also increasing, are a factor is not clear. But there are good reasons for countering those trends as well. To wait for all the evidence to come in would be foolhardy. Experts tend to be linked to a limited set of concerns, in their research/academic appointments and publications. Yet this is a subject for a multisectoral approach, the sor Nightingale showed could be done on the (albeit simpler) issue of soldiers health and has begun to show results on tobacco-related deaths.

Solutions to obesity and its related diseases will require coordinatio across different sectors, involving governments at all levels, with regula tions and taxation, food manufacturers, advertisers, and teachers. Possibl actions include the requirement to provide clear information on total suga content for a standard unit on food and drink packages, with warnings fo amounts exceeding a fixed quantity or proportion. There could be regu lations on permitted sugar content itself. Schools and community center could ban products exceeding a certain level. Advertising could be regu lated, including a ban on advertising sugar-added products above a certai level to children.

To reduce the use of high-sugar drinks, water fountains are needed i public places. Physical education classes in schools, previously availabl and even compulsory in places, could be reinstated or initiated where nc had before. All this means engaging the political sector, at all levels of gov ernment. Changes brought in, in any sector, must be monitored for thei effects and reported.

Nightingale stressed housing as a major determinant of health status and that applies here, too, although more by way of city planning than th quality of the housing itself. People in the suburbs disproportionally depen on car transportation, given the lack of public transit, sidewalks, and bicycl paths—and do, in fact, have greater rates of obesity. Suburban homes ma meet high standards on ventilation, pure water, and light, but encourage sedentary lifestyle. Again, a problem of this size with such complication needs a complex, coordinated, approach.

American nurses have recently joined in pressing for action on child hood obesity (Berkowitz & Borchard, 2009), while Canadian nurses hav published clinical "best practice guidelines" (Registered Nurses Associatio of Ontario, 2014).

OCCUPATIONAL HEALTH AND SAFETY

In Nightingale's time, there was virtually no regulation of workplace safet or health. Laws to protect children were gradually brought in, and partic ularly unsafe workplaces, like mines, were regulated. Factory condition were notoriously bad, even in relatively prosperous countries like th United Kingdom.

Nightingale, again without using the current term, was a subscriber t "human resource theory." It would be economically sound, as well as mor

humane, to have healthier, safer workplaces. It took money to train workers, she frequently pointed out, so that their loss or disability cost the firm,
or the army, as well as the individual and his or her family.

In her paper, "Sick nursing and health nursing," she proposed that
workers themselves should seek improvements:

> As for the workshops, work people should remember that health
> is their only capital, and they should come to an understanding
> among themselves not only to have the means, but to use the
> means, to secure pure air in their places of work, which is one
> of the prime agents of health. (Nightingale, 1893, pp. 190–191, in
> McDonald, 2004, p. 211, in Part II, Chapter 12)

In advocating the addition of a question on health status in the census,
Nightingale sought a means for tracking disease and injury by occupation.
Her recommendations on hospital forms similarly included data on occupa-
tion, so that comparisons by occupation could be made.

Nightingale told an 1867 Parliamentary committee investigating cubic
space in workhouse infirmaries that hospitals had a duty as employers to
ensure a safe workplace. This appears in the excerpt in Part II, Chapter 11,
that "every employer of labour is bound to provide for the health of the
workers." Furthermore, any organization that professed to "provide for
sick," at the expense of the lives of nurses and doctors, proved that "providing for the care of sick is not its calling." She explained further that the
arrangements needed for the care of the sick were the same as to ensure "the
health of nurses" (Nightingale, 1867, in McDonald, 2004, pp. 386–387, Part
II, Chapter 11).

NIGHTINGALE'S ENVIRONMENTALISM

Britain, as the world's leader in industrialization, was early to see losses
in species and suffer from serious air and water pollution. This prompted
a study of the causes and advocacy to counter them. It is no coincidence
that environmental experts emerged early in the United Kingdom, and had
some early, if partial, successes. Organizations were formed, studies conducted, and results published. The environmentally conscious Nightingale
was in touch with leaders on all of these issues.

One expert with whom she worked was Scottish chemist Robert Angus
Smith, a specialist on disinfection based in Manchester. She sent him her
Notes on Nursing and *Introductory Notes on Lying-in Institutions*, the latter

with an apologetic dedication that it was "not much in his line," but was "a tiny tribute of respect and gratitude for his most important sanitary discoveries" (dedication dated July 1872, Johns Hopkins University, Welch Library). Dr. Smith sent her his reports.

Nightingale consulted him in 1865 on an "urgent request" from the Indian Sanitary Commissions to find out "the best methods of finding out how much dirt there is in the water they drink" (letter, October 30, 1865, in Vallée, 2006, p. 878). Dr. Smith did the work, but kept changing his mind on conclusions. However, although fifteen versions of his report went through her and Dr. Sutherland's hands, she declared his final water analysis "worth all the trouble," although he was "more difficult to manage than all the Government of India" (letters, November 18 and 26, 1865, in Vallée, 2006, pp. 879–880). She considered him the "only man in Europe" who could have done it. She had tried her "military hygiene" contacts at Netley, notably Dr. E. A. Parkes, who could not.

Having judged Angus Smith's water paper to be "useful," it had to be circulated. To get enough copies, she had it printed at her own expense, 100 copies for herself, 200 for Dr. Smith (letter, December 7, 1865, in Vallée, 2006, pp. 880–881).

Angus Smith also did research on the amount of carbon dioxide in hospital wards, but Nightingale did not think it helpful, as she told the Cabinet minister Gathorne Hardy who had set up the inquiry on cubic space (letter, July 25, 1866, in McDonald, 2009a, pp. 591–592.).

Nightingale appreciated the pioneering research on acid rain conducted by Angus Smith and Robert Rawlinson (Reed, 2014). Acid emissions from the "alkali works" were then not only blackening the English countryside, but had reached the French wine country. Rawlinson sent Nightingale their first report. He and Angus Smith worked together later also as inspectors on river pollution (letter, June 17, 1865, Boston University 1/3/46). The following year, Angus Smith wrote Nightingale about progress made on extending the provisions of the Alkali Act (Smith letter, June 22, 1866, British Library Add Mss 45799 f261). The Alkali Acts were the first laws in the world to require abatement measures. Nightingale understood their importance.

That Nightingale gave nursing a strong environmental focus is well known. It was influential for some time, but increasingly, however, treatment-oriented nursing took over. It was only with the emergence of the environmental movement in the 1970s that her focus on the biophysical environment again came into favor. A report of the Institute of Medicine shows this reemergence. It was produced at the request of a consortium of federal agencies, and Nightingale herself was quoted extensively on key points (Pope, Snyder, & Mood, 1995, p. 49).

> *Florence Nightingale founded modern nursing on the tenet that the role of the nurse was primarily to modify the environment in ways that enhanced health and healing.*
>
> —Pope et al. (1995, p. 13)

QUESTIONS FOR DISCUSSION

1. How does Nightingale's definition of health compare with those by later nurse theorists? What are the comparative advantages and disadvantages of having such a short, positive definition?
2. To what extent do health promotion/disease prevention measures result in economic benefits, such as reduced expenditure to governments, lower absenteeism to employers? Are these advantages good selling points for health promotion?
3. Tobacco-related diseases: How high do they rank in your jurisdiction as preventable causes of death? What measures are in place to reduce smoking rates, and how adequate are they? What evidence is available to make these judgments? (Smoke-free work and public places, taxes, advertising and sponsorship bans, cessation programs? With what effectiveness?)
4. Obesity and food issues: What programs are available to people seeking assistance on weight concerns? What public measures are in place to promote healthy eating (information displayed on fats, sugar, and additives? Restrictions in advertising to minors? Or other restrictions in advertising? Restrictions or bans on unhealthy foods in schools?) How successful have they been? Are data collected to monitor the effectiveness of interventions?

REFERENCES

Berkowitz, B., & Borchard, M. (2009, January). Advocating for the prevention of childhood obesity: A call to action for nursing. *Online Journal of Issues in Nursing, 14*(1). doi:10.3912/OJIN.Vol14No1Man02

Calkins, B. M. (1989). Florence Nightingale: On feeding an army. *American Journal of Clinical Nutrition, 50*, 1260–1265.

Centers for Disease Control and Prevention. (2016). Surgeon General's report: E-Cigarette use among youth and young adults. Retrieved from https://www.cdc.gov/tobacco/data_statistics/sgr/e-cigarettes

Collins, N. (2012, February 20). Florence Nightingale approach "could help fight infection in modern hospitals." *The Telegraph*.

Cunningham, C. (1996). *Smoke and mirrors: The Canadian tobacco war*. Ottawa: IDRC ISBN: 155250025X.

Gibson, A. (2012). BBC History website. Retrieved from http://forum.lowcarber .org/archive/index.php/t-448107/html

Gilmore, J. (2000). *Report on smoking prevalence in Canada, 1985 to 1999*. Ottawa, Canada: Statistics Canada. No. 82F0077XIE-No. 01.

Hays, J. (2009). Smoking in Japan. Retrieved from http:// factsanddetails.com/ japan/ cat19/sub125/item665.html

Henderson, V. A. (1990, June). National health insurance: If not now, when? *Public Health Nursing, 7*(2), 59. doi:10.1111/j.1525-1446.1990.tb00612.x

Jha, P., Ramasundarahettite, C., Landsman, V., Rostron, B., Thun, M., Anderson, R. N.,...Peto, R. (2013). 21st-century hazards of and benefits of cessation in the United States. *New England Journal of Medicine, 368*, 341–350. doi:10.1056/NEJMsal121128

McDonald, L. (Ed.). (2003). *Florence Nightingale on society and politics, philosophy, science, education, and literature*. Waterloo, Canada: Wilfrid Laurier University Press ISBN: 0-88920-429-2.

McDonald, L. (Ed.). (2004). *Florence Nightingale on public health care*. Waterloo, Canada: Wilfrid Laurier University Press. ISBN: 0-88920-446-2.

McDonald, L. (Ed.). (2009a). *Florence Nightingale: Extending nursing*. Waterloo, Canada: Wilfrid Laurier University Press. ISBN: ISBN: 978-1-55458-170-2.

McDonald, L. (Ed.). (2009b). *Florence Nightingale: The Nightingale School*. Waterloo, Canada: Wilfrid Laurier University Press. ISBN: 978-1-55458-169-6.

McDonald, L. (Ed.). (2012). *Florence Nightingale and hospital reform*. Waterloo, Canada: Wilfrid Laurier University Press. ISBN: 978-0-88920-471-3.

Ng, M., Freeman, M. K., Fleming, T. D., Robinson, M., Dwyer-Lindgren, L., Thomson B.,... Gakidou, E. (2014, January 8). Smoking prevalence and cigarette consumption in 187 countries, 1980-2012. *Journal of the American Medical Association, 311*(2) 183–192. doi:10.1001/jama.2013.284692.

Nightingale, F. (1858, September 25). Hospital construction: Wards. *The Builder 16*(816), 641–643.

Nightingale, F. (1860). *Notes on nursing: What it is, and what it is not*. London, UK: Harrison

Nightingale, F. (1862). *Army sanitary administration and its reform under the late Lord Herbert*. London, UK: McCorquodale.

Nightingale, F. (1867). *Suggestions on the subject of providing training and organizing nurses for the sick poor in workhouse infirmaries* (pp. 64–76). London, UK: Her Majesty's Stationery Office.

Nightingale, F. (1883). Nursing the sick. In R. Quain (Ed.), *A dictionary of medicine* London, UK: Longmans, Green.

Nightingale, F. (1892, November 25). Miss F. Nightigale on local sanitation. *The Times*, 10A.

Nightingale, F. (1893). Sick nursing and health nursing. In A. Burdett-Coutts (Ed.) *Woman's mission: A series of Congress papers on the philanthropic work of women* (pp. 184–205). London, UK: Sampson, Low, Marston.

Nightingale, F. (1894). *Health and local government. Introduction to Report of the Bucks Sanitary Conference October 1894* (pp. i–ii). Aylesbury, UK: Poulton.

Pope, A. M., Snyder, M. A., & Mood, L. H. (Eds.). (1995). *Nursing, health and the environment: Strengthening the relationship to improve the public's health.* Washington, DC: National Academies Press.

Reed, P. (2014). *Acid rain and the rise of the environmental chemist in nineteenth-century Britain: The life and work of Robert Angus Smith.* Farnham, Surrey: Ashgate. ISBN: 978-1409457756.

Registered Nurses Association of Ontario. (2014, May). *Primary prevention of childhood obesity.* (2nd ed.). Toronto, ON, Canada: Author.

Taylor, P. (2014, June 4). The country where nearly two-thirds of men smoke. *BBC News Magazine.* Retrieved from http://www.bbc.com/news/magazine-27677882

United Nations. Declaration of Alma Ata. (1978, September). International Conference on Primary Health Care. Retrieved from http://www.who.int/publications/almaata_declaration_en.pdf?ua=1

Vallée, G. (Ed.). (2006). *Florence Nightingale on health in India.* Waterloo, Canada: Wilfrid Laurier University Press. ISBN: 10-0-88920-468-3.

Wilkinson, R., & Marmot, M. (2003). *Toronto Charter for a Healthy Canada.* Toronto, ON, Canada: Community Services Committee.

World Health Organization. (2002). *World health report: Reducing risks promoting healthy life.* Geneva, Switzerland: Author.

World Health Organization. (2015, December). *Health and Human Rights.* Fact sheet No. 323. Geneva, Switzerland: WHO Media Centre.

World Health Organization. (2017, July 19). WHO report finds dramatic increase in life-saving tobacco control policies in last decade. Retrieved from http://www.who.int/mediacentre/news/releases/2017/tobacco-report/en

Xu, J., Murphy, S. L., Kochanek, D., & Arias, E. (2016). Mortality in the United States, 2015. NCHS Dagta Brief No. 267. Retrieved from https://www.cdc.gov/nchs/products/databriefs/db267.htm

Ethics has been a central concern of modern nursing since the time of Florence Nightingale.

—Chaska (2001, p. 65)

This chapter opens with the challenge Nightingale and her close colleagues faced in establishing nursing as a profession when the ethical standards of the existing (secular) nurses were (generally) so low. The ethical issues she had to deal with in her own school, soon after it opened, are discussed—three thorny problems with appointments.

ETHICAL CHALLENGES IN THE NEW PROFESSION

Anyone reading Nightingale's writing on nursing will be struck by how often and how forcefully she insisted on high ethical standards. Although the term "ethics," however, appears nowhere in her writing, the message itself is clear. The terms that she used were discipline, or self-discipline, morality, goodness, forbearance, and respect for patients, especially their privacy and autonomy. Altogether, this meant putting patients' needs first. Her public "addresses" to nurses are full of moral content, intended to inspire commitment and idealism. They were first read at the school's annual meeting at St. Thomas' Hospital, and then circulated in print (McDonald, 2009b, pp. 755–881; Nash, 1914).

The reason for the emphasis on ethical standards is obvious enough in the task Nightingale faced in raising the new profession from its disreputable past. As noted in Chapter 1, the "cardinal sin" of old-style, unreformed nursing was demanding bribes from patients—worse even than the drunkenness for which nurses were notorious. Training at St. Thomas' Hospital accordingly stressed moral qualities at least as much as technical skills and knowledge. It is telling that, before requiring expertise in dressings, students were rated as to their being "sober, honest, truthful, punctual, quiet, trustworthy, cleanly, neat, and orderly." To make this quite clear to Sarah E. Wardroper, the nursing director (then termed "matron" or "superintendent"), Nightingale stipulated that "the first dereliction under the three first columns, 'sobriety,' 'honesty,' 'truthfulness,' ensures her dismissal" (letter, June 26, 1860, in McDonald, 2009b, p. 149).

Nightingale never relented on this ethical emphasis. In her "Nursing the sick" article for Quain's *Dictionary of Medicine* in the 1880s and 1890s, she modified the list slightly. Ten qualities were on her list in 1883, preceded by the statement that "a really good nurse must needs[sic] to be of the highest class of character." Heading the list was "chaste," meant as the word was used in the Hippocratic oath, not implying sexual conduct. She linked that with the Sermon on the Mount with its "blesseds" for those who hunger and thirst for righteousness, are merciful, are pure in heart, and are peacemakers (Matthew 5).

On the adapted list the next qualities after "chaste" were:

> (2) sober, in spirit as well as in drink, and temperate in all things (3) honest, not accepting the most trifling fee or bribe from patients or friends (4) truthful, which included paying attention to observe truly (5) trustworthy, in carrying out medical orders (6) punctual and orderly (7) quiet, yet quick, discreet; no gossip (8) cheerful, hopeful, not allowing herself to be discouraged by unfavorable symptoms (9) cleanly to the point of exquisiteness (10) thinking of her patients and not of herself. (Nightingale, 1883, Vol. 2, p. 1049, in McDonald, 2009b, p. 751, in Part 2, 3)

"Discipline," in Nightingale's understanding, had a positive, dynamic, quality. In rewriting her Quain's nurse training article for 1894, she said that it was "not drill, or 'standing at attention,' but learning how to develop physically, intellectually, spiritually, all the powers, illustrated by the teaching given by the Laws of Nature" (Nightingale, 1894, in McDonald, 2009b, p. 735).

In her "Sick nursing and health nursing" paper, for a world congress in Chicago, Nightingale set out a number of characteristics:

The nurse must have method, self-sacrifice, watchful activity, love of the work, devotion to duty (i.e., the service of the good), courage, coolness of the soldier, tenderness of the mother, and absence of the prig (Nightingale, 1893, p. 195, in McDonald, 2004, p. 215).

ETHICAL ISSUES AT THE NIGHTINGALE SCHOOL

Three thorny ethical issues emerged in 1868 to 1872 that Nightingale had to deal with as head of the Nightingale Fund, the fund raised in her honor for her work during the 1954 to 1956 Crimean War, which paid for the school.

A Breach of Confidentiality

The first occurred in 1868, soon after the arrival of Lucy Osburn with a team of nurses sent from St. Thomas' Hospital, at Sydney, Australia, to start trained nursing there. The Queen's son, Prince Alfred, who was in Sydney in command of a ship, was wounded in an assassination attempt. The newly arrived nurses looked after him at the governor's residence. Osburn, as nursing director, visited the prince regularly, details of which she wrote in a gossipy letter to a relative in England. He had the letter set in print for convenient distribution. Nightingale feared that it would appear in the press, revealing such a breach of patient confidentiality as to jeopardize the whole nursing project. She recruited her brother-in-law, Sir Harry Verney, to call on the relative and persuade him to give up his copies, which he did. Osburn realized what an error she had made, and offered her resignation. The damage, however, had been averted, and so Nightingale told her to withdraw the letter, which she did (letter to Henry Parkes, October 9, 1868, in McDonald, 2009a, pp. 420–423).

A Lapse in Trustworthiness

The second issue arose from the aberrant behavior of Mrs. Wardroper, the head of both hospital nursing and of the training school, who began to favor morally suspect nursing students over better ones for appointments, Nightingale thought. One good student left the school as a result. The matter came to light when Nightingale learned, late in 1871, that a ward sister and a nurse had taken advantage of a valuable document left by a deceased patient, worth a substantial £700 at the time. The two visited the family together and "asked more or less directly for a reward." The family's solicitor, however, had managed to get the money without the document. The family paid the nurses' fares and expenses for making the trip. The story got back to St. Thomas' and Nightingale was scandalized. She reminded Henry Bonham Carter, her cousin and secretary of the Nightingale Fund, that *trustworthiness* was placed in the first column of required qualities: "We print that the first offence against *honesty* ensures dismissal. And here is our training sister, the one who is to teach 'trustworthiness,' guilty of a lapse worse than any *I* have ever known, even in the army" (letter, November 24, 1871, in McDonald, 2009b, p. 194).

Further, she was concerned that Mrs. Wardroper did not take the matter seriously, but thought that it would suffice to reprimand the ward sister. Nightingale, however, felt that "fear of discovery" might make only the culprit "more cautious" (letter, November 24, 1871, in McDonald, 2009b, pp. 193–194). Honesty, meaning taking "no advantage, direct or indirect, out of the patients," was a concern going back to the old "cardinal sin": demanding bribes.

Alcohol and Opiate Abuse

The third ethical crisis occurred in 1873, a year after the appointment of the first trained nursing director, Elizabeth Ann Barclay, with a team of Nightingale nurses, at the Edinburgh Royal Infirmary. Barclay's management soon deteriorated noticeably, thanks to her abuse of alcohol and drugs. Hospitals then had no policies on how to deal with such matters, and Nightingale had to balance the needs of the hospital and patients against giving Barclay the opportunity to reform. She met with her at length, dissuaded her from resigning on the spot, and had her go on leave. Barclay did not, in fact, return to the position but resigned while on leave. Nightingale then wrote lengthy letters to the nurses and students at Edinburgh about her departure, encouraging reflection on the matter without condemnation (McDonald, 2009a, pp. 318–338).

Edinburgh, before the Nightingale nurses arrived, was particularly notorious for drunken nurses. It was the duty of junior doctors to carry those unable to walk onto or off the wards. The transition occurred with the appointment of a new medical superintendent, Dr. C. H. Fasson, an army doctor who had had experience in India in hospitals without trained (female) nurses, and then at the Herbert Hospital, Woolwich, with Nightingale nurses. He made the move to get trained nurses from the Nightingale School. Then, when the first nursing director proved to have a substance abuse problem, he had to work with Nightingale and the secretary of the Nightingale Fund to seek a fair solution.

Drug and alcohol abuse were well accepted generally where the "old-style" nursing prevailed. Even in her Harley Street hospital, Nightingale had to dismiss a nurse for "her love of opium and intimidation" (Nightingale, 1970/1854, 3rd Quarter, in McDonald, 2009b, p. 110). Doctors were often not concerned because the early "nurses" were mainly cleaners, not responsible for patient care. However, this became an issue when Rachel Williams, after her appointment as the first trained nursing director at St. Mary's Hospital, Paddington, tried to dismiss a ward sister of 20 years' standing who, as it was told to Nightingale, "takes opium and is otherwise incapacitated!" (letter, October 20, 1876, British Library Add Mss 47747 f38). Some doctors and surgeons signed a letter to dismiss the sister, with a pension, but others protested and Williams had to keep her.

Nurses' abuse of alcohol and drugs would only increase over time. An American Nurses Association (ANA) study estimates that about 10% of nurses (nearly 2 million) are dependent on drugs (Copp, 2009). Another study estimated that 6.9% of American RNs were problem users of prescription drugs (Naegele, 2006, p. 59). This impairment, and theft of drugs to support the habit, is a major cause of disciplinary action brought against nurses (Mahlmeister, 1999, p. 245).

Other Ethical Challenges

Correspondence over the years shows that ethical issues continued to be crucial for establishing professional nursing. A long letter Nightingale wrote in 1879 to a woman seeking to establish training in Vienna, Marie von Miller, contains much material on moral qualities. Nightingale told her: "The very ABC of a nurse is (A) to be sober and chaste (B) strictly honest and true (C) and kind and devoted." Nightingale also explained that hospital life

> requires for women more helps, spiritual and moral, more keeping up to the spirit of their work, more of a good "esprit de corps" and pride in and love of their work, than domestic service or family life, and hitherto has received less. (letter, March 17, 1879, in McDonald, 2009a, pp. 475 and 477)

In a paper for a congress on the "Philanthropic Work of Women" in Chicago, Nightingale repeated her rhetorical question in *Notes on Nursing* as to what it was "to feel a *calling* for anything?" with the same answer: satisfying "the high idea of what is the *right*, the *best*, and not because we shall be found out if we don't do it." This everyone from a shoemaker to a sculptor had to do, but "the nurse has to do not with shoes or with marble but with living human beings" (Nightingale, 1893, p. 193, in McDonald, 2004, p. 213).

PREVENTING PATIENT ABUSE

O, the cruelty which may go on in the best medical-staffed hospital behind the backs of the medical staff.
　　　　—Nightingale (letter, March 17, 1879, in McDonald, 2009a, p. 476)

The term "patient abuse" occurs nowhere in Nightingale's writing, but instances of serious neglect and even cruelty arose on occasion. In 1879,

Nightingale remarked to her correspondent in Vienna on the cruelty that could go on "in the best medical-staffed hospital behind the backs of the medical staff." The nurse "ought to be the patient's defender and keeper." However, in old-style nursing, the patient sometimes had to be defended against the nurse (letter, March 17, 1879, in McDonald, 2009a, pp. 475–476).

Children were especially vulnerable to cruel treatment by nurses, Nightingale held, and they could not complain, risking retaliation by nurses if they did. The practical remedy was to place children's wards where they would be open to passersby, for publicity or public opinion would make it difficult for cruelty to go unobserved. Other points on this issue are made in Chapter 6 on pediatric nursing.

In 1878, Nightingale became aware of severe patient neglect at Buxton Hospital, a small hospital near the family home in Derbyshire. She had sent patients there herself, and was appalled to learn that "two or three of the most crying evils" of nursing occurred at it. There was no professional supervision, but a husband and wife team of managers, both of whom drank excessively (McDonald, 2009a, pp. 282–299). There were no trained nurses, no night nurse, or any help for a patient who required it to go to the toilet at night. Patients who needed special foods did not get them, nor did those who needed help in eating get any. A patient she sent would never recover, Nightingale feared. Twenty-five years earlier, "all nursing" had been as bad as at Buxton, but she doubted if "any specimen quite as bad" could be found then (letter, April 10, 1879, in McDonald, 2009a, pp. 286–287).

Nightingale engaged the help of the Duke of Devonshire, the leading landowner of the district, to have an investigation conducted. This had to be done carefully, for the local, good doctor could be "ruined" for giving infor-mation to an inquiry (letter, April 24, 1879, in McDonald, 2009a, p. 292). The language is more old fashioned than what we use today, and probably the local duke would not be asked to help. However, the description of neglect and the reasons for it appear to be remarkably similar to those that occur today when hospitals cut staff to reduce costs, as in the notorious case of the Mid-Staffordshire Hospital 130 years later (Francis, 2010), discussed in Chapter 8.

There was no recognition in law of "human rights" in the 19th century. People had no "right" to care, apart from minimum subsistence and shelter by entrance to the workhouse, and certainly no right to quality health care. Voluntary hospitals took some "charity" patients, but no one had any right to even basic health care. Some doctors took cases without a fee, but were under no obligation to do so.

Nightingale's own philosophy of care came from her faith: God wanted the best for all people, and had no special regard for the wealthy. Establishing care for the poor was God's work. Jesus's praise of the Good Samaritan for arranging care for an assaulted man left to die was an example for nurses centuries later. When the new Highgate Workhouse Infirmary opened in 1870, for which Nightingale provided trained nursing staff, she wrote to the nursing director a biblical paraphrase. Here she turned Jesus' "I was sick and you visited me" into "I was sick and you nursed me" (letter, November 4, 1870, in McDonald, 2004, p. 443).

Patient abuse was evidently rare, so that the far more frequent need was to stress forbearance on the nurse's part for the sake of the patient. Ending her article "Nursing the sick" for Quain's *Dictionary*, she said:

> The nurse must make no demand upon the patient for reciprocation, for acknowledgment or even perception of her services, since the best service a nurse can give is that the patient shall scarcely be aware of any. . . . The nurse must always be kind and sympathetic, but never emotional. The patient must find a real, not forced or "put on," centre of calmness in his nurse.

It was even "cruel," as well as "useless," to demand that the patient give back to the nurse. It was asking the patient

> to bear your troubles and your anxiety as well as his own. . . . Half the battle of nursing is to relieve your sick *from having to think for themselves at all*—least of all for their own nursing. (Nightingale, 1883, Vol. 2, p. 1049, in McDonald, 2009b, p. 752)

Patient Confidentiality

Nightingale insisted on high standards of respect for patient confidentiality, keen to put behind the casual, slovenly characteristics of the old-style "nurse." Every nurse should be capable of keeping information confidential. The nurse "must be no gossip, no vain talker," and must never answer questions about a patient "except to those who have a right to ask them," she said in a new section in *Notes on Nursing* and *Notes on Nursing for the Labouring Classes* (Nightingale, 1860a, 1860b, 1861, Chapter 13).

Nightingale herself was scrupulously careful about maintaining confidential material, both regarding patients and nurses. Many of her letters are marked "Confidential," some "Confidential. Burn." Obviously not all correspondents respected that demand, since many such letters survive. They invariably include personal information.

THE DEVELOPMENT OF FORMAL CODES OF ETHICS

The first nurse to give comprehensive attention to ethical issues was Isabel Hampton Robb, who knew Nightingale and was greatly influenced by her. Hampton Robb became convinced of the need for a common ethical code while preparing her major nursing book, *Nursing: Its Principles and Practices* (1893). In *Nursing Ethics*, originally published in 1903, she deplored the variation of "vague and indefinite" nursing practice and standards. She saw an "increasing necessity" for a common code, to be a "definite moral force or laws" that would bind nurses together, and which would bring nurses "into more uniform and harmonious relations" (Robb, 1903/1912, p. 24). She produced a paper on ethics for a congress in 1897, then the full book. Nightingale is prominent in the introduction.

Nursing Ethics defines the "science" of ethics and differentiates it from "etiquette," or conventional practices short of the standpoint of "right and wrong" (Robb, 1903/1912, p. 12). Hampton Robb also specified that the teaching of ethics should begin early in training, be the responsibility of the director of nursing, and be integrated with other teaching (Robb, 1903/1912, p. 14). Specific qualities she mentioned were self-reliance, self-restraint, self-possession, sympathy, sentiment, conversation, patience, gentleness, cheerfulness, good temper, habits of exactness, truthfulness, method and order, vigilance, and observation, going on to issues of remuneration and conditions of engagement (Robb, 1903/1912, p. 19). Hampton Robb followed Nightingale on "intelligent obedience." In *Nursing Ethics*, she described the nurse as "assistant," not servant, to the physician.

The "Nightingale Pledge" was another American measure aimed at giving more weight to ethics in nursing. It was not written by Nightingale, nor did she ever comment on it. The writer was Lystra Gretter, of the Farrand Training School, Detroit, her chief source the Hippocratic oath taken by doctors. It was first given at the school in 1893 (Goodnow, 1916). It was typically taken by nurses on graduation, in a formal ceremony:

> I solemnly pledge myself before God and in the presence of this assembly to pass my life in purity and to practise my profession faithfully. I will abstain from whatever is deleterious and mischievous, and will not take or knowingly administer any harmful drug. I will do all in my power to maintain and elevate the standard of my profession, and will hold in confidence all personal matters committed to my keeping and all family affairs coming to my knowledge in the practice of my calling. With loyalty will I endeavor to aid the physician in his work and devote myself to the welfare of those committed to my care. (ANA Florence Nightingale Pledge)

Formal, written, codes of ethics for nurses date roughly from the 1950s. The ANA was the first with its "Code for Nurses" in 1950. Based on Nightingale principles, it opens with: "Florence Nightingale believed that a nurse's ethical duty was first and foremost to care for the patient." The code is said to be "nonnegotiable," each nurse obliged to uphold and adhere to it. There are also "Interpretive Statements" that explicate the goals, values, and precepts in the lengthy code.

The ANA treats health care reform, meaning affordable care, without the exclusion of people for "preexisting" medical conditions, as an "ethical challenge." This means that accessible, quality, health care is in no way a right, although it is desirable, a subject to be returned to in Chapter 9 on policy.

The International Council of Nurses Code of Ethics

The International Council of Nurses (ICN) established its Code of Ethics in 1953, again based on Nightingale principles. It identified four responsibilities: to promote health, to prevent illness, to restore health, and to alleviate suffering. The code asks nurses not only to act ethically themselves, but to challenge unethical practices (Broe, 1954).

The International Council of Nurses did a major revision of its code in 2012, expanding it to a 10-page document. Its preamble calls for respect for human rights, described as "inherent in nursing," which include cultural rights, the "right to life and choice" (an ambiguous pairing), "dignity, and the right to be treated with respect," and no restrictions by age, color, creed, culture, disability, illness, gender, sexual orientation, nationality, politics, race, or social status. Nurses are said to render services to the individual, family, and community, and coordinate those services with "those of related groups," unspecified. Doctors are nowhere mentioned and presumably nurses have no special obligation to them.

The ICN code requires nurses to maintain their competence by "continual learning" and to be "active in developing a core of research-based professional knowledge that supports evidence-based practice." Nurses are to "sustain and protect the natural environment" and be "aware of its consequences on health," a reference that reflects back to Nightingale's environmental focus in *Notes on Nursing*, now in more modern language (International Council of Nurses, 2012).

The ICN also tracks national codes from its 130 member organizations. Perusal of the various national codes shows great similarity in language, with values and principles set out, often as if uncontested and in place. Many codes state that nurses "do" various things, that clearly not all do.

Canadian nurses used the international code until adopting their own in 1980, written by a Roman Catholic nurse/nun, Simone Roach, and approved by the Canadian Nurses Association (CNA) Board of Directors (Roach, 1980). It lists what one would expect about care, the priority of the client's needs, and respect for confidentiality. Like many codes, it called on nurses not only to maintain "personal" ethical behavior, but also to "challenge actions which are contrary to acceptable health care goals."

While neither abortion nor birth control is explicitly mentioned in the Canadian code, human life is referred to as having a "sacred and even mysterious character." The wording clearly provides justification for nurses refusing any involvement in procedures for either: "The nurse as a moral person has the ethical responsibility to refuse to participate in programs, treatments, or procedures, and to withdraw from situations which are contrary to his or her informed moral conscience" (Roach, 1980, pp. 4-5).

The code also reflects the progressive social teaching of the Roman Catholic Church (and other churches), giving responsibility to the profession as a whole as well as to individual nurses: "The profession has an obligation to examine its own goals and the service it offers in the light of existing health problems." At the time it was written, there was no national provision for health care in Canada. The CNA original code goes on boldly to affirm responsibility as well to the international community: "Since health is a basic condition for human development, and as no one nation or country can develop its potential in isolation, the interests of the profession transcend national boundaries."

The code as revised in 1990 listed eight items, all but the last of which are in line with Nightingale's approach. This last, protecting clients from incompetent members of the health care team, implies a level of organization not present earlier. Nightingale herself, of course, was an accomplished whistle-blower and worked assiduously, behind the scenes, to prevent or correct incompetent care. Key items of the eight given in the CNA code of 1990 are:

1. *Obligation.* The client's perceived best interest must be a prime concern of the nurse.
2. Respect for client choice.
3. Confidentiality.
4. Dignity, personal modesty. Obligation to intervene when failure to respect.
7. Cooperation with "other disciplines."
8. Protecting client from incompetent "health care team." (CNA, 1991)

The code was expanded to 57 pages in 2008 with a glossary. The edition of 2017 is largely the same. The first part of both edition lists as core responsibilities for all registered nurses in Canada:

1. Providing safe, compassionate, competent, and ethical care
2. Promoting health and well-being

3. Promoting and respecting informed decision making
4. Preserving dignity
5. Maintaining privacy and confidentiality
6. Promoting justice
7. Being accountable

The second part of both documents, "Ethical endeavors with respec to broad societal issues," as in the original version of 1980, calls on nurses to address societal inequities as part of ethical practice. Thus, nurses are tc "make fair decisions about the allocation of resources under their control" and to "advocate for fair treatment and for fair distribution of resources." They are to support a climate that "encourages questioning the status quo" and tc support those who speak out to address concerns in good faith, for example whistle-blowing. The code's second part again calls for advocacy "for changes to unethical health and social policies, legislation, and regulations," including "a full continuum of accessible health care services," which include "healtl promotion, disease prevention" as well as diagnostic, restorative, and palliative care. The "social determinants of health" are mentioned; nurses are tc advocate for policies and programs that address them. Nurses are to suppor "environmental preservation and restoration" and advocate for initiatives tha "reduce environmentally harmful practices in order to promote health anc well-being" (CNA, 2008, p. 20).

The 2017 version is more explicit on the need for "improving systems anc societal structures to create greater equity" than any previous code. Its firs item calls for nurses to advocate "for publicly administered health systems that ensure accessibility, universality, portability and comprehensiveness ir necessary health-care services" (CNA, 2017, p. 8). The wording—hardly a coincidence—repeats the core elements of Canada's national medicare system. That is, for provinces to receive federal funding for health care, they must respect those five requirements.

FROM "INTELLIGENT OBEDIENCE" TO LICENSING STANDARDS

Most jurisdictions in which nurses work have licensing or registratior regulations that set legally binding standards for their work, as opposec to ethical codes that set out unenforceable ideals. Nurses can be reprimanded, fined, suspended temporarily, or have their license permanently revoked, depending on the infraction. In the case of acts of willful harm causing death, a prison sentence may result, quite apart from professiona discipline, probably permanent license revocation in the case of a willfu overdose.

What Nightingale set as the standard for nurses of her time, "intelligent obedience" to medical orders, required the trained nurse to use her professional judgment, and not act when the order appeared to be wrong. Now a nurse is legally required to refuse an order by a physician or surgeon or a person "lawfully authorized to prescribe," which could include pharmacists and nurses as well.

There are cases of nurses being disciplined, for example, for administering penicillin to a patient, as per the doctor's orders, without checking on possible allergies on the part of the patient, the nurse's responsibility. The nurse should have known to check, a failure in competence.

Professional training has been modified with the growing complexities of ethical issues. A three-volume collection of papers on ethical issues shows the diversity of views currently in play (Johnstone, 2015). Some universities have centers specializing in nursing ethics. One, the International Centre for Nursing Ethics at the University of Surrey, Guildford, publishes an international journal, *Nursing Ethics*.

Nonetheless, the core ethical challenges of Nightingale's time remain, centered on the patient's needs, for which her ideas remain relevant. And, while "patients' rights" and "human rights" are later concepts, her precepts are obvious enough under nurses' and hospitals' responsibilities.

ETHICS AND PROSELYTIZING RELIGIOUS BELIEFS

Many nurses, as Nightingale herself, were motivated by their Christian faith to become nurses. Some felt strongly a duty to convert patients, especially dying patients, for the good of their souls. Clearly this poses a dilemma, which some took to Nightingale for advice. She herself believed that conversion was a good thing, but that the nurse's duty and function was to heal the body. Counseling had to be strictly limited. One means was to bring in an appointed chaplain.

When Nightingale was looking after a dying patient at Kaiserswerth, a Lutheran deaconess establishment, she consulted the pastor about counseling the man on the state of his soul. Pastor Fliedner encouraged her to talk with him, a matter pursued in Chapter 7, on palliative care.

Nightingale was asked by a Swedish nurse, Alfhild Ehrenborg, then about to return home to establish a nursing school, about opportunities to speak about her faith as a "missionary" (Ehrenborg letter, December 1, 1883, British Library Add Mss 45807 f111). Nightingale's reply allowed that a nurse could give a reason for her faith "a word in season," a quotation from the Book of Proverbs (letter, December 3, 1883, in McDonald, 2009a, p. 449).

However, one always had to respect patients' right to their own beliefs, and to holding none at all. Healing the body was the nurse's first duty.

Yet Nightingale's addresses to nursing students often had frank religious content. Her last such address, in 1900, shows the faith base of her own nursing:

> The old Romans were in some respects I think superior to us. But they had no idea of being good to the sick and weak. That came in with Christianity. Christ was the author of our profession. We honor Christ when we are good nurses. We dishonor Him when we are bad or careless nurses. We dishonor Him when we do not do our best to relieve suffering—even in the meanest creature—kindness to sick man, woman, and child came in with Christ. They used to be left on the banks of the great rivers to starve or drown themselves. Lepers were kept apart. The nation did not try to avert or to cure leprosy. (in McDonald, 2009b, p. 880)

NEW ETHICAL AND LEGAL CHALLENGES

Ethical issues have become immensely more complicated with advances in medical science. Issues such as religious objections to blood transfusions, end-of-life care, assisted suicide, abortion for sex selection (and other purposes) simply do not appear in Nightingale's writing for obvious reasons. Longer life spans mean that many more patients suffer from dementia, resulting in many more situations with unclear or inadequate patient instructions. Hospitals in Nightingale's day did not have ethicists on their staffs. Doctors did not have medical malpractice insurance and they and hospitals were seldom sued.

In Canada, there is now a recognized right to access to "dying with dignity," or physician assistance for death, in the case of terminal patients enduring great suffering with no prospect of recovery. In practice, this means, or can mean, nurses assisting patient suicides. What right they or doctors have *not* to be required to provide services contrary to their religious or ethical code is under discussion. The Hippocratic oath, still taken by some doctors, requires them to "do the sick no harm." In the past, this would have unequivocally excluded assisted suicide; now, in many places, the failure to assist desperate patients is considered unethical. This is a whole new area, in which there will be developments.

QUESTIONS FOR DISCUSSION

1. At your institution, what measures are taken to prevent patient abuse? How adequate are they? How are they investigated and reported?
2. At your institution, how are issues of substance abuse handled? What weight is given to assisting a nurse to recover versus ensuring patient safety? Can both be promoted at the same time?

REFERENCES

Broe, E. (1954, April). Florence Nightingale and her international influence. *International Nursing Review, 1*(1), 17–19.

Canadian Nurses Association. (1991). *Code of ethics for nursing.* Ottawa, ON, Canada: CNA ISBN: 0920381839.

Canadian Nurses Association. (2008). *Code of ethics for nursing* (Centennial ed.). Ottawa, Canada: Author. ISBN: 978-1-55119-182-9.

Canadian Nurses Association. (2017). 2017 code of ethics for registered nurses. Retrieved from https://www.cna-aiic.ca/~/media/cna/page-content/pdf-en/code-of-ethics-2017-edition-secure-interactive.pdf?la=en

Chaska, N. L. (Ed.). (2001). *The nursing profession: Tomorrow and beyond.* London, UK: Sage. ISBN: 978061919438.

Copp, M. A. B. (2009, April 1). Drug addiction among nurses: Confronting a quiet epidemic. *Modern Medicine Network* online. Retrieved from http://www.modernmedicine.com/modern-medicine/news/modernmedicine/modern-medicine-feature-articles/drug-addiction-among-nurses-con?page=full.

Francis, R. (2010). *The Francis report: Briefing 1—Key recommendations and early response.* Retrieved from https://www.lexology.com/library/detail.aspx?g=fd341164-118c-4409-bb56-14978478258e

Goodnow, M. (1916). *Outlines of nursing history.* Philadelphia, PA: W. B. Saunders.

International Council of Nurses. (2012). *The ICN code of ethics for nurses: Revised 2012.* Geneva, Switzerland: Author. ISBN 978-92-95094-95-6.

Johnstone, M. J. (Ed.). (2015). *Nursing ethics* (3 vol.). Oxford, UK: Sage.

Mahlmeister, L. (1999). Legal issues in nursing and health care. In B. Cherry & S. R. Jacob (Eds.), *Contemporary nursing: Issues, trends, and management* (pp. 237–301). St. Louis, MO: Mosby. ISBN: 9780323101097.

McDonald, L. (Ed.). (2004). *Florence Nightingale on public health care.* Waterloo, Canada: Wilfrid Laurier University Press. ISBN: 0-88920-446-2.

McDonald, L. (Ed.). (2009a). *Florence Nightingale: Extending nursing.* Waterloo, Canada: Wilfrid Laurier University Press. ISBN: 978-1-55458-170-2.

McDonald, L. (Ed.). (2009b). *Florence Nightingale: The Nightingale School.* Waterloo, Canada: Wilfrid Laurier University Press. ISBN: 978-1-55458-169-6.

Naegele, M. (2006, November–December). Nurses and matters of substance. *NSNA Imprint*, 3(4), 58–61.

Nash, R. (Ed.). (1914). *Florence Nightingale to her nurses: A selection from Miss Nightingale's addresses to probationers and nurses of the Nightingale School at St. Thomas's Hospital.* London, UK: Macmillan.

Nightingale, F. (1860a). *Notes on nursing: What it is, and what it is not.* London, UK: Harrison.

Nightingale, F. (1860b). *Notes on nursing: What it is and what it is not.* New ed., rev., enlarged. London, UK: Harrison (library standard version).

Nightingale, F. (1861). *Notes on nursing for the labouring classes.* London, UK: Harrison.

Nightingale, F. (1883). Nursing the sick. In R. Quain (Ed.), *A dictionary of medicine.* London, UK: Longmans, Green.

Nightingale, F. (1893). Sick nursing and health nursing. In A. Burdett-Coutts (Ed.), *Woman's mission: A series of Congress papers on the philanthropic work of women* (pp. 184–205). London, UK: Sampson, Low, Marston.

Nightingale, F. (1894). Nurses, training of. In R. Quain (Ed.), *A dictionary of medicine* (Vol. 2, pp. 231–237). London, UK: Longmans, Green.

Nightingale, F. (1854/1970). *Florence Nightingale at Harley Street: Her reports to the governors of her nursing home, 1853-54.* London, UK: J.M. Dent & Sons.

Roach, M. S. (1980). *CNA code of ethics: An ethical basis for nursing in Canada.* Ottawa, Canada: Canadian Nurses Association. Retrieved from http://ethics.iit.edu/codes/CNA%201980.pdf

Robb, I. H. (1893). *Nursing: Its principles and practice for hospital and private use.* Philadelphia, PA: W. B. Saunders.

Robb, I. H. (1912). *Nursing ethics: For hospital and private use.* Cleveland, OH: E. C. Koeckert. (Original work published 1903).

Chapter 5: Infection Control

Every nurse ought to be careful to wash her hands very frequently during the day.

—Nightingale (1860, Chapter 11)

This chapter begins by recounting Nightingale's own experience of dealing with infection control during the Crimean War (1854–1856) at her own hospital. It goes on to show how precisely she learned the lessons of the high death rates there by research after the war. Her first major publications reported that analysis.

The chapter then takes up how Nightingale applied what she learned both in advising on hospital design and in setting up her nurse training school. Both became lifelong quests. Both had to be applied to civil hospital nursing, and the military.

The chapter next covers the significant contribution Nightingale made to infection control in midwifery nursing, through her pioneering study of maternal mortality postchildbirth. Finally, how her ideas can be applied in clinical practice today is considered.

INFECTIOUS DISEASES IN CRIMEAN WAR HOSPITALS

Nightingale's pioneer work in infection control is still well recognized. For example, numerous examples of specific procedures that date back to her are noted in *Infection Control in Clinical Practice* (Wilson, 1995, p. 287). That her bold and influential ideas date back to the lessons of the Crimean War is also recognized (Oztekin, 2007).

When Nightingale arrived at the Barrack Hospital, Scutari, in November 1854, after the genteel experience of her small Harley Street institution for women, she faced as bad hospital conditions as ever existed. The "hospital" was then the largest in the world, but never intended to be a hospital. Its name explains it, the "Barrack Hospital," meaning simply the living quarters for Turkish soldiers. Its defective sewers and drains were the great culprits, while the soldiers arrived weak from poor nutrition, lack of winter clothing and shelter, and overwork.

The experience was formative for Nightingale, for she had to deal with enormous numbers of patient deaths; she saw the death rates brought down when strict sanitary measures were introduced. This experience—that applying the best scientific knowledge in practice brought results—equipped her for the rest of her life. In the worst month, the death rate at the worst Crimean War hospital exceeded 40% of admissions. Yet the Crimean death rates were reduced to 2% to 3% in the second year of the war.

A complication must be confronted, that her role in infection control has been exaggerated in the secondary literature. Important and pioneering as Nightingale's work was, some authors have exaggerated her achievements on infection control during that war. She has been credited with the "isolation of patients with antibiotic-resistant pathogens, avoidance of cross-contamination, routine cleansing of all patient areas, aseptic preparation of foods, ventilation of wards, and disposal of human and medical wastes" (Gill & Gill, 2005, p. 1804). She did indeed improve procedures in all those respects, mainly after the war, after reflecting on the poor practices she had to confront, and seeing the difference made with what improvements could be made. She was not authorized to take on the needed structural renovations, nor had she means to do so. This took considerable work, directed by a top ranking engineer, with experienced "nuisance inspectors" brought from Liverpool, plus hired local workers.

The British government had not anticipated the war lasting into the winter when they began to send out troops to "the East" in the spring of 1854. In fact, they remained for two full years. The British Army had not fought a well-equipped army for half a century. They were able to conquer technically less advanced enemies, but, while the Russian Army had less sophisticated weapons, it had vast numbers of soldiers and good engineering support.

The suffering that British soldiers endured was the result of lack of preparation. Yet the situation was turned around in a matter of months. The French Army, by comparison, had lower death rates in the first year of the war—they were better prepared for it—but they did not bring in the concerted reforms the British did, and their death rates nearly doubled in the second year. Significantly, the members of the two crucial commissions, Dr. John Sutherland and engineer Robert Rawlinson of the Sanitary Commission, and Sir John McNeill of the Supply Commission, became Nightingale's close colleagues in making great reforms postwar.

Post-Crimea, Nightingale could get questions on virtually any hospital or health care matter answered promptly by a top expert. Dr. Sutherland did even more for her, often drafting material, both for letters she had to answer and publications. This did much to make up for Nightingale's lack of medical education.

The impact of Nightingale's reforms at Scutari during the war "were so obvious and well publicized that the treatment of hospitalized and infected patients was forever changed." Her analysis postwar proved that the majority of deaths were due to preventable diseases (Gill & Gill, 2005, p. 1801). Most of the deaths were indeed preventable, but again, this is exaggeration. She herself credited the Sanitary and Supply Commissions for making the great difference.

The term "infection control" was not part of the medical or public health lexicon in Nightingale's day. Yet the fact of substantial incidents of disease and death were a reality in regular hospitals, war hospitals, schools, prisons, and private homes, even those of the wealthy. The terms used were "hospital disease," "hospital-generated disease," "hospital gangrene," and "hospitalism."

How diseases were spread was not understood in this prebacteriology era. The surgeon who pioneered antiseptic surgery, Joseph Lister, thought that the mode was entirely air-borne, hypothesizing "something in the atmosphere" or "floating particles," and hence devised a disinfectant spray as a remedy (Lister, 1867). Nightingale's then adherence to miasma theory was more effective in practice, for the "filth" it aimed at removing could be in liquids (blood, pus), solids, including fingers (requiring frequent handwashing), floors, curtains, walls, and clothing (hence strict rules for nonabsorbent materials and general cleanliness), or air (good ventilation). In a dictionary article, Nightingale noted that "cuffs and sleeves" were "possible carriers of contagious material" (Nightingale, 1883, Vol. 2, p. 1047, in McDonald, 2009b, p. 745).

Faulty sewers and drains, inadequate ventilation, and poor hospital design continued to be issues for Nightingale over the next decades, both in civil and army hospitals. Even the new St. Thomas' Hospital, state-of-the-art when it opened in 1871, had flaws that caused sickness and death.

Nightingale also soon realized that her student nurses faced risks in coming to train. There were no deaths in the first class, but periodic deaths occurred subsequently. When writing her "Notes on Hospitals" in 1858, Nightingale examined the data on nurse deaths to conclude that nurse deaths were higher than they should be, and advised that hospitals track those rates.

INFECTIOUS DISEASES IN CIVIL HOSPITALS

In building or extending a hospital, it is to be taken for granted that the object in view is to benefit and not injure the sick.
—Memo from Nightingale (September 30, 1859,
Buckinghamshire Record Office)

Death rates at regular civil hospitals were high when Nightingale set to work. Data from London teaching hospitals, presumably as good as could be found, averaged 10 percent of admissions when Nightingale's school opened ("Statistics of the General Hospitals of London," 1862) and deaths postsurgery were often as high as 50%. Bringing those death rates down was an ongoing struggle. Since comparable data stopped being available, the success of the improvements is not known. Experts are vague about when and how progress came about. One hospital expert would only say that it was "much later" that "hospital patients could be reasonably certain of dying from the disease with which they were admitted," as opposed to one they acquired in hospital (Abel-Smith, 1964, p. 125).

Soon after the Crimean War, Nightingale persuaded the Colonial Office to collect data on disease and deaths in native colonial schools and hospitals. The results duly came in, with many flaws and omissions, but enough for her to see something of the same pattern as before: "By far the greater part of the mortality is the direct result of mitigable or preventable diseases. . . . The mortality statistics of these hospitals show a very high death rate upon the numbers treated" (Nightingale, 1863b, pp. 479–480, in McDonald, 2004, pp. 172, 174). She, however, gave up pursuing colonial institutions when she could not get them to act, to concentrate on endeavors where she could have more effect, especially in India.

Nightingale worked on getting the best measures in her own years of hands-on practice. She purchased "finger stalls," the early version of surgical gloves, for her Harley Street hospital. She later obtained them for workhouse infirmary nurses. However, these proved not to be effective and use was discontinued. Some nurses and student nurses fell dangerously ill of "blood poisoning," or septicemia. Maria Machin, who pioneered trained nursing in Montreal, was an unhappy example, ill for months during her training period.

Even at the new St. Thomas' Hospital, there were lapses in infection control. In 1878, an increase in septicemia led to new rules on handwashing being instituted. Nightingale insisted that these rules be clear for nurses, as well as for doctors. A memorandum on procedures to avoid "finger poisoning" was drawn up and added to the student nurses' list of duties, reproduced in Exhibit 5.1. Washing instructions were detailed, complete with the requirement to carry carbolic soap and permanganate of potash, both disinfectants, with them. The last item, No. 17, was a caution against going on duty without having a meal first.

Nurses evidently learned the new antiseptic procedures at St. Thomas' Hospital, so that when the first trained nurses began work at the Montreal General Hospital in 1875, Jane Styring could report that she was "quite an authority" thanks to the experience she had had at St. Thomas' notes from a meeting (May 1883, in McDonald, 2009b, p. 373).

EXHIBIT 5.1   MEMORANDUM FOR PROBATIONERS ON BEGINNING WARD WORK, JULY 1878

Each probationer will carefully study and attend to the following instructions:

1. Take care to pare the finger nails close: to keep them, as well as fingers and hands generally, scrupulously cleaned.
2. Look upon anything which has soiled the fingers as a possible source of contagion or infection to others and to yourself.
   No nurse who, being warned, poisons her finger is fit to be a nurse. If she cannot take care of her own cleanliness, how can she take care of her patient's?
3. Look upon a hangnail, or crack or scratch or pin puncture, as likely to prove a poison nest to others or to self—even more than an open wound or sore.
4. Such poison nests must be rendered harmless by first washing with pure water; secondly, by the application of styptic colloid; thirdly, by being covered with an India rubber fingerstall.
5. Immediately *before* any dressing, and in every case *after* a nurse has *touched* her patient, whether in dressing wounds, rubbing in applications, administering enemata, internal syringing, washing out eyes, ears, nose, mouth—the nurse to dip her hands into watery solution of carbolic acid, 1 to 80; then to wash hands and nails carefully with carbolic soap. "Dressing forceps" or syringe, or whatever is used, has to be dipped in solution of carbolic (1 to 80) *before* use as well as *after*. The teeth and joints of the "dressing forceps" must also be brushed clean.
6. You are desired to remove soiled dressings with "dressing forceps," and not with your fingers: and on no account to scratch up adhesive plaster or other adhering dressing with your nails.
7. With all "internal" cases, the nurse is to keep her nails short, to fill the same with carbolic soap, and anoint carefully the fingers she is about to use with carbolic oil, 1 in 20. She is to oil the tube or nozzle, and the like, to be used for any internal application, with carbolic oil, 1 in 20. Otherwise the appliance used might convey contagious matter from one patient to another.
8. You are always to use *two* basins in washing wounds.
9. Catheters must be cleansed and disinfected, first with a stream of warm water, and then with a stream of watery solution of carbolic acid, 1 to 40. Catheters of other material than silver should *not* be *soaked* in carbolic acid solutions, as the acid injures varnish and gum.

A nurse is never to "blow down" toward the eye *first* instead of last: for so she always succeeds in effecting some lodgment at the bottom.

10. You are never to fail in taking your own carbolic soap, with which you will be provided, in your own soap tin, into the ward each morning and evening in your pocket. But you are to take it out before beginning "dressings," as otherwise you would put a dirty hand into your pocket.

11. After offensive cases, the nurse is to blow her nose and expectorate, and to rinse mouth and throat with Condy and water: or with permanganate of potash, a few grains in water.

12. Cleaned fingers and hands should always be dried on towels which have *not* been used for any other purpose.

13. You are to look upon cuffs and sleeves and stuff dresses as possible carriers of contagious or infectious matter. No nurse should eat or drink until she has changed the apron and oversleeves which she has worn in the wards.

14. If you discover that you have any scratch or crack or hangnail or sore or wound, you are desired to report it immediately to the matron, or in her absence, to the home sister.

15. When you have been breathing in an offensive air, you are recommended to ask immediate advice on the subject from the ward sister.

16. You are desired to learn on entrance the nature of contagion and infection, and the distinctions between disinfectants and antiseptics.

17. You are especially cautioned against going on duty in the morning without having taken a meal.

Source: McDonald (2009b, p. 753).

BETTER HOSPITAL DESIGN

I know no class of murderers who have killed so many people as hospital architects.

> —Nightingale (letter, 1877, in McDonald, 2012, p. 823)

Soon after the Crimean War, Nightingale turned to better hospital design as a means to reduce rates of disease and death from cross-infection. The French had pioneered the "pavilion" style of hospital architecture, which featured cross-ventilation in the wards and careful separation of the wards, which reduced the numbers exposed to the same atmosphere and disease pathogens. Nightingale, with reform-minded doctors, architects, and engineers, promoted the pavilion model in England. The "new" St. Thomas' of 1871 soon became the pavilion exemplar, considered the best civil hospital of that design, and the Herbert Hospital in Woolwich the model pavilion army hospital. Other major pavilion examples are, in Britain, the Edinburgh Royal Infirmary; in the United States, Johns Hopkins University Hospital; in Canada, the Royal Victoria Hospital, Montreal; in Germany, the City Hospital, Berlin. A whole volume in the *Collected Works of Florence Nightingale*, *Hospital Reform*, reports progress made on hospital design (McDonald, 2012). The pavilion model dominated hospital architecture into the 20th century.

Another safety measure was to keep administrative offices physically separate from wards. Failure to do so meant the diffusion of "a common atmosphere" throughout the building, in pregerm theory language. It exposed "both sick and administrators to very unnecessary risks," and "a danger that should never be incurred on any plea of economy" (Nightingale, 1863a, Chapter 4, Improved hospital plans).

INCREASING PRECAUTIONS FOR INFECTION CONTROL

Nightingale continued to track antiseptic and aseptic procedures, getting briefings by surgical nurses and keeping up with medical developments. Her 1883 *Dictionary of Medicine* article required nurses always to have chlorinated soda to wash their hands, "especially after dressing or handling a suspicious case." She quoted a surgeon that it might "destroy germs at the expense of the cuticle," but, "if it takes off the cuticle it must be bad for the germs" (Nightingale, 1883, Vol. 2, p. 1045).

Nightingale often gave nurses a book, usually of their choice, on finishing their nursing program or on departure for a post. In 1892, a nurse about to leave for Bangkok asked for a microscope instead, which she thought all the nurses would enjoy (letter from E. S. Shakespeare, October 25, 1892, British Library Add Mss[1] 45811 f176). The request shows the increasing awareness of bacteriology on the part of nurses.

Notes Nightingale made from an interview with a St. Thomas' ward sister in 1892 specified that they wash their hands "between each case," and keep "patients and all instruments and utensils antiseptically" (notes, May 21, 1892, in McDonald, 2009b, p. 444).

---

[1] Further references to Add Mss (Additional Manuscripts) are also to the British Library.

In 1896, a nurse gave Nightingale further specifics about best practice, including sterilizing instruments in boiling water containing 1 p.c. bicarbonate of soda after use, then emptied straight into carbolic lotion (1 in 20). Procedures by then included handing the sponge to the surgeon with forceps, "to prevent germs from contact," throwing away sponges after use (notes, August 1896, in McDonald, 2009b, p. 484).

A Finnish nurse, also in 1896, gave Nightingale a list of 16 precautions taken in surgical cases. These included details on sterilizing and storing the various products used. Doctors in the operating theater wore "sterilized white linen aprons," and nurses wore short sleeves in the surgical wards, although not in the medical. There were separate operating theaters for "semi-infectious" cases and purely noninfectious cases. Patients' clothing was taken to a separate building; they wore only clothing supplied by the hospital. A special bathroom was provided for new patients. After a death or case of infection, the bedding was sterilized by baking or heated to a high temperature (Nightingale, notes, 1896, British Library Add Mss 45813 ff186–87).

Later advice specifies that doctors and nurses should wear washable garments, and the hospital should be responsible for washing them.

Nightingale joked to Henry Bonham Carter in a letter in 1897 that "aseptic" could be briefly defined as "*boiling* yourself and everything within your reach, including the surgeon" (letter, January 9, 1897, in McDonald, 2004, p. 577).

MIDWIFERY NURSING AND MATERNAL MORTALITY

Nightingale did pioneering research on maternal mortality postchildbirth when her midwifery ward at King's College Hospital was closed, discussed in Chapter 2. She never agreed to a reopening, for she could never be sure that having such a ward would not result in unnecessary deaths. She continued to be asked for her advice on midwifery, and she continued to track issues of infection control related to it for the rest of her working life.

When the King's College midwifery ward opened in 1861, the lessons of Ignacz Semmelweis's Vienna experience were available, but not known to Nightingale or her colleagues. He had made his great breakthrough in reducing maternal deaths in 1847 to 1848 by requiring doctors and medical students to follow a strict handwashing procedure, using a disinfectant solution, on entry into the midwifery ward. The admission procedures at the Vienna General Hospital provided, in effect, a controlled experiment on handwashing. There were two clinics, one staffed by medical doctors and medical students, the other by midwives. The death rates were higher in the medical clinic, for doctors and medical students conducted autopsies on dead mothers. Midwives, who were less well trained, did not. Mortality decreased in the medical clinic when Semmelweis made disinfectant hand-washing on entry a requirement (Semmelweis, 1983).

In Paris, the well-trained midwives, all women, conducted autopsies, usually the prerogative of (male) doctors. The death rates of these highly trained midwives were high. These facts Nightingale learned only second hand, through a publication by a French doctor who collected comparative statistics (Le Fort, 1866). She used them in her own pioneering study, *Introductory Notes on Lying-in Institutions* (Nightingale, 1871, in McDonald, 2005).

The title is telling, "Introductory Notes," or even more tentative than her usual "Notes on." She was enormously apologetic about the analysis. She had worked hard to collect good comparative data (home births, workhouse infirmaries, and hospital wards), but realized that much more was needed. When she sent the book to colleagues, including leading obstetricians, she stressed the preliminary nature of the results and asked for advice. She hoped that Dr. Sutherland would produce a more definitive edition later. He did not, nor did she.

Nightingale learned the lessons on infection control. Careful measures were needed to keep maternity visits separate from visits to sick patients. In the organization of district nursing, or home nursing, she advised a strict separation of duties between the two different types of cases.

There is a warning against women giving birth, "lying-in," in hospitals in her 1890 item on hospitals: "The continuous use of wards for this purpose appears to be very dangerous to the patients." She again noted that there were fewer deaths of birthing mothers in workhouse infirmaries than in other hospitals, and why "lying-in at home is safer than either" (Nightingale, 1890, p. 806, in McDonald, 2012, p. 916).

When she revised her article on nursing practice in Quain's *Dictionary of Medicine* for 1894, she added a short explanation that midwifery nursing differed from regular hospital nursing in that the patient was not, "or ought not to be, sick." She stipulated that "midwifery and general cases should not be attended by the same nurse. No ordinary precautions will secure the lying-in case from danger arising out of this practice." Midwifery cases required hygienic precautions similar to those for surgery (Nightingale, 1894, Vol. 2, p. 247, in McDonald, 2009b, p. 736).

As late as 1896, Nightingale was concerned about combined midwifery and regular visiting to sick patients in Lincolnshire. Each nurse should have knowledge of the other field, but the work had to be kept separate (letter, September 8, 1896, in McDonald, 2009a, pp. 846–847).

Doctors, at the same time, were advising a similar separation, some stipulating a change in clothing before going to a maternity case from a regular sick patient.

INFECTION CONTROL NOW

Hand hygiene is the primary measure to reduce infections.
—World Health Organization [WHO] (2009, Foreword)

Despite 150 years of progress in the grounding of infection control, unnecessary disease and deaths occur. Antibiotics have made an enormous difference in death rates, but after decades of their use antibiotic-resistant bacteria, such as methicillin-resistant *Staphylococcus aureus* (MRSA), severe acute respiratory syndrome (SARS), *Clostridium difficile*, and Ebola, have evolved.

Estimates of people affected by hospital-acquired diseases in 2010 are as high as 20 million worldwide, with 7 million deaths, roughly 35% of those who fell ill (Daniels, 2011). "Proper hand hygiene is the primary method for reducing infections" (Gawande, 2004), or another instance of how Nightingale's measures are still valid.

A doctor protested use of the term "nosocomial or hospital-acquired infection" (nosocomial is Italian for hospital), arguing that "health-care associated infections" would be more appropriate. These were "by far the most common complications affecting hospital patients." Between 5% and 10% of patients admitted to acute care hospitals acquire one or more infections, "and the risks have steadily increased during recent decades. . . . In the United States, roughly 2 million patients each year suffer such adverse effects" (Burke, 2003, p. 651).

Citing Burke and Nightingale, and noting the costs to health care, a nurse concluded "hand hygiene is the single most important factor for infection control." Yet monitoring found that it was performed only one third to one half as often as it should be (Maxworthy, 2008), an old story, now.

WHO has taken up hand hygiene in earnest in its many publications, guidelines, and joint publications with other agencies (The Joint Commission, 2009; WHO, 2009).

Hospitals today put up signs urging handwashing, make spot checks, install cameras, and award prizes for good practice, but still there are lapses in compliance and patients fall ill and some die from infections acquired while being treated. Hospital designers are trying such measures as placing a wash basin at the patient's bed, at the same spot in every room, to make handwashing easier, desirably absolutely routine. Doctors urge their teams to do better, yet acknowledge mistakes. One surgeon, who credited Nightingale with leadership on the subject, referred to "130 years of doctor's plagues" caused by inadequate cleansing. He referred to two leading specialist journals, *The Journal of Hospital Infection* and *Infection Control and Hospital Epidemiology*, for reading "like a sad litany of failed attempts to get us to change our contaminating ways." He flagged the introduction of a ci culating nurse in surgery to keep operators from "contaminating patients, to be an extra set of hands for "unanticipated instruments." He acknow edged that, in an intensive care unit on his floor, a member of his team (possibly himself?) gave their patient a killing infection (Gawande, 200 pp. 1284–1285).

> *Are not great surgeons proverbially careless about infection?*
> —Nightingale (letter, December 10, 1890, in McDonald, 2009b, p. 438)

QUESTIONS FOR DISCUSSION

1. How can nurses in today's hospitals and other health care facilities determine the adequacy of measures to prevent cross-infection? What data are available?
2. How can nurses know if cross-infection rates are as low as possible, that is, by comparison with other like institutions?
3. What literature is available reporting innovative measures for preventing cross-infection?

REFERENCES

Abel-Smith, B. (1964). *The hospitals 1800-1948: A study in social administration England and Wales.* London, UK: Heinemann.

Burke, J. P. (2003, February 13). Infection control: A problem for patient safety. *Ne England Journal of Medicine, 348,* 651–656. doi:10.1056/NEJMhpr020557

Daniels, R. (2011). Surviving the first hours in sepsis: Getting the basics right (a intensivist's perspective). *Journal of Antimicrobial Chemotherapy, 66*(2), 811–82 doi:10.1093/jac/dkq515

Gawande, A. (2004). Notes of a surgeon: On washing hands. *New England Journal Medicine, 350,* 1283–1286. doi:10.1056/NEJMp048025

Gill, C. G., & Gill, G. (2005, June 16). Nightingale in Scutari: Her legacy re-examine *Clinical Infectious Diseases, 40*(12), 1799–1805. doi:10.1086/430380

The Joint Commission (2009, December 6). Measuring hand hygiene adherenc Overcoming the challenges. Retrieved from http://www.jointcommission.org

Le Fort, L. (1866). *Des maternités: étude sur les maternités et les institutions charitabl d'accouchement à domicile dans les principaux états de l'Europe.* Paris, France: Masso et fils.

Lister, J. (1867, September 21). On the antiseptic principle in the practice of surger *Lancet, 90*(2299), 353–356. doi:10.1016/S0140-6736(02)51827-4

Maxworthy, J. C. (2008, May 27). The dirty hands of health care: What would Florence think? *Reflections on Nursing Leadership, 34,* 2.

McDonald, L.. (Ed.). (2004). *Florence Nightingale on public health care.* Waterloo, Canada: Wilfrid Laurier University Press. ISBN: 0-88920-446-2.

McDonald, L. (Ed.). (2005). *Florence Nightingale on women, medicine, midwifery and prostitution.* Waterloo, Canada: Wilfrid Laurier University Press. ISBN: 0-88920-466-7.

McDonald, L. (Ed.). (2009a). *Florence Nightingale: Extending nursing.* Waterloo, Canada: Wilfrid Laurier University Press. ISBN: 978-1-55458-170-2.

McDonald, L. (Ed.). (2009b). *Florence Nightingale: The Nightingale School.* Waterloo, Canada: Wilfrid Laurier University Press. ISBN: 978-1-55458-169-6.

McDonald, L. (Ed.). (2012). *Florence Nightingale and hospital reform.* Waterloo, Canada: Wilfrid Laurier University Press. ISBN: 978-0-88920-471-3.

Nightingale, F. (1860). *Notes on nursing: What it is, and what it is not.* London, UK: Harrison.

Nightingale, F. (1863a). *Notes on hospitals* (3rd ed.). London, UK: Longmans, Green.

Nightingale, F. (1863b). Sanitary statistics of native colonial schools and hospitals. *Transactions of the National Association for the Promotion of Social Science,* 475–488.

Nightingale, F. (1883). Nursing the sick. In R. Quain (Ed.), *A dictionary of medicine* (Vol. 2, pp. 1043–1049). London, UK: Longmans, Green.

Nightingale, F. (1890). *Hospitals. Chambers's encyclopaedia: A dictionary of universal knowledge* (New ed., Vol. 5, pp. 805–807). London & Edinburgh, UK: W. & R. Chambers.

Nightingale, F. (1894). Nursing the sick. In R. Quain (Ed.), *A dictionary of medicine* (Vol. 2, pp. 237–244). London, UK: Longmans, Green.

Oztekin, S. D. (2007). Florence Nightingale in Turkey: Genesis of modern infection control. IFIC Conference in the Shadow of Florence Nightingale: 150 Years Later. *International Journal of Infection Control, 2,* 21–24.

Semmelweis, I. P. (1983 [1861]). *The etiology, concept, and prophylaxis of childbed fever* (K.C. Carter, trans). Madison: University of Wisconsin Press.

Statistics of the General Hospitals of London. (1862, September). *Journal of the Statistical Society of London, 25*(3), 384–385.

Wilson, J. (1995). *Infection control in clinical practice.* London, UK: Baillière Tindall. ISBN: 97807027611

World Health Organization. (2009). *WHO guidelines on hand hygiene in health care: A summary.* Retrieved from http://www.who.int/gpsc/5may/tools/who_guidelines-handhygiene_summary.pdf

Chapter 6: Pediatric Nursing

The human baby is not an invalid, but it is the most tender form of animal life.
—Nightingale (1893, in Part II, Chapter 12)

This chapter begins with the case Nightingale made, well supported by mortality data of the time, that children were at greater risk than adults at all stages of becoming ill from an infectious disease or from bad external conditions, and had lower ability to fight infection and to recover after the acute stage of the disease. Next comes a concerted debate for and against children's hospitals, which were only beginning to become popular charities in her day. The special conditions Nightingale thought necessary for them, including space requirements (with gardens), higher staff–patient ratios, and measures to prevent abuse are all noted.

The chapter continues with comparison of the use of separate hospitals for children against having separate children's wards within regular general hospitals, and for mixing children with adults in such hospitals. The problems of institutional care of children in large orphanages are next reviewed, with observations from trusted colleagues who saw children at and from them.

Finally, as Nightingale always preferred preventive measures to treatment after the fact, the special requirements for disease prevention she thought necessary for children are related.

NIGHTINGALE'S OWN EXPERIENCE OF GIVING CARE TO CHILDREN

Nightingale's views on pediatric care are largely taken from advice she obtained from colleagues and the research literature, for she herself never worked in a children's hospital or children's ward. She had nursed children, briefly, in 1851, at Kaiserswerth, and got some experience there by assignment to the orphanage and infant school. There were, occasionally, children at her small hospital on Harley Street.

Nightingale's fondness for children is evident in her own relations with them. Colleagues often wanted their children to meet her and she (sometimes) obliged. Evidently she could put children at ease, adept at telling stories (a sandstorm on the Nile and the heroic dog "Bob" on an Arctic expedition did the trick). There is charming correspondence over many years with the grandchildren of Sir Harry Verney, her sister's husband.

Nightingale took a particular interest in the children's ward at St. Thomas' Hospital, named, with the Queen's permission, Victoria Ward. She routinely sent presents, toys, games, and greenery for Christmas to this ward, and often to other hospitals as well. She treasured meetings with the ward sister, sometimes following up by asking how a particular child was doing. This interest only heightened in her own old age.

Despite her minimal direct experience of pediatric nursing, Nightingale was frequently asked for advice on the care of children and on children's hospitals. To respond, she sought out advice from more experienced nurses. St. Thomas' had a children's ward and children were also treated in adult wards, so that she did not lack sources of information.

THE SPECIAL VULNERABILITY OF CHILDREN

The life duration of babies is the most "delicate test" of health conditions.
—Nightingale (1893, in Part II, Chapter 12)

Death rates before age 5 years were high in Nightingale's day. The statistic is still one used as an indicator of the quality of life and health care available. Epidemics were worse in children's hospitals, a fact Nightingale knew. She gave the example of a one in five death rate, from 1804 to 1861, at the Paris Enfants Malades, "the greatest and oldest child's hospital in the world" (Nightingale, 1863, Chapter 6, in McDonald, 2012, p. 175), later recognized as the first pediatric hospital in the world. *Notes on Nursing* emphasized that children were "much more susceptible than grown people to all noxious influences." They were "affected by the same things, but much more quickly and seriously," by all the problems from lack of fresh air to improper food and dullness of light: "One can, therefore, only press the importance as being yet greater in the case of children, greatest in the case of sick children, of attending to these things" (Nightingale, 1860, Conclusion, in Part II, Chapter 10).

When medical statistician William Farr began work on a paper on child mortality in 1865, he enlisted Nightingale's assistance in getting background information. She wrote to Mary Jones, director of nursing at King's College Hospital, for help, explaining that he had been collecting "very valuable tables from all over Europe as to child's death rates. The thing is now to ascertain why these death rates are so high" (letter, December 12, 1865, in McDonald, 2005, pp. 170–171).

In her much later paper for the Chicago congress, Nightingale remarked sardonically that "everybody must be born," yet there was "probably no knowledge more neglected than this....how to feed, wash, and clothe the baby, how to secure the utmost cleanliness for mother and infant." Raising healthy children was essential "to make a healthy nation" (Nightingale, 1893, p. 445, in McDonald, 2004, p. 207, in Part II, Chapter 12).

To build health and prevent disease in children required, in addition to all the conditions of adequate housing, cleanliness, and nutrition, special knowledge of early child care. Nightingale thought that midwives, both nurses and women doctors, should teach new mothers the basics of feeding and washing their infants and general infant care. Few did. She regretted that, as women (still in small numbers) entered the medical profession, they would not take this on as a responsibility. Some told her that this would cause them to "lose caste" with their male colleagues (Nightingale, 1893, in McDonald, 2004, p. 207, in Part II, Chapter 12).

In her day, women of means employed a "monthly nurse" for a month after giving birth, who looked after both the mother and the child. These untrained "nurses," however, gave no instruction on infant care. Nightingale hoped that monthly nurses, trained to give such advice, would become accessible to poorer women.

In the library standard edition of *Notes on Nursing*, Nightingale quoted extensively from a published lecture of Dr. Charles West, of the Hospital for Sick Children, on sudden deaths in infancy and children (West, 1859). Sudden deaths, in the great majority of cases, were by accident, "not a necessary or inevitable result of any disease" from which the infant or child was suffering (*Notes on Nursing*, Conclusion).

Next, the following year, Nightingale added a chapter, "Minding Baby," for a new edition, with simplified language, *Notes on Nursing for the Labouring Classes*, 1861. This chapter is fully devoted to non-professional home care, including that given by older sisters to young infants and toddlers. The "health at home" and "home missioners" material Nightingale wrote decades later continued to stress the need.

THE CASE FOR AND AGAINST CHILDREN'S HOSPITALS

Children...suffer to such an incredible degree from being in hospital that they ought not to be kept an hour longer than medical or surgical treatment is constantly and strictly necessary.

—Nightingale (McDonald, 2004, p. 532)

Children's hospitals were a fashionable charity in Nightingale's day, but she herself remained wary. Whether or not they should be built was an empirical question: If treating children in children's wards in regular hospitals, or by mixing them in with adult patients, resulted in lower death rates, they should be preferred to children's hospitals.

When asked for advice on particular plans for a children's hospital, however, Nightingale obliged. This happened as early as 1860, when Prince Albert asked her to assist with the Lisbon Children's Hospital, which was to be named after the Queen of Portugal; it still exists as the Dona Estefania Hospital. Nightingale corresponded with the architect and gave detailed advice on the plans. She included a full chapter on children's hospitals, with material on Lisbon, in the final edition of *Notes on Hospitals* (Nightingale, 1863, in McDonald, 2012, pp. 524–532).

In 1874, Nightingale was approached by Emily Gregory, a Nightingale nurse who later became a missionary, to meet with Dr. K. A. Rauchfuss, a distinguished Russian pediatrician visiting London. He was then director of the children's hospital in St. Petersburg, commissioned to plan one for Moscow, which became the Vladimir Children's Hospital. Nightingale evidently sent him comments on his plans, but he wanted to meet her in person, which was arranged by another nurse, Maria Machin, then the home sister at the Nightingale School.

Nightingale was not happy with the nurses at Dr. Rauchfuss's hospital being supervised by the doctor/director, but did meet with him. The timing proved to be useful, because Dr. Rauchfuss's views on Russian winter conditions gave her ideas for advising on the Montreal General Hospital (letter, January 4, 1875, in McDonald, 2012, p. 804–805). The Vladimir Hospital, 180 beds, built on the favored pavilion principle, on a substantial plot of land, was opened in 1876. It was later awarded a gold medal as the best children's hospital in Europe.

Nightingale never got over her skepticism as to the desirability of separate children's hospitals. Hospitals continued to be dangerous places, even with gradual improvements. Children were even more vulnerable than adults to hospital-acquired diseases. In an unpublished note, she even strengthened her general advice of "not a day longer" in hospital for adults, to make it "not an hour longer" for children:

> It is now a well known rule: keep no patient in hospital a day longer than is absolutely necessary for hospital treatment and nursing. And even this may be many days too long. The patient may have to recover not only from illness or injury but from hospital. But for children one *may*, nay one *must* say: keep no child an *hour* longer in hospital than is positively needful. (undated note, Add Mss[1] 45820 f112, in McDonald, 2004, pp. 8–9)

When children's hospitals were built, numerous special features were needed. There had to be space for exercise, gardens, and schooling. "Physical exercises, in and out of doors, are a part of its treatment, in all but acute cases. Bathing also. Teaching also," Nightingale wrote the architect: "A large garden ground, laid out in sward and green hillocks and such ways as children like (*not too pretty* for the children to be scolded for spoiling it) must be provided for" (letter, December 24, 1860, in McDonald, 2102, pp. 528–530).

Advice for a Children's Hospital in Manchester

The requirements were no less onerous when Nightingale gave advice on a possible children's hospital for Manchester in 1866. The letter was to her brother-in-law, Sir Harry Verney, who was acting as an intermediary:

> Have they considered what are the essentials of a children's hospital? The baths, the exercises of all kinds, in a garden (not too pretty to spoil—with plenty of green sward), in covered sheds for bad weather, in playrooms for very bad weather—the exercises, including gymnastic exercises (which ought to be superintended by…a professor—otherwise the children will hurt themselves more than benefit themselves)…Singing exercises in chorus—all these form an important part of the medical treatment of children. Then, there must be classes for instruction, which, again, must be carefully regulated in reference to your children's health.…Then, the proportion of nurses to children ought to be considerably more than double that of nurses to adults in a hospital. And you must have nurses to your baths, to your exercising grounds, etc., so that no children should be left alone. (letter, October 15, 1866, in McDonald, 2004, p. 530–531)

---

[1] Further references to Add Mss, Additional Manuscripts, are also to the British Library.

Another stricture, "however large and good the grounds" of a children's hospital, "it must have a convalescent hospital, desirably at the seaside. This was even more important for a children's hospital than for a regular acute-care hospital" (letter, October 15, 1866, in McDonald, 2004, p. 532).

Adequate grounds in no way could make up for sanitary defects. The "Enfant-Jésus," the Paris orphanage that merged with the Enfants-Malades, was "the most complete children's hospital in the world," the same letter explained. It had "large and capital grounds," but "the mortality among the children is still so alarmingly high." Scrofula was responsible for a large number of children's disease.

In the same letter on the Manchester proposal, Nightingale warned of cruelty to children in hospital, unknown to people who have "*not* passed their lives in hospitals." Public opinion was needed to "keep down cruelties and neglects in hospitals, and there can be *no* public opinion in children's hospitals" (letter, October 15, 1866, in McDonald, 2004, p. 532). Children could not complain, or faced retaliation if they did.

Getting good children's nurses, in sufficient numbers was difficult, and not at all obviated, as was sometimes thought, by having religious orders to do the nursing: "Children are so utterly at the mercy of their nurses (be they nuns or seculars)" (letter, October 15, 1866, in McDonald, 2004, p. 531).

The Manchester hospital was not, either in construction or situation, what was wanted "to put children into," Nightingale wrote. It had "all the disadvantages of the adult hospital with none of the advantages of the children's hospital. (And I could tell you terrible experiences which have been made in these children's wards.)" Altogether, Nightingale concluded, there were only two valid objects for "founding a *children's* hospital: (1) to keep the children innocent of what they must see and hear in an adult hospital; (2) to secure all the essentials enumerated above, which are quite different for a children's hospital from what are essentials for an adult hospital." If not secured, "I do not hesitate to say that children are better off in the female wards of an adult hospital," workhouse infirmaries excluded (letter, October 15, 1866, in McDonald, 2004, p. 531).

Children should never be workhouse inmates, the same letter asserted. A child born in a workhouse, as soon as "weaned and out of arms...ought to be removed from the workhouse walls, never to re-enter them." Workhouses then had "union schools," which gave some basic instruction, an advantage before state schools were provided for all children. Such schools for workhouse children, Nightingale said, "ought to be in the country, entirely under different administration, separate from the workhouse and ought to include its sick children's infirmary" (letter, October 15, 1866, in McDonald, 2004, p. 531).

The next year, 1867, after giving her advice related earlier, Nightingale was notified that she was elected an honorary governor of the new Clinical

Hospital and Dispensary for Children, and sent its rules. She declined (letter, July 12, 1867, with note of reply, London Metropolitan Archives, H1/ST/NC2/V26/67). However, when the new hospital was built, outside Manchester at Pendlebury, and in full operation, she called it "the best there is." An article in a later medical journal acknowledged that the location was outside the city, for the sake of "more room and more salubrious surroundings." No children's hospital anywhere was "more admirably constructed and more advantageously located upon ample grounds" (Kelley, 1893, p. 587).

A Children's Hospital for Staffordshire

In 1876, answering an inquiry from Staffordshire on children's hospitals, Nightingale stated that she had not "modified the opinion" she had given in *Notes on Hospitals*. Rather, she was "confirmed in it" every year from what she heard:

(1) an experienced matron or head nurse, whose "opinion" is really valuable, tells you "never put sick children in an adult ward; they disturb the other patients." You inquire, and you find her experience to be that of a ward of forty beds, where throughout the winter there have never been less than twenty severe children's cases, chiefly burns, and twenty "heavy" adult cases, all of them too serious to think of anything but themselves, or to be able to take any other interest in a child than to be disturbed by its moans and cries....

(2) An equally experienced matron or head nurse whose "opinion" is as valuable as that of No. 1 tells you, "Never put your sick children except in an adult ward; they do the other patients so much good, and the other patients nurse them." You inquire, and you find her experience to be that of a ward of thirty two beds, with five or six (or even more) children in it, a clever sister (head nurse) placing each next [to] an adult whose own woes are capable of alleviation by alleviating the child's. (Nightingale, 1876)

Nightingale remarked also that she was not aware of any children's hospital that gave good nurse training. She hoped to get further information on the subject, but was stymied by lack of comparative data. As she continued:

It would be exceedingly interesting to find out the relative rate of mortality and duration of sickness in children's cases, otherwise *similar*, placed in "general" or "children's" wards or hospitals, but unfortunately hospital statistics are not sufficiently well kept to ascertain this. (Nightingale, 1876)

Advice for a German Children's Hospital

When the Grand Duchess of Baden in 1879 asked for her help on plans for a new children's hospital in Heidelberg (letter, March 31, 1879, in McDonald, 2005, p. 839), Nightingale started looking for plans of "the best children's hospitals in England." She wrote numerous nursing directors and doctors for plans of their hospital. Most of those elicited had serious defects, she thought, including hospitals where she was in frequent touch with the nursing director. Her excellent collaborator, Dr. John Sutherland, assisted by revising the Heidelberg plans. Nightingale wondered about "warning" the Grand Duchess's architect on the cautions needed (letter, May 24, 1881, in McDonald, 2012, p. 862).

On Children's Hospitals for an Encyclopedia

Nightingale, in writing on children's hospitals in 1890, for *Chambers's Encyclopaedia*, did not debate the pros and cons of having such institutions, but offered qualifications "if you have a children's hospital." She repeated a point she had made when giving her first advice on a children's hospital for Lisbon, that sick children could not be "left alone for a moment." As a result, "one might almost say a nurse is required for every child." Thirty years laters, he repeated the admonition: "In all hospitals (in a child's hospital much more than in others) the patient must not stay a day longer than is absolutely necessary" (Nightingale, 1890, p. 807, in McDonald, 2012, p. 916). She never published the "not an hour longer" warning.

Children's hospitals remain today popular charities, even as some have become big business operations. The Hospital for Sick Children in Toronto, for example, engages in massive fund-raising by lotteries (widely advertised); its executives are richly remunerated, and junk food is readily available to its visitors. Perhaps Nightingale's not-an-hour longer advice is no longer needed.

SPECIAL REQUIREMENTS FOR PEDIATRIC NURSING

The high standard of observation required in caring for children appears in Nightingale's writing from *Notes on Nursing*:

> In the case of infants, *everything* must depend upon the accurate observation of the nurse or mother who has to report. And how seldom is this condition of accuracy fulfilled. It is the real test of a nurse whether she can nurse a sick infant. (Nightingale, 1860, Chapter 13, in Part II, Chapter 10)

By the 1880s, in her nursing practice article for Quain's *Dictionary of Medicine*, the requirements for a pediatric nurse had become more stringent.

> She will be required to make these observations [pulse, secretions, breathing, sleep, wounds]—if possible still more accurately—for child patients, who cannot tell what is the matter with them; to understand the management of sick children and children's wards, which need a yet more exquisite cleanliness. And children show a much more rapid change of symptoms for life or for death generally than adults. Children are the best air test, the best test of sanitary conditions. (Nightingale, 1883, Vol. 2, p. 1048, in McDonald, 2009, p. 749)

Nightingale's advice on children's hospitals stressed female control. She did not explicitly mention the risk of sexual abuse, but clearly the stipulation that there be the fewest male employees as possible, and none sleeping in, suggests that concern.

Finally, Nightingale thought that children's nurses needed special qualities. In the children's hospital section of *Notes on Hospitals* she stated:

> There must be a real genuine vocation and love for the work, a feeling as if your own happiness were bound up in each particular child's recovery. Nothing else will carry you through the perpetual wear and tear to the spirits, of the fretfulness, the unreasonableness of sick children—not that I think it is greater than that of many sick adults—but it is more wearing, because the strain is never off you for a minute. (Nightingale, 1863, Chapter 6, Children's hospitals, in McDonald, 2012, p. 172)

In her second last "address to nurses," Nightingale noted yet again the difficulties of providing good care and the need for "love for children" to do it:

> Children require the most observing and best nursing because they cannot tell you what they feel, and, what is more, a fretful complaining child is by no means always the most suffering. Still, you must not neglect fretfulness. *Love* for *children* is a necessity in a children's ward....

They must be either "those dear little souls" or "those tiresome dirty things" (Nightingale address, 1897, in McDonald, 2009, p. 873).

OTHER INSTITUTIONAL CARE OF CHILDREN

Children who were destitute and orphaned were often placed in "homes," some small, and some for as many as 300, as in the Gibraltar Training Ship for Destitute Boys in Belfast. Nightingale came to consider such institutional care to be defective, from the numerous reports she received on it from Jessie Lennox, nursing director at the Belfast Children's Hospital, where the boys were sent when ill.

Nightingale told her sister, then involved in planning for another institution for destitute boys, the Gordon Boys' Home, that the matron of the Belfast Children's Hospital disapproved of the training ship. With "no mothers," it was against "God's laws."

Lennox told Nightingale that a nurse "mother" would be a "blessing" on the ship (Lennox letter, September 14, 1889, Add Mss[1] 47751 f195).

Lennox once got a lady to live in the hold for 3 months to nurse the boys. When she gave a sick boy a pat, another moaned, asking for a pat "like his'n" (letter, September 25, 1885, in McDonald, 2003, p. 239). Another letter from Lennox said that the boys placed on a training ship suffered from depression (letter, June 21, 1890, Add Mss 47751 f218).

Nothing had changed by 1892 when Lennox, in a meeting with Nightingale, recounted that the boys who came into her hospital from the training ship were "surprised to receive individual care—they came in so depressed in body and mind" (notes, February 2, 1892, in McDonald, 2003, p. 241).

Nightingale had these concerns in mind when she was approached for help in planning for the Gordon Boys' Home, to be a memorial to General Gordon, who had been assassinated in Khartoum, and who himself had earlier looked after orphan boys. She and her colleagues at one point had to protest the use of a former prison as the home!

There were the usual concerns about ventilation and adequate space. Boys needed as much cubic space as men, she explained (letter, June 12, 1889, Add Mss 68886 f59).

Nightingale wrote Gordon's cousin, Amy Hawthorn, with her concerns about care. Experience gained over the previous 30 years had shown "that health, morals, and discipline" had to be obtained "in huts or small pavilions, not in a large building containing 300 cells." She asked whether the boys appeared "to need a (motherly) matron's care." Without a "motherly woman" much that was unhealthy took place. Bullying evidently was a problem: "And some boys get depressed and others become tormentors—some are devourers and some devoured." She asked whether they were subdivided enough or all together. "And do they live enough in the open air? And do they look happy and look you in the face? Are their quarters in the fort dark or unairy?" (letter, May 18, 1886, in McDonald, 2012, p. 479).

Nightingale worked closely with the committee both on the selection of the nursing head and the physical planning. She kept in touch with the person selected, St. Thomas' trained Lydia Constable. She went from asking questions about the home to faulting its regime. It relied excessively on "authority," "no sympathy—nothing like a home or a family" (letter, February 11, 1892, Add Mss 47751 f239).

DISEASE PREVENTION FOR CHILDREN

For Nightingale, the best approach for care for children, as for adults, was prevention: to establish health rather than resort to hospital, of whatever kind, after they become ill. As she asserted in *Notes on Nursing*, "The causes of enormous child mortality are perfectly well known: they are chiefly want of cleanliness, want of fresh air, careless dieting, and clothing" (Nightingale, 1860, Introductory). She would continue to make these points in correspondence from then on.

In 1889, Nightingale was alerted to the issue of infantile blindness in Egypt, from poor sanitary practices. A doctor at the Women's Hospital in Cairo wrote her about it, noting its frequency among both Muslim and Coptic children (Sandwith letter, Add Mss 45809 f210). However, there is no information on any follow-up.

The subject was brought to Nightingale again in 1894 by Charlotte Smith, who was neither a nurse nor a doctor, but the author of a paper at a meeting of the British Institution of Public Health. This set off an exchange of information, which culminated in Nightingale pulling together instructions on the prevention of infantile blindness, which she sent back to Smith and also to the medical officer of health for Buckinghamshire, for use in his rural health visiting program.

> Prevention of blindness. After a newly born child is washed, great care should then be taken to clean the inside of the eyelids of each eye, as any collection of matter within the eyelids is very dangerous and must be removed. The outside of the eyelids should be well cleaned, and the eyelids separated and the edges cleaned. Each lower eyelid should be pulled gently down on the cheek and some water dropped on the inner surface, the eyelid should then be allowed to close. The water will thus wash the eyes. This should be done twice a day for a month. (Note [March 1895], in McDonald, 2004, p. 575)

In a paper of 1894, for a conference on rural health in Leeds, Nightingale discussed disease prevention in children, ending with a succinct list of concerns:

> *Management of Infants and Children*. How to feed, clothe, and wash. Nursing, weaning, hand feeding, regular intervals between feeding, flatulence, thrush, convulsions, bronchitis, croup. Simple hints to mothers about healthy conditions for children. Baths. Diet: how to prevent constipation and diarrhea. What to do in sudden attacks of convulsions and croup. Deadly danger of giving "soothing syrups" or alcohol. Made foods not wholesome. Headache often caused by bad eyesight. Symptoms of overwork at school—headache, worry, talking in the sleep. Danger to babies and little children of any violence, jerks, and sudden movements, loud voices, slaps, box on the ear. Good effects upon the health of gentleness, firmness, and cheerfulness. (Nightingale, 1894, p. 55, in McDonald, 2004, pp. 615–616)

The section ends on a delightful note, with which this chapter ends:

> No child can be well who is not bright and merry and brought up in fresh air and sunshine and surrounded by love—the sunshine of the soul. (Nightingale, 1894, p. 55, in McDonald, 2004, p. 616)

QUESTIONS FOR DISCUSSION

1. To what extent today are the risks of hospitalization on hospital-acquired infections greater for children than adults; what age groups are at greatest risk? What data are available to address this question?
2. To what extent is child abuse, sexual or physical, a reality in hospitals known to you? How is it reported? What special measures are in place to prevent it? What are the institutional barriers to reporting? Are nurses and other employees legally required to report observed abuse in your area?

REFERENCES

Kelley, S. W. (1893). Some other cities and citizens of Great Britain. *Cleveland Medical Gazette, 9*, 584–590.

McDonald, L. (Ed.). (2003). *Florence Nightingale on society and politics, philosophy, science, education, and literature*. Waterloo, Canada: Wilfrid Laurier University Press. ISBN: 0-88920-429-2.

McDonald, L. (Ed.). (2004). *Florence Nightingale on public health care.* Waterloo, Canada: Wilfrid Laurier University Press. ISBN: 0-88920-446-2.

McDonald, L. (Ed.). (2005). *Florence Nightingale on women, medicine, midwifery and prostitution.* Waterloo, Canada: Wilfrid Laurier University Press, p. 1085. ISBN: 0-88920-466-7.

McDonald, L. (Ed.). (2009). *Florence Nightingale: The Nightingale School.* Waterloo, Canada: Wilfrid Laurier University Press. ISBN: 978-1-55458-169-6.

McDonald, L. (Ed.). (2012). *Florence Nightingale and hospital reform.* Waterloo, Canada: Wilfrid Laurier University Press. ISBN: 978-0-88920-471-3.

Nightingale, F. (1860). *Notes on nursing: What it is, and what it is not.* London, UK: Harrison.

Nightingale, F. (1861). *Notes on nursing for the labouring classes.* London, UK: Harrison.

Nightingale, F. (1863). *Notes on hospitals* (3rd ed.). London, UK: Longmans, Green.

Nightingale, F. (1876, January 22). Letter. *The Staffordshire Advertiser.*

Nightingale, F. (1880). Hospitals. In *Chambers's encyclopaedia: A dictionary of universal knowledge* (Vol. 5, pp. 805–807). Edinburgh, Scotland: W. & R. Chambers.

Nightingale, F. (1893). Sick nursing and health nursing. In A. Burdett-Coutts (Ed.), *Woman's mission: A series of Congress papers on the philanthropic work of women* (pp. 184–205). London, UK: Sampson, Low, Marston.

Nightingale, F. (1894). Rural hygiene. *Official Report of the Central Conference of Women Workers, 46–55.*

West, C. (1859, January). Lecture on sudden death in infancy and childhood. *Medical News and Library, 17*(193), 4–11.

Chapter 7: Long-Term and Palliative Care

How many so-called incurables are curable!
—Nightingale (letter, October 7, 1896, in McDonald, 2009a, p. 403)

Long-term and palliative care are both fields that have changed enormously since Nightingale's days. Neither term was then in use, although both types of care were given. Rather, a brutal term for long-term care facilities appears, "hospital for incurables."

There were, then, no separate institutions for "palliative care," but it was recognized that some patients were at the end of their lives and no cure could reasonably be expected. This meant, instead of preventing and curing disease, "smoothing the path of the dying and the incurable" (Nightingale, 1880, p. 1). Obviously there was an overlap between care for "incurables," infirm or chronic cases, and the dying.

This chapter begins with Nightingale's challenge to the very concept of "incurable" patients. It next relates Nightingale's own experience of giving palliative care, both during the Crimean War and before it. A sample letter she wrote is included for each. Messages she sent to dying persons, later in life when she could not visit, are described.

The pros and cons of deathbed conversions are briefly described, picking up from a concern first raised in the chapter on ethics. Finally, a succinct statement is given for applying Nightingale's principles on care of the dying.

The challenges for Nightingale on long-term and palliative care seem to have been very much like what they are today. Nursing care was needed, but not the same scale as for acute-care hospitals. Resources were frequently inadequate. Long-term care institutions could not have a nurse training school, nor did they have a medical school. Their nursing positions were professionally less desirable than in acute-care hospitals.

CHALLENGING THE "INCURABLE" CONCEPT

Nightingale challenged the use of the term *incurable*. In a letter of 1880, she asked rhetorically, "how many would be cured by proper attendance, appliances, and trained nursing," with the benefit also of being able to leave the workhouse infirmary and so be "taken off the rates," or tax rolls (letter, July 9, 1880, in McDonald, 2004a, p. 475). Many patients were incurable as they were then treated, or not treated.

Again, in 1892, she found the line between incurable and treatable to be unclear. A letter to Mary Jones, the Anglican nun then running a small incurables home, noted that the two agreed that some patients "linger on for years," while others, "under good care," recover. In this same letter, Nightingale regretted, even that there was "perhaps nothing sadder in the whole world" that an incurable child could be cured, and then find that "nobody wants it back" (letter, July 3, 1892, in McDonald, 2005, p. 1028).

As the population ages, long-term care facilities are increasingly needed, but in many places they are still the poor cousins of hospital care. Nightingale examined the excuse for poor care in her own day, that the "infirm and aged" did not require "such careful nursing" as "hospital sick." This was a "mistake," she said, for many were helpless, or "dirty" cases (Nightingale, 1867, in McDonald, 2004a, p. 387, in Part II, Chapter 11).

LONG-TERM CARE, "INCURABLES," AND CONVALESCENTS

Hospitals for "incurables" at that time tended to be small, some in people's homes. Convalescent homes and small hospitals also served for long-term or "incurable" patients, patients not needing acute care. As noted in Chapter 2, Nightingale made (small) financial contributions to a number of such small institutions. A favorite was the Ascot Convalescent Home, which also took incurable patients, run by Anglican nuns in the Sellonite order.

The great majority of "incurable" or chronic patients, however, were in the workhouse infirmaries. In her entry on hospitals for *Chambers's Encyclopedia*, she described them as "chronic, not acute, cases, and incurables" (Nightingale, 1890, p. 806, in McDonald, 2009b, p. 915).

Nightingale was aware that "incurable" and "chronic" hospitals lacked the glamor of acute-care and children's hospitals and had difficulty raising funds. She became an avid supporter of the "London Infirmary for Diseases of the Legs, Ulcers, Varicose Veins," a charity that served many old soldiers. Her name appeared as a patron for years in its fund-raising advertisements, numerous in *The Times* from 1857 to 1872. One listed the Earl of Shaftesbury and Lord Bishop of Ripon after her, noting that she was "well aware of the sufferings of our brave soldiers in the Crimea from this disease" (*The Times*, 1860).

Nightingale routinely made distinctions in the care needed of those lumped together in the workhouses, among sick, infirm (long-term), lunatics, and children (letter, February 11, 1868, in McDonald, 2003, p. 153).

She was pleased when Lady Lothian took up the workhouse issue in 1880, telling her that the "great thing wanted" was "to transform the workhouse infirmaries," where most of these patients were. The workhouses should not be "supplementary hospitals to the great London and county hospitals, but rather hospitals in all respects fitted to receive to nurse and to cure those for whom the voluntary hospitals are not suitable." The great difficulty was "in making voluntary aid heartily cooperate with state aid, and thereby promoting the comfort and cure of thousands and hundreds of thousands of our fellow creatures, the poor sick, and old paupers" (letter, July 9, 1880, British Library Add Mss 45806 f51).

In 1881, Nightingale was asked to assist with plans for a new building for the Hospital for Incurables, Putney, later the Royal Hospital for Incurables, and still later renamed the Royal Hospital for Neuro-disability. Her friend and colleague on the matter was Dr. T. Graham Balfour, an able statistician and former secretary of the Royal Commission on the Crimean War. Nightingale was keen to oblige such a valuable colleague. She was a subscriber to the institution, which meant that she paid dues, but declined to be on the committee.

Nightingale also succeeded in getting an excellent nursing director for them, Ulrike Linicke, who was keen to move from her hospital in Dublin, Sir Patrick Dun's, fed up with its bureaucracy. As head of its training school, she had to deal with two boards, a ladies' committee, medical staff, house surgeon, nurses, both private and hospital, nursing students, and servants (letter, May 15, 1881, in McDonald, 2009a, p. 169).

When asked for advice about a new hospital for "dying incurables" in 1881, Nightingale knew of only one, run by a Miss Stephenson in her own home (letter to Henry Bonham Carter, February 6, 1881, in McDonald, 2009a, p. 52).

Mary Jones and other Anglican sisters, after leaving King's College Hospital and their order, founded a home for incurables/convalescents in Kensington, London. Nightingale contributed money and encouragement. She sent greenery and mince pies for Christmas (e.g., December 21, 1876, London Metropolitan Archives HI/ST/NC1/76/3). Still, she would have much preferred Jones to take on the nursing at a workhouse infirmary.

In 1888, Nightingale regretted not being able to find a "thoroughly-hospital-trained" person for their home; by then they had only one trained nurse among them (letter to Sister Frances Wylde, February 1, 1888, in McDonald, 2005, p. 1022).

She was also asked for advice on plans for hospitals for incurables, and complied as much as she could, as for other types of hospital. In 1862, she was asked to advise on plans for a hospital for incurables in Malta, which she did. The civil servant in charge duly informed her that "almost all" of her suggestions had been attended to (Inglott letter, August 15, 1862, London Metropolitan Archives H1/ST/NC2/V19/62). The plans are in *Notes on Hospitals* (Plan No. 9, in McDonald, 2012, p. 163). She advised also on a plan for an asylum for the aged and infirm in Malta (Plan No. 8).

Nightingale was always practical in giving advice on care facilities, aware of the limitations of resources. She routinely sought the most cost-effective way to provide good care. When the Diocese of Durham asked for her advice in 1887, she told them that trained district nursing (home visits) saved expenses, as it made it possible "to nurse incurable cases at home, which otherwise go into the workhouse infirmary." Such nurses would also serve to tide cases over "a temporary illness," set them on foot "so that they need not go either into hospital or infirmary at all" (letter, December 2, 1887, in McDonald, 2009a, pp. 801–802).

NIGHTINGALE'S OWN EXPERIENCE OF GIVING PALLIATIVE CARE

Both [Dr] Newton and [Dr] Struthers, it may be a consolation to their friends to know, were tended in their last moments, and had their dying eyes closed, by Miss Nightingale herself.

—(*The Times*, 1855)

For large numbers of soldiers during the Crimean War, 1854 to 1856, Nightingale could give no more than (cursory) palliative care, although the term "palliative" was not then used. She had learned care of the dying in her very first nursing experience, in 1851, at the Kaiserswerth hospital (McDonald, 2004b, pp. 518–553), and had looked after dying patients as well at her Establishment for Gentlewomen in Harley Street, 1853 to 1854. Palliative care is an essential component of nursing care still, especially now when so many people spend their last days in a hospital or long-term care facility.

Care of the Dying at Kaiserswerth

At Kaiserswerth, Nightingale learned how to counsel the dying and how to "lay out" the dead for viewing by the family before burial. At Harley Street, she made arrangements for funerals. Later, in advising on hospital design, she was sensitive to the needs of families visiting the mortuary or "deadhouse" to see their deceased family member. For the children's hospital in Lisbon, she advised that a separate entrance be provided so that families would not have to use the one used by doctors doing autopsies (letter, December 24, 1860, in McDonald, 2012, p. 530).

Nightingale had two dying patients to look after at the hospital at Kaiserswerth, which was, as noted in Chapter 4, a Lutheran institution run by the pastor. Pastor Fliedner told her, when she asked his advice on counseling a dying man, that the patient would talk more openly to her than he would to a pastor. Fliedner suggested that she inquire kindly into the patient's feelings, if his case were death, and what grounds of confidence he had that he would be saved, if he knew the commandments and had kept them, what his relations were with others. It was best to talk to the patient alone. If the man would

> not believe that he is dying, show him that it is good for him to be converted at all events—he may afterwards live. Do not be always trying to convert your patient, but tell him a story, a parable, the history of a conversion that he may say she does not want to convert me, but she comes and tells me something pretty. (note, July 28, 1851, in McDonald, 2004b, p. 580)

What Nightingale said to this patient is not known, but her journal notes that she later said prayers "with the dying man" and that she read to him the next day.

Several days later, Nightingale recorded having gone to read to him. When she saw that he was dying, she sought another deaconess's help: "When I came back, the cold sweat was already on his forehead. The preacher came and prayed." Her journal next recounts that she

> sat with him till his death, which came quite quietly about 8 p.m. The struggling moon shone on the bed of the dying man and, when he was gone, I sat on the window sill and looked out on the busy, lighted town. Death is so much more impressive in the midst of life. (note, September 4, 1851, in McDonald, 2004b, p. 537)

The other person who died while Nightingale was on duty at Kaiserswerth was a deaconess, Sister Amalie, who made her think it "beautiful to be so sure of a speedy death, and yet able to work till the last" (note, August 22, 1851, in McDonald, 2004b, p. 533). A few weeks later, soon after the death of the male patient related in this section, she noted that Sister Amalie had "broken a blood vessel and was dying. I was soon summoned, but she was insensible; she was galvanized, mustard poultices laid on her legs, but no sign of life. I remained with her till 11 a.m. when she became cold." Later in the day, Nightingale laid out her body and said prayers for her (note, September 6, 1851, in McDonald, 2004b, pp. 537–538).

Palliative Care at Harley Street

Nightingale's Harley Street hospital preferred not to admit convalescent patients, but did keep patients past the normal 2-month term, if there were some "prospect either of improvement or of death." Thus, patients could stay if on a "downward path, even if slow," might be "softened in such an institution as this" (letter, November 25, 1853, in McDonald, 2009b, p. 86). Of their 10 patients, her quarterly report stated, five were "without hope of recovery...awaiting their end at periods varying from a few days to many months" (Nightingale, 1970/1854, 4th quarter, in McDonald, 2009b, p. 111).

In the case of a woman who died at her Harley Street hospital, Nightingale went well beyond what would be expected of a nurse. The patient was a German governess named Von Raven, who had been seduced by a nobleman. She subsequently gave birth to an illegitimate son. How she came to be in England is not clear, but Nightingale "fished her out of the Middlesex Hospital," to look after her at Harley Street (letter, May 27, 1872, in McDonald, 2001, pp. 810–811). The woman lacked friends and family who could assist her, apart from one Miss Welch, to whom Nightingale wrote a short time later (see Exhibit 7.1).

Von Raven died later that day, and Nightingale made arrangements for her burial and attended the funeral, held 2 days later. Years later, she was asked to procure a "Certificate of Death or of Burial," for which she asked Dr. Bence Jones to check his records (letter, May 27, 1872, in McDonald, 2001, pp. 810–811).

Von Raven had evidently asked Nightingale to assist with the arrangements for her son's care. She had 100 guineas from her mother set aside for him. Nightingale asked a competent friend in Berlin to help (letter, September 19, 1854, in McDonald, 2005, pp. 776–777). Again, today, these are responsibilities well beyond those expected of a nurse; Nightingale was exceptional in her sympathies, and was able, through her own means and network, to do much more, as evidenced by the care she gave, including staying with the dying woman, administering prescribed painkillers, reporting on her condition to a nearby friend, and attempting to ascertain others who should be notified of her coming death.

Palliative Care of Soldiers and Nurses During the Crimean War

During the Crimean War, Nightingale often could do no more than give palliative care to soldiers, many of whom were dying when they were admitted

EXHIBIT 7.1   LETTER OF FLORENCE NIGHTINGALE REGARDING A DYING PATIENT

April 27, 1854

I think I ought to tell you that I think most seriously of Miss v. Raven's case, and I should never be surprised if twenty-four hours end the scene in this world. She has been since 2 o'clock yesterday morning in a state of alternate frantic delirium and complete stupor.

I sent for Dr Bence Jones and Dr Weber last night at 11 o'clock and, by their orders, I was all night pouring brandy and laudanum alternately down her throat. About 5 o'clock this morning she became sensible and asked me to pray in German, which I did. If there are any friends to be let known, there is no time to be lost.

I would not let Madame Lauenstein see her last night because she was then asleep. We are ordered to keep her strictly quiet and in the dark. I therefore should be afraid of letting anyone see her. I have never left her and I am now writing in haste to know whether you think of any friends in Germany to be written to. She *may* last some time, but not likely.

Source: Letter, April 27, 1854 (in McDonald, 2009b, pp. 89–90).

to the hospital (some died while being carried in from the dock). The observations made by a former patient, a private soldier who recovered and subsequently accompanied her often on her rounds, are revealing. He described her sitting up all night with patients (Robinson, 1861). Nightingale kept no journal at this time and there were far too many patients and crises for her to have made notes by case. The chef Alexis Soyer saw her at this task one night around 2 a.m., with young Robinson holding the lamp for her as she penciled down the soldier's "last wishes to be despatched" to his friends or relations, with his watch and a few trinkets (Soyer, 1857, p. 142).

Other Nightingale acts on behalf of the dying are known from the many letters she wrote to family members relaying the soldier's last words, sometimes on disposing of his last wages and goods. Many of these letters were preserved and circulated, for they gave great comfort to the family. Certainly officers of the British Army did not write bereavement letters of such sympathy. A fine example is one Nightingale wrote to the mother of a private soldier, published in the *Derby Mercury* (see Exhibit 7.2).

EXHIBIT 7.2   LETTER OF FLORENCE NIGHTINGALE TO THE MOTHER OF A DEAD SOLDIER

Barrack Hospital, Scutari
April 12, 1855

I am very sorry to have to communicate to you the illness of your poor son, Private John Cope, 95th Regiment, No. 2884. He was admitted here about ten days ago suffering from diarrhea. He was immediately attended to by surgeons, by one of my nurses, and myself. He was fed in small quantities and frequently with port wine and arrowroot.

He wished very much to have a letter written to you, and two or three times I went to him for the purpose, but he was always too weak and put it off, and once he wandered and said it was done. He often murmured, "dear, dear mother!" and tried to say many things to you—that he was well cared for and wanted for nothing—that he had no wish for anything. I sent for the chaplain, who came twice, and both times he was quite sensible and prayed fervently, and said he was quite happy in mind and could follow all that was said. He spoke little after this, and sank rapidly and died at 2 o'clock on the morning of Easter Sunday, quite quietly and without pain, in the full hope of a resurrection with Him who rose again on that day.

I remain with true sympathy for your grief,

yours sincerely

Florence Nightingale
P.S. I would have sent you something of his, but he left nothing.

Source: Nightingale (1855, in McDonald, 2010, p. 438).

The letter shows what Nightingale saw as her responsibility as a nurse: to give what food and drink the patient could take, to summon the chaplain when requested, and to communicate his last words and wishes sympathetically to the family.

A Crimean War nurse, Winifred Sprey, a Roman Catholic Sister of Mercy from Liverpool, died suddenly of cholera, only hours after falling ill, at the General Hospital, Balaclava. Nightingale related to the mother superior

> that everything was done that could be done, two R.C. doctors, two priests, for whom I telegraphed from headquarters, were with her. I did not leave her till after her death, and attended

her body to the grave with the whole sisterhood next day, to a secluded spot chosen by themselves. (copy of a letter, Bundle 306, Claydon House Archives)

Deaths of Nursing Students and Nurses

Post–Crimean War, as the director of the Nightingale Fund, which funded the school (the money was raised in her honor for her war work), Nightingale felt a particular responsibility to ensure that nursing students who died while in her school were well looked after in their last days, and a proper burial provided. That is, she made her own inquiries about the dying student, offered extras, and checked with the family about burial. Some families wanted assistance, some not. She typically sent a wreath and wrote a condolence letter. She wanted families to know that the student nurse was appreciated.

On the death of a young nurse, Martha Rice, a member of the first set of trained nurses sent to Montreal, Nightingale recounted her noble sacrifice in her next address to nurses and students (address, April 28, 1876, in McDonald, 2009b, p. 838).

In 1888, a young night nurse, Jessie Craig, died of typhoid fever at her post at St. Thomas', a year after her training. The nursing director, Angelique Lucille Pringle, kept Nightingale posted on her illness and care (Pringle, 1888, 1889). Nightingale sent a wreath and passages to be read to the family and contributed to the cost of a tombstone. The family evidently appreciated the letter, for they had it copied and circulated (letter, December 7, 1888, London Metropolitan Archives H1/ST/NC1/88/10).

In the case of Helen Jane Preece, who began her nursing studies in 1891 and died of typhoid fever in 1894, Nightingale sent flowers when she became seriously ill and asked the nursing director, L. M. Gordon, if any food or drink would be appreciated. She sent her eau de cologne, which was then used to toughen the skin to prevent bedsores (Gordon letter, August 27, 1894, British Library Add Mss 47737 f180). On Preece's death, Nightingale sent the mother her sympathy, plus money to help with expenses (letter, September 1, 1894, in McDonald, 2009b, p. 460). The nursing director made the arrangements and reported back to Nightingale (Gordon letters, August 30 and September 10, 1894, British Library Add Mss 47737 ff182 and 184).

In the case of the death of older nurses, Nightingale appreciated hearing of their final illness and the care given. She made inquiries when the information was not forthcoming. Often, nursing colleagues knew that she would want to know, and sent details. There are numerous exchanges of letters and last tributes.

Nightingale, of course, also wanted nurse deaths to be the minimum possible, no more than the expected death rate for women of the same age.

In fact, the death rate of nurses was 40% higher, a point she made in *Notes on Hospitals* (Nightingale, 1863, Note A, Table 1, p. 20, in McDonald, 2012, p. 98).

Gill and Gill thought Nightingale's work on palliative care, or what they termed "hospice care," to have been noteworthy. They credit her with having practiced the care of the dying with dignity, long before Kübler-Ross's theory appeared (Gill & Gill, 2005, p. 1803).

Nightingale's Messages to the Dying

For many years, Nightingale was not well enough to visit sick and dying friends, colleagues, or relatives, so she had to make do with messages and gifts. She followed the last illness of those close to her, sending a messenger to their home "to inquire," often with a gift.

The nurse Nightingale most respected when she started nursing, Mary Jones, died in 1887 of typhoid fever. Over the 3 months preceding Jones's death, Nightingale sent her, as "her loving and grateful old friend," 25 letters or notes via another sister (letters, March 29 to June 3, 1887, London Metropolitan Archives, in McDonald, 2002, pp. 218–223). Many of these included practical gifts: fresh eggs, panada [a bread soup], orange jelly, a special meat juice (for irritable stomach), champagne, and port wine. Once Nightingale asked Sister Frances what she could send that would make her friend "less suffering" (letter, March 30, 1887, London Metropolitan Archives HI/ST/NC1/87/6/2). Her last gift was a bottle of old brandy, given to patients who could not ordinarily take brandy, but needed a stimulant (letter, May 15, 1887, in McDonald, 2002, p. 221).

Jones was a devout nun who did not fear death. Nightingale remarked on her soon being in the "Immediate Presence" of God. When she sent a "little panada without sauce or ornament," she noted that it was for one who was "not fed by 'bread' alone but by the Holy Spirit." Another message was: "To inquire after her *body*. The rest I know is all right" (letter, April 11, 1887, in McDonald, 2002, p. 218). When her friend made a brief recovery, Nightingale sent her a newsy letter, describing the survival of nurses from a spectacular shipwreck on return home from Egypt (letter, May 5, 1887, in McDonald, 2002, pp. 219–220). The next day, she sent her "great love" with her note and specified: "Ale twice daily, bacon, etc., for breakfast, fish or meat for dinner; at night milk and biscuits" (letter, May 6, 1887, in McDonald, 2002, p. 220).

The wreath Nightingale sent for the funeral called Jones a "friend of God...taken home by Him who has ascended on high and led captivity captive," a biblical quotation from Ephesians 4:8 (Nightingale message, in McDonald, 2002, p. 224).

For Royal Engineer Sir Douglas Galton, a close colleague married to her cousin, eight notes and envelopes from his terminal illness in 1899 survive. One to her cousin says, "Sir Douglas has excellent nurses. It requires them to persuade a patient to 'take nourishment' every hour. Is there anything we could send him? It would be a privilege" (letter, February 22, 1899, private collection). A cook was duly sent, and Nightingale assured her cousin: "I shall eat all the better if the cook can save *you*" (letter, March 4, 1899, private collection). In his last days—he died on March 10th—he would have known of her concern.

Nightingale's Views on Deathbed Conversions

As a person of Christian faith, Nightingale believed that conversion was a good thing: It was better to meet one's Maker prepared than not, but better still to have converted when still in active life and able to do good. Nightingale's conception of the afterlife was of ongoing activity. She did not believe either in passive absorption or ongoing torment. The sacrifice of Jesus, as Savior, sufficed for all. Unlike the vast majority of Christian believers of her time, Protestant, Roman Catholic, and Orthodox, she simply did not believe in hell fire, purgatory, or other forms of torture. Hence, she did not share the anxiety to convert the dying to rescue them from eternal, or at the least long-lasting, flames. Her conception of a "perfect" God excluded such concepts as eternal punishment, judgment, and heaven and hell (unpublished essay in McDonald, 2002, pp. 66-67).

Nurses who were Christian believers often asked Nightingale if it were permissible to talk to the dying about the state of their souls. She allowed that one could speak "a word in due season," a quotation from Proverbs, as noted in Chapter 4. However, this must always be done with discretion, for the nurse's first task was to *heal* the sick. British hospitals then, as now, had chaplains appointed to them who could be called at the patient's request. Ethical principles required nurses to respect their patients' religious views, or lack thereof.

APPLYING NIGHTINGALE'S EXAMPLE AND ADVICE TODAY

From Nightingale's own practice of palliative care a number of specifics are clear, some of which would not be expected of a nurse at a hospital or care facility today:

- Administer drugs as prescribed by the physician.
- Administer food and drinks directed by the physician, as the patient can manage.

- Procure spiritual assistance from an appropriate chaplain (priest, minister, rabbi, imam) as requested by the patient.
- Provide spiritual comfort and counsel yourself if the patient requests it, such as by prayer or scripture reading.
- Alert family or friends of the patient's coming end.
- If needed, and a more appropriate person is not available, ascertain the patient's last wishes and pass these on to family or friends.
- Watch with the patient till the very end, all night if necessary. Close the deceased person's eyes.
- Write family or friends with any last wishes and give details of the patient's last days or hours.

QUESTIONS FOR DISCUSSION

1. What are the challenges for long-term care patients in your area? How adequate are services? What is available to low-income persons?
2. To what extent do you consider deficiencies in long-term care facilities in your area a matter for public provision? At what level of government?
3. Discuss examples of "incurable" diseases becoming curable, or at least significantly treatable. What were the factors influencing this change for HIV/AIDS?
4. What provisions for palliative care are available in your area? Attached to a hospital or how organized?
5. Are nursing students given explicit instruction on palliative care? How should it differ from other instruction in care?

REFERENCES

Gill, C. G., & Gill, G. (2005, June 16). Nightingale in Scutari: Her legacy re-examined. *Clinical Infectious Diseases, 40*(12), 1799–1805. doi:10.1086/430380

McDonald, L. (Ed.). (2001). *Florence Nightingale: An introduction to her life and family.* Waterloo, Canada: Wilfrid Laurier University Press. ISBN: 0-88920-387-3.

McDonald, L. (Ed.). (2002). *Florence Nightingale's theology: Essays, letters, and journal notes.* Waterloo, Canada: Wilfrid Laurier University Press. ISBN: 0-88920-371-7.

McDonald, L. (Ed.). (2003). *Florence Nightingale on society and politics, philosophy, science, education, and literature.* Waterloo, Canada: Wilfrid Laurier University Press. ISBN: 0-88920-429-2.

McDonald, L. (Ed.). (2004a). *Florence Nightingale on public health care.* Waterloo, Canada: Wilfrid Laurier University Press. ISBN: 0-88920-446-2.

McDonald, L. (Ed.). (2004b). *Florence Nightingale's European travels.* Waterloo, Canada: Wilfrid Laurier University Press. ISBN: 0-88920-451-9.

McDonald, L. (Ed.). (2005). *Florence Nightingale on women, medicine, midwifery and prostitution.* Waterloo, Canada: Wilfrid Laurier University Press. ISBN: 0-88920-466-7

McDonald, L. (Ed.). (2009a) *Florence Nightingale: Extending nursing.* Waterloo, Canada: Wilfrid Laurier University Press. ISBN: 978-1-55458-170-2.

McDonald, L. (Ed.). (2009b). *Florence Nightingale: The Nightingale School.* Waterloo, Canada: Wilfrid Laurier University Press. ISBN: 978-1-55458-169-6.

McDonald, L. (Ed.). (2010). *Florence Nightingale and the Crimean War.* Waterloo, Canada: Wilfrid Laurier University Press. ISBN: 978-1-55458-245-7.

McDonald, L. (Ed.). (2012). *Florence Nightingale and hospital reform.* Waterloo, Canada: Wilfrid Laurier University Press. ISBN: 978-0-88920-471-3.

Nightingale, F. (1855). Clipping of letter from *The Derby Mercury,* Wellcome Ms 5484 f18.

Nightingale, F. (1863). *Notes on hospitals* (3rd ed.). London, UK: Longmans, Green.

Nightingale, F. (1880, September). Hospitals and patients. Unpublished paper for *Nineteenth Century,* 1–4.

Nightingale, F. (1890). Hospitals. In *Chambers's encyclopaedia: A dictionary of universal knowledge* (New ed., Vol. 5, pp. 805–807), Edinburgh, Scotland: W. & R. Chambers.

Nightingale, F. (1970/1854). *Florence Nightingale at Harley Street: Her reports to the governors of her nursing home, 1853-54.* Introduction H. Verney. London, UK: J.M. Dent & Sons.

Pringle, A. L. (1888, December 2 and 1889, April 9), letters, British Library Add Mss 47735 ff172 and 238.

Robinson, R. (1861). Memorandum, British Library Add Mss 45797 ff82-101.

Soyer, A. (1857). *Soyer's culinary campaign: Being historical reminiscences of the late war.* London, UK: G. Routledge.

The Times. (1855, February 8). The sick and wounded fund, 3A.

The Times. (1860, August 22). The London Dispensary for Disease and Ulceration of the Legs, 7D.

Chapter 8: Administration

If Florence Nightingale were carrying her lamp through the corridors of the NHS today, she would almost certainly be searching for the people in charge"
—Gorsky (2013, January)

This chapter begins with Nightingale's experience of nursing administration, both of her reporting to superiors, and her management of nurses at her army hospital and nursing directors under her in other hospitals. It talks about her views on training for administration and her experience of mentoring nursing administrators, both assisting them with decision making and defending them when they got into difficulties with their administrators.

The chapter highlights some spectacular deficiencies found in the administration of Britain's major army hospital, one of which led to a lengthy, formal inquiry. Finally, a recent major scandal, at a National Health Service hospital, is discussed, which shows how far below its standards for nursing administration were from those advocated and practiced by Nightingale.

NIGHTINGALE'S EXPERIENCE OF ADMINISTRATION

Nightingale's only concerted experience of administration was brief, confined to the Crimean War, 1854 to 1856. (In her earlier small hospital, she did the nursing and aftercare arrangements herself, as well as managing the housekeeping and supplies. She got experience in reporting to her superiors, the Ladies' Management Committee, for which she produced detailed, quarterly reports.) During the Crimean War, she supervised both the nurses in her own Barrack Hospital and nursing directors of up to seven other hospitals, the latter by letter and occasional visits. Postwar, she submitted detailed reports to the Army Medical Department on the nurses under her.

When the Nightingale School opened at St. Thomas' Hospital in 1860, the nursing director, Sarah E. Wardroper (1813–1892), was thoroughly experienced in directing ward nursing—indeed that experience and her known high standards were the main reason Nightingale chose St. Thomas' for her school. However, Mrs. Wardroper lacked experience in nurse training and had little interest in it. She was appointed "superintendent" of the training school, with an additional salary (with the two salaries, she was very well paid). Nightingale largely left her alone in the first years. When a major problem arose in the school in 1871, a clear failure in oversight, only then did she begin her active involvement.

That first problem was no less than an embarrassing mini-scandal. The school advertised that classes were given, but the instructor, the resident medical officer, R. G. Whitfield, stopped giving them, and Nightingale was never informed. She only learned of this by a circuitous route. That he had a drinking problem and had become overly familiar with the nurses and students, short of sexual assault, was well-known in the hospital, but not to her. She sent Henry Bonham Carter, secretary of the Nightingale Fund, which financed the school, to obtain Whitfield's resignation. Whitfield's successor as the instructor, Dr. John Croft, who stayed on the job for 20 years, was exemplary and kept in touch with Nightingale to boot.

In 1872, Nightingale set up new measures to oversee nurse instruction, with the appointment of a tutor, called "home sister" as she ran the Nightingale Home, the nurses' residence. She would have preferred a loftier title, "under matron" (the nursing director was then called "matron") or "mistress of probationers," but Mrs. Wardroper refused. Moreover, she did not allow the tutor into the wards. She was confined to attending and taking notes at the classes. This was a key function, given that many students needed her help to prepare for their tests, all conducted by doctors, of course.

The tutor met with Nightingale periodically and kept her informed with regular letters. The third appointee, Mary S. Crossland (1837–1914), a former governess, served the cause well from 1875 until her retirement in 1896. She kept in touch with former students, visited some at their new hospitals, and welcomed many back to the "Home" periodically afterward. Before the existence of nurses' conferences and journals, this was a major means of networking. She also, at times, sent her class notes to Nightingale, to keep her up-to-date on the material covered.

As well as appointing a tutor, Nightingale instituted the practice of meeting with (not all) the students at the end of their first year. She took notes of these meetings, still available, which were used later for writing letters of reference for them. Nightingale invited nurses about to go on to higher positions to keep in touch with her, by letter and occasional visits.

TRAINING FOR ADMINISTRATION

Nightingale was a firm believer in the need for training for administration, albeit via on-the-job experience rather than in any formal program, then not available. A nurse to be appointed to an administrative position would have served for some time first as head of a ward, "ward sister," and thus had been in charge of some 30 patients, with clear responsibility for the supervision of the assistant (untrained) nurses and nursing students in her ward. Desirably, the person to be appointed would also have had some experience in a similar administrative post, perhaps at a smaller hospital, or as an interim when the nursing director was on holiday (holidays were normally a month).

When nurses hailed from countries outside the United Kingdom, Nightingale often arranged for them to spend a month or so at St. Thomas', then go to other British hospitals for further experience. For this, she favored the Liverpool Workhouse Infirmary, the best place, and for some time, the only place to get workhouse experience, and the Edinburgh Royal Infirmary, a large and well-run hospital with an excellent medical school.

Nightingale learned the need for training for administration the hard way. The confidentiality breech posed by Lucy Osburn in Sydney, Australia, was recounted in Chapter 4 for its ethical dimensions. Nightingale and Bonham Carter thought that Osburn was guilty of other poor decisions as well. Most flagrantly, she dismissed all the Nightingale nurses who had been sent with her, at great expense and trouble, and replaced them with Australians, but to no untoward result. She apparently set the nurses against each other, so that there was much rancor and a high turnover rate (Godden, 2006; MacDonnell, 1970).

Osburn, nonetheless, succeeded in making a good start for nursing in Australia. The dismissed nurses found posts elsewhere in the Australian colonies, thus taking Nightingale principles and standards further afield. The profession grew, and Osburn deserves much of the credit for that. She had opposition from a major doctor at her hospital, and her work was a subject (with others) of a public inquiry into the "charities" of Sydney. Nightingale defended her, but she and Bonham Carter remained wary of appointing a nurse at such a senior level without any previous experience of management. They, admittedly, were in a difficult position—pressed by Australians to send nurses from the school, still in its early years—with no one better prepared to send.

The patient abuse at Buxton Hospital, described in Chapter 4, is another example of failure in administration. Adequate oversight certainly would have ensured, if not prevented, the shoddy nursing and/or overt abuse from occurring was caught early on.

MENTORING MAJOR NURSE ADMINISTRATORS

Eva Luckes, director of nursing at the London Hospital, to Nightingale: "It is such a relief to be able to say to you all that comes into one's mind or heart at the moment, and to be so sympathetically understood as to feel the burden lifted and the sense of weight which accumulated worries and anxieties being melted almost peacefully away! I feel now as though I could be 'strong' again, as though I could see clearly the way to go."
—(letter, December 7, 1899, British Library Add Mss[1] 47746 f377)

In Nightingale's day, there were no organizations for mutual support or networking among the nursing directors, so that the support and advice she gave them was important. Those she mentored were mainly women who had gone through her school, but there were others who came to her for support and advice. A major example is Eva Luckes, director of nursing at the largest hospital in London, the (Royal) London Hospital, who was the subject of a House of Lords inquiry on her management.

Nightingale held numerous meetings with Luckes to give her support. Nightingale also enlisted the assistance of her cousin, Sir Lothian Nicholson, a member of the hospital board. He spoke up for Luckes at a meeting, giving both his and Nightingale's view, that the accusations against Luckes "were absolutely without foundation. No one stood higher in nursing circles than the matron of their hospital." The meeting adopted a motion supporting her (*The Times*, 1890).

Nurses leaving for administrative posts often had a last meeting with Nightingale, when she offered, or they asked for, further contact when needed. Some sent her occasional letters with reports of their work. For some, these years of periodic visits and correspondence went on to genuine and long-lasting friendships. Nightingale often assisted the nurse in getting the post in the first place. In some cases, she invited the candidate to stay at her house for interviews. She wrote strong, precise letters of reference.

Typically, Nightingale did her best to find institutional support for a nursing director new on the job. When difficulties arose, she went to enormous trouble for them, writing to the most influential doctors and/or governors at the institution to enlist their assistance. She sent gifts to the person in difficulty—books, roses, coffee, jelly, or partridge.

One unhappy case occurred when Rachel Williams (1840–1908) was appointed nursing director at St. Mary's, Paddington. Nightingale had written a highly flattering letter of reference for her and had her stay at

---

[1] Further references to Add Mss (Additional Manuscripts) are also to the British Library.

her home while applying. She supported her through months of complaints about what she considered to be a misunderstanding about salary. The hospital eventually decided to dismiss her. Nightingale then managed a final maneuver to allow Williams to resign instead. The hospital administration agreed. This conveniently happened just at the time that nurses were needed for military service in Egypt. Rachel Williams was able to leave the hospital with her head held high, wearing the new, smart uniform of an army nurse, which resembled an officer's dress uniform (McDonald, 2009a, pp. 907–908). The nurse's uniform during the Crimean War was drab gray, practical, not at all like an officer's.

Luise Fuhrmann, a German nursing director, whom Nightingale had mentored (she had received English experience at St. Thomas' Hospital), told her of a problem brought on by a senior nurse in England, Florence Lees Craven, speaking ill of her to the Crown Princess of Prussia, turning the princess against her, she thought:

> I felt very sad at heart and I do not know how I should have got on if you had not said those kind and encouraging words when we parted and had not written those dear sweet lines into the two books which make them my most precious property. I am so glad to be able to tell you through my coming and since people know me personally the strong prejudice against me has faded away like a summer cloud and everybody is as good and kind to me as I can wish. (Fuhrmann letter, December 24, 1882, Add Mss 45807 f24)

Nightingale had given Fuhrmann two books on her return to Germany in 1881, a *Dictionary of Medical Terms* and a book on bandaging (Fuhrmann letter, August 24, 1881, Add Mss 45806 f211). Showing her colleagues the positive words Nightingale had written to her undid the damage.

In 1886, the director of nursing at Northern Hospital, London, Izalina Huguenin, informed Nightingale that she had resigned for the second time. The problem was interference by the "medical men" in the selection of nurses and discussing them. Evidently, the nurses were not young or good-looking enough, but Huguenin thought that they were "thoroughly good women who would make good nurses if encouraged." She also raised a new problem, that a (medical) resident smoked in the wards and made it clear he would continue to when she spoke to him about it (Huguenin letter, November 24, 1886, Add Mss 45807 f225). There was nothing for Nightingale to do at this point. It seems they corresponded over possible new posts; a letter Nightingale wrote her a few months later suggested another to try and regretted that she had not yet been successful (letter, May 7, 1887, Add Mss 45807 f260).

Nightingale found these mentoring sessions exhausting, but reserved time for them and gave of her best. Her visitors went away feeling a lot better. Luckes, for example, found it comforting that, "as you approve, it *must* be all right." She appreciated Nightingale's "patient, bright, listening," commenting that there are "as many differences in the ways of listening as in the ways of talking." She left with a gift of "lovely flowers" (Lucke's letter, December 7, 1899, British Library Add Mss 47746 f377).

The Greater Difficulties of Workhouse Nursing

Agnes Jones, the first trained workhouse nursing director, frequently wrote to Nightingale about the difficulties she experienced in introducing professional nursing in the Liverpool Workhouse Infirmary. Words like "anxiety" and "ordeal" appear all too frequently in her descriptions of relations with the workhouse "governor," her superior. However, she was able to report progress, of sorts, after a few months:

> I have seen little of the governor since our "row," but he has been very civil. I am much amused by the way in which I finally get all I ask for—I suggest arrangements, etc.—the governor seems to laugh at them or takes no notice and, long after, I hear this or that is to be. I have been for months urging more "comfort" in the serving of food. On Saturday I received intimation [that] on Sunday so and so begins. (Jones letter, August 31, 1865, Add Mss 47752 f172)

In a letter the following year, Jones reported on the positive impact of the visit to the workhouse infirmary of Nightingale's brother-in-law, Sir Harry Verney, a Member of Parliament and chair of the Nightingale Fund Council. The visit was arranged by William Rathbone, the benefactor and a notable citizen of Liverpool (Jones letter, October 8 [1866], Add Mss 47752 f293).

However, there were still serious shortages the following year, after a difficult winter, as a letter reported to Nightingale. She expected the numbers would soon go down, so that when they took on the sizable female wards (they had started with the men's), the work would not be too much. However, it was a strain when she had scarcely been able to arrange for beds and bedding for their existing patients, at 9 p.m. 20 to 30 newcomers had to be taken in, with no sheets, straw, shirts, or blankets. She wrote:

> 20 to 30 boys packed into 3 or 4 beds, they and even men without shirts for many hours. I have often had 25 shirts to change, 665 patients and even having then washed twice a day you may imagine how long we were in going round. Everything equally

short: stockings, shoes, trousers, chambers, spit cups, bedrests, forms. What the difficulty is in keeping people clean you may imagine, no clean stockings since Xmas, if we send them to the wash they do not come back till it is our turn to be changed—all the head work of all this devolves on me. (Jones letter, April 20, 1867, Add Mss 47752 f301)

Nurses naturally came to Jones with "where can I get this or that?" and she had to decide which ward could best spare what was needed (Jones letter, April 20 [1867], Add Mss 47752 f301).

Another early workhouse nursing director, Annie Hill, at the Highgate Infirmary, also wrote to Nightingale about one of the great challenges of workhouse nursing. They were sometimes "crowded with patients, sick and dying coming in at all hours, many from their own homes." They might have to use the day rooms for them, one letter stated. This letter also reported a troubling case of a workhouse patient assaulting a nurse. The man was "really ill and suffering," as Hill described him. He struck the nurse with his crutch but did not cause serious injury: her scalp was "cut and bruised, but not deeply." The patient was charged, to set an example (Hill letter, January 4, 1875, Add Mss 47749 f380).

Hill could never get away for a holiday that Nightingale had organized for her because their male wards were "filled with beds," with "cases most serious." She had to stay back to watch that the nurses were not overworked (Hill letter, July 20, 1875, Add Mss 47749 f381). There was a problem even when they had "only" 395 patients in the infirmary, instead of 530. She wanted to ask for more probationers but had to wait for the numbers to rise. She would "fail" in making the committee understand that it was "the nature of the cases, and not the number of patients which makes a ward busy" (Hill letter, August 7, 1874, Add Mss 47749 f378).

FAILURES IN ADMINISTRATION IN MILITARY NURSING

Although Nightingale saw it as her duty to defend nursing directors under attack by their superiors, in one case, she had to bow out and accept the dismissal. Jane Shaw Stewart (1821–1905) had served well as the director of nursing at the Castle Hospital, Balaclava, during the Crimean War, and then spent some years getting hospital experience in London, Vienna, and Paris (Nightingale wrote letters to get her entrance). She was appointed the first nursing director at Woolwich Hospital in 1861, then at the Royal Victoria Hospital, Netley, when it opened in 1863, where she was made the superintendent general of army nursing. This made her the first woman to appear on the British Army List.

Shaw Stewart's tenure at Netley, however, was stormy from the beginning, not least because it was the hospital's first use of female nurses. Nightingale had to visit quite often to quiet matters down. She had recommended both Shaw Stewart and the hospital governor, General Wilbraham, for their posts. He was thought to have the right "tact and temper" for the "experiment" of female nursing; however, he soon began to complain, not only to Nightingale but to numerous others, about the matron. Nightingale thought throughout that Shaw Stewart had as much cause for complaint on his conduct as he about hers (letter, September 4, 1863, in McDonald, 2011, p. 162). Moreover, if Shaw Stewart resigned or was dismissed, there was no one qualified to replace her.

Nightingale's Crimean War experience of medical interference with decisions about nurses was strongly negative. She had had to keep a nurse on who had been dismissed by one of her superintendents, "upon quite sufficient cause," by command of a superior officer. The nurse had caused "grievous injury" and had to be dismissed later (letter, ca. August 9, 1866, in McDonald, 2011, p. 174–175).

One of the difficulties was the difference in social status between the commandant, a mere general, and his nursing director, a member of the Scottish nobility, sister of the sixth baronet Sir Michael Shaw Stewart, a Conservative Member of Parliament and an eminent member of his county. When matters came to a head in 1868, Nightingale remarked that "Colonel W.'s mind had constantly been rankling on certain refusals of Mrs. S.S. to come to tea." Furthermore, she had to acknowledge that her high-minded nursing head never "breathed a word against Colonel W." (letter, May 1, 1868, in McDonald, 2011, p. 178). One can imagine what Nightingale must have thought about Shaw Stewart's scruples about drinking tea with the lowly general and his wife, but such refusal could hardly be grounds for dismissal.

Shaw Stewart was not the only eccentric member of her family. Her mother, Lady Shaw Stewart, Nightingale remarked years later, "still wore mourning on the day of Charles I's execution!" (letter, June 4, 1892, in McDonald, 2002, p. 434). She freely acknowledged Shaw Stewart's peculiarities to her inner circle, insisting that, nonetheless, "with all her 'insanity,' she knows her work better than anyone" (letter, February 4, 1864, Add Mss 45762 f27).

Wilbraham "sobered down" in 1864, Nightingale reported to Douglas Galton. She thought that Shaw Stewart would do "capitally if they will but let her alone" (letter, April 16, 1864, Add Mss 45762 f108).

He did not, but subsequently complained that Shaw Stewart was "rough to the sick men." Nightingale, however, observed that the principal medical officer, "the only officer with a right" to make such a complaint, never did. Shaw Stewart could complain of their being rude to her (letter, October

3, 1864, Add Mss 45762 f226). One might wish that she had "the manners of an archangel," Nightingale quipped to Galton, but as to the grounds of the complaints against her, Wilbraham's and the war secretary's, "she could not have acted otherwise than she did" (letter, November 10, 1864, in McDonald, 2011, p. 166).

Nightingale defended Shaw Stewart the following year too on her right to dismiss a nurse (her prerogative) and on the employment of an "underage" nurse, which nursing directors did on occasion, Nightingale well knew, for a "fit object" (letter, January 15, 1865, in McDonald, 2011, p. 170).

The accusations of 1866 were more serious, assault on a nurse, no less, but the situation was complicated. Nightingale thought that the authorities should "reprimand her and give her a further trial as superintendent general" (letter to Galton, August 9, 1866, Add Mss 45763 f215). Nightingale's letter to Mary Jones, then the experienced head of nursing at King's College Hospital, is revealing:

> *Burn.* I have only just averted a public trial. Some nurses informed against her for assault. And, she writes word direct to the secretary of state, that she *has* "beaten nurses," "to make "them subordinate," tho' not *those* nurses!!!! (letter, September 23, 1866, in McDonald, 2011, p. 419)

Shaw Stewart was reprimanded and undertook not to repeat such conduct.

A Formal Inquiry by the Army Medical Department

Nightingale continued to defend Shaw Stewart the following year, judging Wilbraham's accusations against her to be unfounded. However, the final showdown occurred when he laid a formal charge against her in 1868, which led to a 5-day inquiry at Netley. Three of the board members were old Nightingale allies from Crimean days, one of them being Dr. John Sutherland, her long-term and highly supportive collaborator, but another, Professor Thomas Longmore, professor of military surgery, testified against Shaw Stewart. The third, Dr. Maclean, was another Crimean War doctor, but his evidence on Shaw Stewart was largely positive. Rather, he saw "system" problems, but considered the nursing overall a "boon to the sick."

The board issued a 16-page printed report, including the evidence (Add Mss 45774 ff101-16). This evidence ranged from such trivial matters as a corporal and a sergeant stating that Shaw Stewart gave an egg to a patient without medical authority to the very serious. The latter included "unfitness for office from want of control over temper," with examples from both nurses and patients. Nurses complained that she stamped her feet, clapped her hands at them, slammed the door in their faces, and "jumped and raved" at them.

Longmore's evidence included high turnover of nurses, which Nightingale considered "unfounded," as reports showed that fewer nurses left than at the civil hospitals.

Altogether, the evidence shows that some of the complaints were serious. Nightingale did not try to rescue Shaw Stewart, who did not ask a single question herself at the inquiry. When the decision went against her, she recommended a nurse who would be "most suitable" to take over as (temporary) superintendent, but who would not be fit, she said, for the general duties of superintendent general (Add Mss 45774 f114, Appendix D). In 1869, Nightingale feared that Shaw Stewart would commit suicide, and wondered if she should apprise her brother (note, ca. February 5 1869, Add Mss 45753 f184). Nothing came of this.

Shaw Stewart, it seems, never worked again, although she gave her occupation in the subsequent censuses as a "hospital nurse." She continued to correspond with Nightingale, from lodgings in Sussex, until 1888. She also corresponded with the acting director of nursing at the Herbert Hospital, Woolwich, and sent information on it to Nightingale. She wanted to publish an account of her experiences, which Nightingale discouraged. She dropped the subject on Nightingale's strong "disapprobation," although intimated that she might publish while noting Nightingale's "nonparticipation" (Shaw Stewart letter, July 30, 1870, Add Mss 45774 f202). She never did. Unfortunately, she burned Nightingale's letters to her; although, Nightingale kept her lengthy and convoluted letters and reports.

Further Administrative "Failures" in Army Nursing

Shaw Stewart was replaced as "superintendent general" by Jane C. Deeble (1828–1913), widow of an army medical officer, as Mrs. Wardroper had been. The process of selection was difficult. Henry Bonham Carter told Nightingale that she was "seemingly the best candidate" (Bonham Carter letter, November 4, 1868, Add Mss 47716 f19). Nightingale liked her and was always sympathetic to "poor Mrs. Deeble," yet considered her less able and devoted than Shaw Stewart. She presumably also met Mrs. Deeble's "celestial" child, whose existence made for another dilemma, as the superintendent general had to be ready to leave at any time to go to war or a foreign posting.

General Wilbraham continued to act badly. Nightingale had to agitate for Deeble's salary, as for many others. She thought that the War Office failed to recognize the "rise in the market price of nursing" since its regulations were first drawn up (letter, November 7, 1868, in McDonald, 2011,

p. 187–188). Furthermore, army nurses engaged "for life" and work in a military hospital lacked the advantages of a civil hospital. She felt that there should be compensation for this.

What Deeble's failings were is not entirely clear in the surviving correspondence. In 1874, she was mentioned with Barclay and Osburn as examples of the "dreadful failure" resulting from an appointment after only the minimal year's training. One year's training at St. Thomas' was "*no trial*," Nightingale told her colleagues (letters, February 12 and October 20, 1874, in McDonald, 2009a, p. 282 and McDonald, 2009b, p. 191). Certainly, Mrs. Deeble had much against her with the commandant, General Wilbraham, and the existing nurses at Netley. Nightingale condemned his "inclination to be a matron," which post, he showed by experience (in the gap after Shaw Stewart left) he did not fill "successfully," yet he was "wild" to direct the nursing (letter, June 30, 1869, in McDonald, 2011, p. 195).

Deeble remained as the superintendent general from 1869 until her resignation in 1890. She led the nursing during the Zulu War, in 1883 winning, along with Nightingale, one of the first Royal Red Crosses, an award established by Queen Victoria to honor war nurses.

The early decades of work to establish professional nursing included failures, even "dreadful experiments" in Nightingale's terms, setbacks certainly, before the lessons were fully learned. However, even those instances of mistaken appointments had their good features. Osburn did much to establish professional nursing in Australia, and Deeble oversaw much progress in army nursing. The exception is Barclay, who was felled by alcohol and opiate abuse. Keeping medical and military superiors from assuming day-to-day control over the nursing was a core problem and an ongoing challenge for Nightingale.

THE MID-STAFFORDSHIRE HOSPITAL SCANDAL

It is appropriate to echo a statement made by Florence Nightingale 150 years ago, It may seem a strange principle to enunciate as the very first requirement in a hospital that it should do the sick no harm. Unfortunately, this requirement has not been met at Stafford Hospital.

—Franics (2010)

Still, today, when things go wrong in hospital care, the principles of Florence Nightingale are often called up. This occurred during the ground-breaking Griffiths inquiry into the National Health Service (NHS), which was instituted by the U.K. government during the first Thatcher administration

(Griffiths, 1983). The inquiry found "institutional stagnation" to be a major feature of the system, and called for a "more thrusting and committed style" of management. The best-known phrase from the report was its reference to "searching for the people in charge,"featured in the epigraph at the beginning of this chapter. The inquiry, in fact, led to massive changes in NHS administration.

The "searching for the people in charge" phrase was repeated in 2013, on the release of findings described as "the biggest scandal in NHS history" at the Mid-Staffordshire NHS Hospital (Francis, 2013, executive summary, p. 54). Commenting in the House of Lords, a peer cited Griffiths's earlier remark about Nightingale "searching for the people in charge," adding that "she would have been more concerned today about finding someone in charge of the care of the patients in the corridors of the Mid-Staffs hospital. She would have been looking for anyone able to explain what had been happening to the patients for so long and would have found no one" (Turnburg, 2013).

What would be called "the biggest scandal in NHS history" took place at the Mid-Staffordshire hospital between 2005 and 2009, and involved gross failures in patient care, including "unnecessary" deaths. Two inquiries were held. The first, by the Healthcare Commission in 2009, produced an estimate of 400 to 1,200 unnecessary deaths; the second, a lengthier, public inquiry, chaired by Robert Francis, produced a three-volume report in 2013 detailing the failure in administration in the hospital and oversight from regulatory bodies outside it.

Briefly, between 2005 and 2009, "appalling conditions" were the norm at what was the main hospital for Stafford and district, prompted by cutbacks in service. These were instituted by the hospital to obtain "foundation trust" status, which would give it greater autonomy in its operations. It succeeded, but, in the course of cutbacks, it ignored complaints by the families of patients. Complaints that families took to their members of parliament also failed. A staff nurse is credited for whistle blowing in 2007, for reporting on failures in the hospital's Accidents and Emergency Department. However, although these were judged to be "serious and substantial," her complaint was "not resolved by trust management," nor did the trust report it "to any external agency." It was known to the Royal College of Nursing (RCN), "because of its involvement with the personnel involved" (Francis, 2013, executive summary, p. 42). It took a noticeably higher mortality rate, compared with similar hospitals, to spur an investigation. The nurse whistleblower continued to agitate, was a major witness at the public inquiry, and was honored with an Order of the British Empire (an award given for the performance of a worthy services in the United Kingdom) in 2014.

The Francis report brought out numerous conditions oddly reminiscent of those encountered by Nightingale and her nurses more than a century ago. Specifics include gross defects in fundamental care:

- Patients left in excrement in soiled bedclothes, for lengthy periods
- Assistance not provided to those needing help to eat
- Water left out of reach so that desperate patients drank from a flower vase
- Patients not helped to the toilet, in spite of persistent requests
- Privacy and dignity denied, even in death
- Patients and friends treated with "callous indifference."
- Lack of basic care across many wards and departments. (Francis, 2013, 1:19 and executive summary, 1:13)

The defects in the administration, or "how the failures occurred and why they were not brought to light sooner," included:

- Culture at the trust "not conducive to providing good care or a supportive working environment for staff"
- Atmosphere of "fear of adverse repercussions," low morale
- High priority placed on the achievement of targets
- Acceptance of poor standards
- Management thinking dominated by financial pressures, achieving foundation trust status, to the detriment of quality of care
- Failure to remedy long-known deficiencies in staff and governance
- Absence of clinical governance
- Preference for statistics and reports over patient experience data
- Failure of external organizations. (Francis, 2013, executive summary, 1:13)

Francis too found that all the normal regulatory and oversight bodies had failed. General practitioners did not notice the problems until the inquiry was called, although they should have been obvious. The RCN was found to be "ineffective both as a professional representative organization and as a trade union. Little was done to uphold professional standards among nursing staff or to address concerns and problems being faced by its members." This was partly due, Francis said, to the dual status of the RCN as both a professional organization and a trade union, which still applies.

The finding of "higher than average" mortality rates in Accidents and Emergency, by the Healthcare Commission, raises another issue—lack of consensus on how to count deaths. Actual numbers of deaths are not published for any NHS hospital, but only "standard mortality ratios," based on "observed minus expected" deaths.

The hospital trust acknowledged "unacceptable" neglect and mal-treatment (Francis, 2013, executive summary, p. 65). It was charged crimi-nally in the case of four deaths, including one of a diabetic patient not given prescribed insulin. A 3-year police investigation, however, led to a decision not to prosecute. No manager, doctor, or nurse ever had to answer to a crim-inal charge. In the case of the diabetic patient who died, the trust pleaded guilty to a violation of health and safety laws.

Two nurses were disciplined for misconduct. The chief nurse, who made the nursing cuts and long denied the evidence, retired early and agreed to be taken off the Nurses' Register. The trust itself was dissolved in 2014.

The Francis report revealed the pressures on the trust from government policy to achieve "foundation" status, which required reductions in spend-ing. Savings were made by cutting staff, although the hospital had already been shown to have "serious problems in delivering a service of adequate quality and complying with minimum standards. No thought seems to have been given as to the potential impact on patient safety and quality" (Francis, 2013, executive summary, p. 42). The trust had been criticized in the first report "for not undertaking sufficient impact or risk assessments before making significant changes."

The section of the report on "why things were not discovered sooner" repeated the material on trust failings, adding points on "regulatory gaps." A large number of organizations had some involvement in hospital over-sight, but no one acted. Failure to put the patient first applied to them all. Francis pointed to the NHS Constitution, which "should be the first refer-ence point for NHS patients and staff," but clearly was not (Francis, 2013, executive summary, p. 65).

APPLYING NIGHTINGALE'S PRINCIPLES ON ADMINISTRATION TODAY

Anyone familiar with Nightingale's principles on management would won-der how such basic requirements of care could be neglected. The NHS is a far larger and more complicated organization than any she had to deal with, so that her work is hardly a source to go to in today's world. However, fol-lowing her advice and practices would have prevented most of the abuse from occurring and/or would have enabled its prompt discovery. Key requirements in Nightingale nursing are as follows:

- Changes in management or treatment should be tried first on small num-bers and evaluated before being applied more widely. This would have shown early that the staff cuts had serious, harmful, consequences.

- The director of nursing should visit all the wards daily, sometimes at unexpected times, which would have revealed that patients were lying in excrement and lacked drinking water.
- Handover procedures between shifts should serve to identify the ongoing concerns, which, if done, would have revealed that some patients were unattended because of lack of staff.
- Nurses should be the patient's defender and advocate; one nurse was brave enough to report defects, but this was insufficient; the chief nurse identified with management and its objectives.

Nightingale also believed that public opinion could help to prevent abuse. In the case of Mid-Staffordshire, public opinion did, eventually, but it was ignored for a long time. Restaurant owner Julie Bailey, who saw her mother's negligent care and even moved into the hospital to provide care herself, founded "Cure the NHS" and led the public campaign. Bailey was subsequently honored by being named "Commander of the British Empire." A retired risk assessor who had conducted a hygiene inspection became a whistleblower, again an "outside agitator." His findings were initially sat on.

The Mid-Staffordshire tragedy points to the consequences of not having functioning safeguards for administrative goals. The reference to Nightingale's advice on administration is simply to make the point that nurses and hospital administrations have abandoned an out-of-date source for none at all. This is not to argue to bring back Nightingale's advice, as she always advocated best practice, which would now be different. However, change must be monitored carefully for unintended consequences, which was not done. Is it too much to ask, when safeguards are dropped as unneeded, to monitor the results carefully?

QUESTIONS FOR DISCUSSION

1. What formal training at the university or college level is provided for administrative positions in nursing in your area? At what level (undergraduate, junior year, senior year, graduate)?
2. What encouragement are nurses given to qualify for and move into administrative positions? Would mentoring be helpful to you or your colleagues? Are mentoring relationships facilitated?
3. To what extent is public opinion an effective safeguard against abuse in hospitals? What public accountability measures are in place in your area? What role does reporting play, in newspapers, radio, and television, to publicize hospital abuses or inadequate care?

REFERENCES

Francis, R. (2010). *The Francis Report: Briefing 1—Key recommendations and early response.* www.lexology.com/library/detail.aspx?g=fd341164-118c-4409-bb56

Francis, R. (2013). *First report of the Mid-Staffordshire NHS Foundation Trust public inquiry.* London, UK: Her Majesty's Stationery Office.

Godden, J. (2006). *Lucy Osburn: A lady displaced: Florence Nightingale's envoy to Australia.* Sydney, Australia: Sydney University Press. ISBN: 9781920898397

Gorsky, M. (2013, January). "Searching for the people in charge": Appraising the 1983 Griffiths NHS Management Inquiry. *Medical History, 57*(1), 87.

Griffiths, R. (1983). *NHS management inquiry.* London, UK: Department of Health and Social Security.

MacDonnell, F. (1970). *Miss Nightingale's young ladies: The story of Lucy Osburn and Sydney Hospital.* Sydney, Australia: Angus & Robertson.

McDonald, L. (Ed.). (2002). *Florence Nightingale's theology: Essays, letters and journal notes.* Waterloo, Canada: Wilfrid Laurier University Press. ISBN: 0-88920-371-7.

McDonald, L. (Ed.). (2009a). *In Florence Nightingale: Extending nursing.* Waterloo, Canada: Wilfrid Laurier University Press. ISBN: 978-1-55458-170-2.

McDonald, L. (Ed.). (2009b). *Florence Nightingale: The Nightingale School.* Waterloo, Canada: Wilfrid Laurier University Press. ISBN: 978-1-55458-169-6.

McDonald, L. (Ed.). (2011). *Florence Nightingale on Wars and the War Office.* Waterloo, Canada: Wilfrid Laurier University Press. ISBN: 978-1-55458-382-9.

The Times. (1890, September 4). The London Hospital. *The Times,* 12.

Turnburg, L. (2013, March 11). Hansard, Parliamentary Debates.

Chapter 9: Research and Policy Development

Get the best information available.

—Nightingale

The passionate statistician.

—Cook (1913)

Good research was crucial for Nightingale's whole mission. Her calling was to save lives, but whether any particular action did so had to be ascertained by research. Nightingale was numerate as well as literate and wanted to save more lives rather than fewer. Statistics would be key in ranking the issues for intervention. As she had an acute fear of the possibilities of unintended consequences, an ongoing verification and monitoring would be essential.

In this chapter, we begin with the manner in which Nightingale conducted research and then moved on to policy application. Her major published reports with good, hard data, are listed. Her "methodology," although she never reports it such, is set out, which an experienced researcher today will see remains a useful example. The chapter then takes up a competing paradigm that treats numerous "ways of knowing" as equal in worth to the data acquired by empirical research. The contention that Nightingale subscribed to alternative "ways of knowing" is contested.

Finally, Nightingale's approach to research and policy formulation is applied to a problem she never had to consider: climate change. Many nursing organizations now acknowledge that it is one of, if not the, most pressing problem contemporary society has to face. The way Nightingale's example can be applied here is an excellent test of her ongoing relevance.

GOOD RESEARCH: THE FOUNDATION FOR POLICY

Effective health policy requires careful, thorough research. Nightingale was early recognized as an expert methodologist. In 1858, she was elected the first woman fellow of the Royal Statistical Society, and, in 1874, was made an honorary member of the American Statistical Association. She was a sound analyst of available government documents, from the census to hospital reports and mortality data. She was an expert in questionnaire design, of institutional data, mainly of hospitals, rather than mass surveys. She routinely debriefed experts returning from India for the latest data and context on their reports.

For Nightingale, the same kind of laws apply in both the natural and social worlds, for God was the creator of both. The laws of both worlds were open to human discovery by induction from research results. The social and natural worlds interact, so that the quality of air, water, soil, and forests help to determine health status. One important difference between the social and physical spheres was that some components of the natural, such as the solar system, cannot be modified by human action, while the social system can be and obviously is modified. For a solar eclipse, humans can predict the time, but not affect it, although for educational attainment and health status, people can both predict and, to some extent, influence them. Nightingale made these comparisons in a journal article (Nightingale, 1873, in McDonald, 2002, p. 29).

Practically, Nightingale learned how to research by analyzing what went wrong in the Crimean War of 1854 through 1856. Soon after her return from it, she undertook a major piece of research, using official War Office statistics, aided by the top medical statistician in Britain, Dr. William Farr. The field of applied statistics was changed by their joint work.

The happy story is that the appalling Crimean War death rates were brought down drastically in the second year of the war, both those of patients in the war hospitals and men in camp. The credit for the reduction of mortality must go chiefly to the Sanitary and Supply Commissions, which were empowered to make actual changes. Thus, Nightingale learned that applying the best knowledge (both commissions were led by highly capable experts) could work. There is no simple explanation, such as that there were no battles in the second year, for such would also apply to the French Army, whose death rates nearly doubled.

Figure 9.1 demonstrates this powerfully by showing the comparative death rates of the two armies for the first and second winters.

Nightingale gained confidence from this experience: highly favorable results from acting on the best science. Few people have seen such massive changes brought about by instituting better measures, in this case in hospital cleanliness, sewers and drains, food, shelter, clothing, workload, and

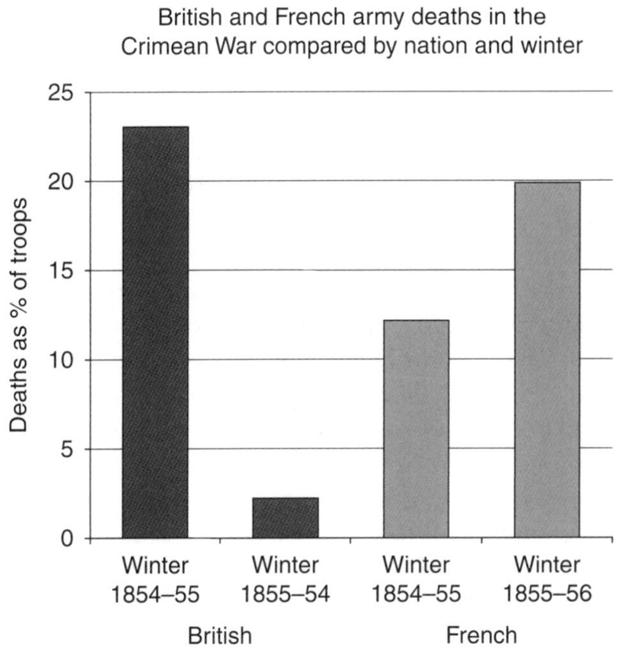

British and French army deaths in the
Crimean War compared by nation and winter

FIGURE 9.1 British and French mortality rates.
Source: Chenu (1870, p. 131).

recreation. That she would be so bold in her vision for health care reforms goes back to that experience.

Nightingale, however, maintained a healthy skepticism about instituting change. All new programs and any substantially modified should be carefully followed up to ascertain their actual results.

She made decisions based on evidence. After the closing of her midwifery ward at King's College Hospital in 1868, Nightingale was asked about its reopening, and advice on other midwifery wards. She never did agree to reopen the King's College ward, for she could never be sure that bringing birthing mothers together for the sake of instructing midwifery nurses would not risk excessive maternal deaths. "Excessive" meant a rate higher than would be expected for birthing in the safest situation, home births. She had also learned that workhouse infirmaries had lower death rates than general hospitals, despite the poor health status generally of their patient inmates and the inferior amenities of the institutions. The term Nightingale used was the "normal death rate." She continued to be reticent in giving advice on other midwifery wards, stressing the hazards.

All too often, Nightingale's attempts to get good data collected and applied came to no satisfactory end. In 1860, she got approval from the International

Statistical Congress for her proposal for a uniform collection of hospital data. The resolution in support was passed unanimously (Nightingale, 1860a). However, in practice, hospitals did not follow up. There is more comparative data on hospital death rates per admissions for the period before, showing rates at around 10% of admissions (Statistics of the general hospitals of London, 1862). For decades, she worked mightily to get pavilion-style hospitals built precisely to reduce cross infection, and deaths. However, there is no hard evidence as to the effect of pavilions versus the usual hospital design, which lacked cross ventilation and required large numbers of people to breathe the same air. There are no data on the effect of the move to high-rise hospitals away from pavilions in the 20th century.

As noted in Chapter 3, Nightingale was unsuccessful in getting questions on housing and illness added to the census form for 1861 (McDonald, 2003, Proposals for the 1861 Census). The very project shows how far ahead of her time she was. Housing would become a major component of census questions and remains so. Illness has seldom made it into any national census but is typically pursued with major special surveys. The data on both subjects are much used in social and health care planning.

In *Notes on Hospitals*, Nightingale argued that nurses' health was a good indicator of the health of the hospital itself (Nightingale, 1863a, Note A, On the Mortality of Hospital Nurses) so that hospitals should keep data on nurse death rates. They did not oblige.

Nightingale's analysis of colonial hospitals and schools (Nightingale, 1863b), noted in Chapter 5, showed unnecessarily high rates of sickness and death, but her recommendations for follow up were not heeded.

Exhibit 9.1 lists major examples of Nightingale's quantitative work.

Nightingale was also adept at formulating questionnaires for administrative purposes, sizing up the dimensions of the situation. In 1859, she drafted a questionnaire to be used by newly established hospitals (letter, September 24, 1859, in McDonald, 2003, pp. 76–79). In 1873, she prepared a questionnaire of workhouse schools for Jane Senior, the first woman to hold a major public service appointment, as Poor Law inspector (letter, January 28, 1873, in McDonald, 2009, pp. 640–642).

THE NIGHTINGALE METHOD

We do not want a great arithmetical law; we want to know what we are doing in things which must be tested by results.
    —(letter, January 3, 1891, in McDonald, 2003, p. 110)

A report is not self-executive, and when the report is ended, the work begins.
    —Nightingale (letter to J. McNeill, July 9, 1863, in Vallée, 2006, p. 220).

EXHIBIT 9.1   NIGHTINGALE'S QUANTITATIVE RESEARCH

1858: Notes on Matters Affecting the Health, Efficiency, and Hospital Administration of the British Army (Nightingale, 1858b, in McDonald, 2010, pp. 575–888)

1858: Answers to Written Questions (Nightingale, 1858a, in McDonald, 2010, pp. 889–972)

1859: *A Contribution to the Sanitary History of the British Army* (Nightingale, 1859, in McDonald, 2012, pp. 333–359)

1860: Note as to the number of women employed as nurses in Great Britain. In *Notes on Nursing: What It Is and What It Is Not* (library standard, Nightingale, 1860b)

1862: Note on the Supposed Protection Afforded Against Venereal Disease (Nightingale, 1862, in McDonald, 2005, pp. 428–435)

1863: Note A: On the Mortality of Hospital Nurses. In *Notes on Hospitals* (Nightingale, 1863a, in McDonald, 2012, pp. 97–99)

1863: Sanitary Statistics of Native Colonial Schools and Hospitals (Nightingale, 1863b, in McDonald, 2004, pp. 163–183)

1869: Memorandum Regarding Sanitary Progress at Home and Foreign Military Stations and in India (Nightingale, 1869, in McDonald, 2011, pp. 482–489)

1871: *Introductory Notes on Lying-in Institutions* (Nightingale, 1871, in McDonald, 2005)

1879: Irrigation and Water Transit (Nightingale, 1879, in Vallée, 2006, pp. 843–860)

Nightingale's principles of research are still valid for use, by nurses and doctors as well as social scientists, in the 21st century. She never set out anything identifiable as a "Nightingale method," but the rules set out in Exhibit 9.2 are evident from her work.

Reports must not only be adequate in their content but must also be carefully considered for application. A report is not "self-executive," as Nightingale pointed out to Harriet Martineau in a letter on implementing the recommendations of the Indian Sanitary Commission. It had taken three days of tough convincing to get the necessary "working commission" established (letter, May 19, 1863, in Vallée, 2006, p. 434). It was essential to designate a person to be in charge of implementation, specify the resources required, including a reporting structure. Care must be given to means to publicize the report, persuade those in a position to act on it. Legislators must be approached, and key legislators given special attention to get them

EXHIBIT 9.2   THE NIGHTINGALE METHOD

1. Get the best information available; use government reports and statistics wherever possible.
2. Read and interview experts as well as use printed data.
3. If the available information is inadequate for the purpose, collect your data, for which you must first:
   Draw up a questionnaire
   Consult experts on it (practitioners who use the material)
   Test the questionnaire with suitable persons or institutions before sending it out
4. When using quantitative data, including full tables, identifying sources. Report a range of sources if more than one set is available, and explain any differences among them.
5. Where possible, present quantitative data in a chart as well as a table, to make contrasts visible.
6. Provide other visual documentation as appropriate, such as plans or elevations of hospitals; catchment areas, maps, charts, and photographs.
7. When using written documents, organize them well. A chronology, with dates, author, and source may be needed.
8. When writing for a general readership, include stories of individuals as examples.
9. After writing up the research results, send out a preliminary draft to experts for review before publication.
10. Any new treatment, program, hospital design, educational measure, or drug must be subjected to an ongoing review of its effectiveness, or not, to ascertain any unintended, negative consequences. Whenever possible, conduct a follow-up study.

onboard. Academic journals must be contacted for reviews, to give the report's recommendations credibility.

Recommended actions have to be followed up to ascertain their actual results, as harmful unintended consequences are always possible. All this, of course, applies today as much as when Nightingale learned the ropes of research and advocacy.

Some new programs and policies require new legislation, so that advocates must be familiar with the relevant legislative process, and know, in federal systems, which level of government is appropriate. Both congressional systems, as in the United States, and parliamentary systems, as in Britain and Canada, have committee stages where interventions from outside experts and organizations can be made. Advocates of a new law must track it through the whole process, working with the bill's sponsors. Good provisions can be weakened by amendments if the bill's sponsors are not on their toes. Provisions may also be strengthened by amendments.

Nightingale was skilled in this process, as can be seen in her tracking of the Metropolitan Poor Bill in Parliament in 1867. This was the law that provided for the appointment of professional nurses in the workhouse infirmaries (she wanted this to be a requirement for these institutions, which did not happen, but at least opened up the possibility). When the bill was in the House, she had three Members of Parliament she could count on to support it and press for stronger measures. Her brother-in-law, Sir Harry Verney, moved a motion in the committee to add a provision for the training of nurses, which was agreed on (Hansard, 1867). John Stuart Mill, the great advocate for the vote for women, spoke twice in the committee in favor of strong central administration for the Poor Law hospitals, noting the defects in the current system. (Nightingale signed his petition for the vote for women in 1866; here he is supporting her great concern.) The former (Liberal) minister, C.P. Villiers too supported this petition.

"WAYS OF KNOWING" AND SCIENTIFIC METHOD

Nurses of the 21st century are much better educated, especially in science, than those belonging to Nightingale's time, when few had anything close to a secondary school education. Now, a university degree is a basic requirement in many places, and nursing academics and other profession leaders often have higher degrees. "Evidence-based" health care, which Nightingale practiced, now has a wide following, with conferences and journals in support. A number of nursing authors, for all their superior education, denigrate science, in favor of multiple "ways of knowing," making empirical research, or evidence-based conclusions, merely one of the several options.

Carper (1978) advanced a typology of four "patterns of knowing": empirical, personal (self-understanding and empathy), ethical (attitudes and knowledge), and aesthetic (awareness of immediate situation). It was a reaction to what was considered "overemphasis on just empirically derived knowledge, so-called 'scientific nursing.'" In other words, empirically derived knowledge is not good enough, and "scientific" nursing is demoted to "so-called." The article, when checked for this book, had been cited 2,289 times.

Chinn and Kramer (2008), using Carper, treated "every pattern" of knowledge as "equally valid," from the "empiric" to ethics, personal, and aesthetics. (It is not clear here if "empiric" refers to the results of actual empirical research, or simply the casual use of what worked before.)

Carper's typology was taken further in an article arguing that Nightingale, much earlier, had used "multiple patterns of knowing" in her "practice, research, and social reform efforts." The four types were all set out in detail, following Carper, with an assertion that Nightingale was "not definitively viewed as a nurse theorist" (Clements & Averill, 2006, p. 273). However, the sources the authors used to make that point omit entirely her mature work on nursing. They cite her *Notes on Nursing*, along with her philosophical work *Suggestions for Thought*, which was written before *Notes on Nursing*. Nightingale is mistakenly said to have written her nearly 1,000-page book on the Crimean War while still at Scutari, for which the reference is a children's book (Gorrell, 2000). Even a cursory look at Nightingale's massive volume would reveal its date, 1858, 2 years after the end of the war. Further, its detail and complexity would be obvious, the product of having had the assistance of leading medical scientists and statisticians.

Nightingale would be amazed that the authors have attributed a "care/cure dichotomy" to her, assigning "Nightingale nursing" to caring, while "the more valued and prestigious half of the dichotomy" went to medicine (Treiber & Jones, 2015). Not nursing and medicine both? Nightingale drew firm distinctions between the two fields, but never of that sort. Nursing was always both an art and science, as was medicine. Both were required in giving care, both employed to facilitate (but not guarantee) a cure.

Nightingale's observations on a cholera inquiry in India, in a letter to *The Lancet*, show how she regarded the relationship between theory and fact, without any reference to alternative ways of knowing. "Jenner first started a theory," she stated, referring to Edward Jenner's pioneering of smallpox vaccination in 1796, but it was not put into law, the Vaccination Acts until his theory "had become a fact of long experience." Vaccination was only made compulsory in England in 1853.

"Saving lives" was the object of the cholera inquiry in question in 1870, as it was in Jenner's day, not quite the ethics, personal knowledge, and aesthetics of the typology. Meanwhile, decisions had to be made, notably on expenditures on treatment and prevention. Nightingale hoped that the new cholera inquiry would help to tell if the public's money was well spent, or not, on the means employed (Nightingale, 1870).

The distinction between empirical/scientific and any of ethics, aesthetics, and the personal might better be dealt with by acknowledging what is called, in the social sciences, the "fact/value" distinction. Beatrice Webb gave a succinct definition of it, specifying that science (any science) can only deal with "means or process," not the purpose. Medical science can tell "how to kill or cure" someone, but not "whether you want to kill or cure him" (Webb, 1906). Webb is also an excellent source of a related issue, the separation of quantitative and qualitative aspects of research into two, opposed research methods. She asserted that they "must go hand in hand": "Statistical inquiry without personal observation lacks all sure foundation, during personal observation unless followed by statistic inquiry, leads to no verified conclusion" (Webb, 1906).

Can we have it both ways: evidence-based research and multiple ways of knowing? How can the results of a careful piece of research (or even a careless piece of research) be compared with one's ethical views or aesthetic judgments? They are not the same thing.

Nightingale was a committed follower of the scientific method and, in her early years, keen on the history of science. It is clear throughout her writing that knowledge must always be the object of research, although the researcher must be scrupulously modest in claiming reliable results. Science advanced, with reversals. Scientists draw inferences from data that are later disproved. She was anti-Darwin when he first published the theory of natural selection, but later came to accept it. Similarly, she changed her mind on germ theory, as solid evidence for it became available.

Nightingale cited the eminent scientist, Sir John Herschel when writing to Francis Galton in 1891 on founding a course in "social physics" at Oxford University. (The term "social physics" was Quetelet's, and meant what would now be called social science.) She gave an example of studying the effects of legislation for the punishment of crime, that one should "put down what you expect from such and such legislation after __ years, see where it has given you what you expected and where it has failed. But you change your laws and your administration of them without inquiry" (letter, February 7, 1891, in McDonald, 2003, p. 113). The reference is to Herschel's comments on Quetelet. Nightingale herself had read Quetelet thoroughly and commented on him while learning the material (McDonald, 2003, Nightingale's Quetelet, pp. 11–68).

Nightingale cited Herschel again in 1895 when insisting on the use of evidence, instead of "a priori" or preconceived opinion in making a scientific judgment. The subject was a syllabus on rural hygiene, which taught, she thought, faulty material on the treatment of burns. They should ask: "Has this been tried? What was the result?" Yet they did what Herschel said we all did, namely, to enunciate "opinions a priori, without the slightest inquiry: has 'this been tried? What was the result?'" (letter, March 10, 1895, Wellcome Ms 9015/32).

However, she always understood that facts gained from inquiry were provisional; new programs or treatments should be carefully tested before being extended. She had learned from Quetelet how easy it was to go wrong.

Nightingale had read the great scientist Herschel when young and possibly met him when her father took her to meetings of the British

Association for the Advancement of Science at Oxford University in 1847. Her paper "Rural Hygiene" has been cited as "validating the aesthetic way of knowing" (Clements & Averill, 2006, p. 270). The actual content of "Rural Hygiene" is anything but: filth, foul water, and the saddened lives that follow, with her call to action to prevent such diseases.

APPLYING NIGHTINGALE PRINCIPLES TO CURRENT CHALLENGES

Nightingale's mission was to save lives, for which nursing was one of the available means. Safer hospitals, better public health measures (especially clean air and water and decent housing), and famine prevention and relief were other ways to save lives on which she worked. Access to quality care for the poorest was a concern throughout her working life.

Applying Nightingale's principles to today's conditions, we would ask what are the greatest causes of death, related sickness, malnutrition, and so on, that can be prevented. Preventable mortality from cigarette smoking (an estimated 6–7 million deaths per year worldwide) was discussed in Chapter 3. The other diseases for which substantial reductions in mortality could be achieved are malaria, tuberculosis, and HIV/AIDS, but the numbers rank lower than for tobacco and are decreasing. Lack of access to health care is known to cause substantial numbers of deaths, estimates themselves varying considerably, and estimates even vary for hospital-acquired infections.

The issue to be pursued here is climate change as a major health issue, with much more problematic data, but undoubtedly increasing in threat, including substantial species losses as well as the threat to human health. Estimates are much shakier but are sufficient to raise the alarm. Available sources are examined in the light of Nightingale's principles of saving lives by using the best research results available.

Climate Change as a (Macro) Health Issue

Climate change is now recognized as a major health threat, with increased deaths and morbidity already evident in the most affected parts of the world. At meetings of the UN Framework Convention on Climate Change at Durban, December 2011 (Conference of the Parties 17), more than 200 international health leaders from more than 30 countries called on negotiators to push for the most ambitious commitments possible, warning that the lives of billions of people worldwide were at risk. At its Global Climate and Health Summit, it issued a Declaration and Call to Action, for a legally binding agreement on climate change, without delay, with urgent action to replace energy sources based on fossil fuels with clean, renewable sources.

Fossil fuel combustion causes immense harm both to the climate and human health. The Durban conference report urged that countries contribute equitably to a green climate fund to assist adaptation and mitigation The goal set at the Durban meetings was to limit the global average tem perature rise to 2°C above the preindustrial levels. The Paris meetings ir 2015 (Conference of the Parties 21) went on to recommend that the goal be to limit the rise to 1.5°C.

A study published in *The Lancet* in 2009 called climate change the "great est global health threat of the 21st century." Effects of climate change or health will affect most populations in the following decades and will pu the lives and well-being of billions of people at an increased risk. Vector borne diseases will expand their reach and death tolls, especially among the elderly, will increase from heat waves. Extreme climate events, like floods and forest fires, are likely to have the biggest effect on global health Moreover, there will be indirect effects causing decreased food security Climate change effects will exacerbate the inequities between the global rich and poor (Costello et al., 2009, p. 1693).

Health professionals argue that just as "early aggressive treatment fol lowing acute injury makes a huge difference to the patient's chances ol survival," so the time for action on climate change is now. "Delay is fatal Climate change is delivering an acute injury to humanity which will become much worse in the future, and we have already used up many precious minutes of our 'golden hour'" (Haines, 2009, p. xviii).

Food emergencies have already increased with rises in global temper ature. Rising temperatures are expected to reduce basic food crops such as rice and maize. In addition, although rising temperatures might increase yields in high-latitude countries and possibly West Africa; crops, forests, livestock, fisheries, and aquaculture are all threatened elsewhere. Sea-level rises and flooding of coastal lands salinate agricultural lands and destroy nursery areas for fishing.

Climate change impacts on health also occur through the decreased availability of clean water. In 1995, almost 1.4 billion people lived in water-stressed regions, making them vulnerable to diarrheal and other diseases caused by biological or chemical contaminants. Depleted aquifers, such as in Mexico City, are the result of overexploitation and result in the need to import water (Costello et al., 2009, pp. 1704–1705).

Extreme weather events, on the increase from global warming, affect health through the breakdown of clean water supply systems. Of the 238 great natural catastrophes that occurred between 1950 and 2007, two thirds resulted from extreme weather, mainly floods and windstorms. Population growth increases the competition for scarce food and water resources, resulting in greater degradation of arable land (Costello et al., 2009, pp. 1706–1707).

Climate Change as a Concern for Nurses

Climate change is a new subject for nurses. Sattler and Lipscomb's *Environmental Health and Nursing Practice* (1993) was billed, in 2002, as the "first book on how environment affects nursing practice" (Sattler & Lipscomb, 2002). It covers numerous subjects from asthma to environmental toxins, lead poisoning, and hospitals as causes of pollution. Climate change did not make it into the book, indicating that the knowledge on this issue is very recent. Global warming was addressed by scientists in the 18th and 19th centuries, but the first report of the Intergovernmental Panel on Climate Change dates only to 1988, and the Earth Summit, in Rio de Janeiro, which adopted the UN Framework Convention on Climate Change, to 1992.

Some nurses' organizations have taken on climate change, developing a policy for government action, at all levels, and liaising with other health care professions to press the case. The American Nurses Association (ANA), for example, in 2015 had delegates meet with members of Congress on climate change. The RNs noted that they were accustomed to advising people to eat nutritious food, but could not say, "be sure and breathe clean air today" (ANA, 2016). They were here referring to deaths caused by burning fossil fuels in air pollution, an immediate, measurable impact, and yet far short of the devastation that will happen if greenhouse gas emissions are not significantly brought down.

The Alliance of Nurses for Healthy Environments (ANHE) was formed in 2008 by American nursing leaders to develop a "strategic plan for environmental health nursing." It saw the formation of a national organization, which issues fact sheets, including climate change as a health issue itself, facilitates blogs, and sponsors work groups directed at research, practice, and policy advocacy. It urges nurses to take "the Nurses' Pledge to green their nursing practice."

The Canadian Nurses Association (CNA) has been (comparatively) early and vigorous in tackling climate change. In 2009, before the UN Copenhagen conference, it joined with the Canadian Medical Association, an environmental foundation, and a medical students organization to urge that the Canadian prime minister "Put Global Health at the Centre of UN Climate Summit," which he did not. The brief sensibly argued that "voluntary action by individual Canadians is not enough to solve the problem of climate change," and called for government policies and programs. "The prime minister must sign on to a fair, ambitious, and binding global agreement in Copenhagen," stated the CNA president (CNA, 2009).

The CNA, for a 2007 project marking its centennial as an organization, surveyed Canadian nurses to identify their awareness of environmental health issues, education about environmental exposures, use of teaching resources with patients or clients, and their "perception of the sustainability of the health system in which they work." The study, funded by the Government of Canada, showed substantial gaps in knowledge on environmental issues. It omitted such a serious concern as climate change to focus on more visible matters of air pollution and hazardous wastes. It advocated a focus on environmental health in nursing curricula, undergraduate and graduate, and opportunities for nurses in the work force. The study was optimistic about the ability of nurses to play a more active role, with training, "in reducing or preventing the health consequences of environmental hazards" (CNA, 2007). When the climate crisis specifically is considered, grounds for this optimism disappear.

The Registered Nurses Association of Ontario (RNAO) has gone further than the CNA on climate change, with several comprehensive, well-argued briefs. It came out in favor of a carbon tax for Canada, as a simple, quick, effective way of putting a price on carbon, without "gaming and cheating," an allusion to the many ineffective cap-and-trade schemes. When the Ontario government, however, opted for cap-and-trade instead, the RNAO endorsed it, although reminding the government, in a 20-page brief, of the reasons for preferring a carbon tax (RNAO, 2015, p. 2).

Ontario nurses have also formed their organization to work for action on climate change and other environmental concerns. Ontario Nurses for the Environment is a prime example of such an "interest group," which can be joined when a nurse or student nurse joins the RNAO.

In the United Kingdom, nurses have recently joined medical organizations in calling for action on climate change, but clearly, medical groups have been well ahead. *The Lancet* to date has launched two commissions on the subject. Its second endeavor called on the health professionals to "mobilize and lead against climate change," as they had previously on tobacco and HIV/AIDs (Lugsdin & Hook, 2016; Watts, Stott, & Rafferty, 2015). The "Health Professional Alliance to Combat Climate Change" includes the British Medical Association, Climate and Health Council, eight royal colleges (one of them the Royal College of Nursing), and such medical journals as the *British Medical Journal* and *The Lancet* (British Medical Journal, 2015).

The Canadian Medical Association established a policy on climate change in 2010. In 2016, it made climate change the focus of its General Council meetings, with an expert on climate change, Dr. James Orbinski, as its keynote speaker. The message was thorough and tough, the best so far from a medical or nursing organization (Collier, 2016).

Nurses, doctors, and any health professionals who take on the climate crisis are, whether they know it or not, following Nightingale in her taking on the greatest challenges of her day. For her, they were health care for the poorest, and famine in India. She was following the example of her grandfather, who took on the greatest challenge of his day, the abolition of the slave trade and slavery.

FINAL OBSERVATIONS AND REFLECTION

One has to agree with the American nursing professor who concluded that "few people" recognized and emulated Nightingale's research ability, or used their findings "as leverage for social action or as a basis for nursing practice" (Halloran, 1995, p. 267). No can one dispute his observation that, in spite of the rise in research in nursing, Nightingale, who never attended college, "did more with her statistical studies" both to influence hospital care and, as measures for prevention, the living conditions of British soldiers "than any nurse of today has accomplished for comparable groups of citizens through implementation of his or her recommendations based on research" (Halloran, 1995, p. 300).

Halloran's assessment of Nightingale's ability and effectiveness was highly favorable. However, he greatly oversimplified the process in crediting her with persuading "the British Government to change conditions in hospitals" because she showed "convincingly" that conditions were harmful (Halloran, 1995, p. 301). Indeed, it took a team of superb experts—she deserves credit for bringing them together—plus years of agitation, to effect those changes. For some reforms, laws had to be adopted, with complex regulations to guide their application. For others, spending had to be approved by the official bodies with many competing claims for limited sums. For others, leading members of the medical profession had to be persuaded to support a new project, if not a contradiction to the usual practice, at least a significant modification. In some cases, both doctors and nurses, in a variety of organizations, had to be convinced.

Political action is required for many reforms and it cannot be easily taught. Leadership and administration courses are now offered to many nurses and are compulsory in some places, but these do not, at least so far, include how to change policies and practices through the political system. Knowledge of the purpose and functioning of major political bodies can be taught. So can the basic skills of writing to officials and letters to the editor, as well as writing and presenting a brief. However, one suspects that to learn how to affect policy requires experience and mentoring, which can be done but requires a different process.

Nursing leaders who want to make the kind of difference Nightingale did are invited to ponder what steps they might take in their respective areas. What needs to be done and how vary by country (national legislation and regulations) and area (state or province, and municipality, down to the local hospital or care agency). Even for climate change, although it is a global crisis, the actions needed vary by area.

Formal statements, even the World Health Organization's "framework conventions" are only a means to an end of a healthier population, longer life spans, and lower death rates. Its "Framework Convention for Tobacco Control," 2004, as noted in Chapter 3, won widespread support, with 168 signatory countries. However, tobacco use continues to rise in some countries, especially countries in Asia, and cigarette companies find new smokers to replace those who die or quit. Success must be judged on outcomes, as seen in prevalence and death rates, with hard data.

QUESTIONS FOR DISCUSSION

1. What health care issues are the greatest challenges in your area, such as hospital-acquired infections, drug errors, or lack of access to care?
2. In your area, on what issues might health promotion measures be more effective? Consider cigarette smoking, illicit street drugs, prescription drugs, and bad food options in schools and care facilities.
3. How can existing nursing and health science organizations be more effective in promoting health, preventing disease, and improving care?
4. What interests have to be countered, and how, to bring in reforms in such areas as cigarette smoking and fast foods?
5. What advice and mentoring are available in your area to nurses wanting to become active on policy matters? Does, or can, your professional organization provide this?

REFERENCES

Alliance of Nurses for Healthy Environments. Climate Action Network International. Retrieved from https://envirn.org/about/

American Nurses Association. (2016, December 13). Members take action to reduce effects of climate change. *The American Nurse*. Retrieved from http://www.theamericannurse.org/2015/11/01/members-take-action-to-reduce-effects-of-climate-change

British Medical Journal. (2015). UK health professionals unite for stronger measures to tackle climate change. *Science Daily*. Retrieved from https://www.sciencedaily.com/releases/2015/11/151119095834.htm

Canadian Nurses Association. (2007). Nurses and environmental health: Survey results. Retrieved from https://www.cna-aiic.ca/~/media/cna/page-content/pdf-en/survey_results_e.pdf?la=en

Canadian Nurses Association. (2009, December 1). Prescription for Canada's prime minister: Put global health at the centre of UN climate summit [CNA press release].

Carper, B. A. (1978). Fundamental patterns of knowing in nursing. *Advances in Nursing Science, 1*, 13–24.

Chenu, J.C. (1870). De la mortalité dans l'armé et des moyens d'économiser la vie humaine, extraits des statistiques médico-chiruergicales. Paris, France: Hachette.

Chinn, P. L., & Kramer, M. K. (2008). *Theory and nursing: A systematic approach.* St. Louis, MO: Mosby. ISBN: 0801679478.

Clements, P. T. & Averill, J. B. (2006). Finding patterns of knowing in the work of Florence Nightingale. *Nursing Outlook, 54*(5), 268–274. doi:10.1016/j.outlook.2006.06.03

Collier, R. (2016). CMA GC: Doctors must engage in climate change. *Canadian Medical Association Journal.* doi:10.1503/cmaj.109-5318

Cook, E.T. (1913). *The life of Florence Nightingale* (2 vols.). London, UK: Macmillan.

Costello, A., Abbas, M., Allen, A., Ball, S., Bell, S., Bellamy, R.,...Patterson, C. (2009, May 16). Managing the health effects of climate change. *The Lancet, 373*(9676), 1693–1733. doi: 10.1016/S0140-6736(09)60935-1

Gorrell, G. (2000). *Heart and soul: The story of Florence Nightingale.* Toronto, Canada: Tundra. ISBN: 9780887767036

Haines, A. (2009). Introduction. In J. Griffiths, M. Rao, F. Adshead, & A. Thorpe (Eds.), *The health practitioner's guide to climate change: Diagnosis and cure* (pp. xviii–xix). London, UK: Earthscan. ISBN: 978-1-84407-728-1.

Halloran, E. J. (Ed.). (1995). *A Virginia Henderson reader: Excellence in nursing.* New York, NY: Springer Publishing. ISBN: 0826188303.

Hansard. (1867, March 11). *Parliamentary debates,* col. 1623.

Lugsdin, J., & Hook, C. (2016, January 30). Climate change and health. *The Lancet, 387*(10017), 431. http://dx.doi.org/1016/S0140-6736(16)00172-0

McDonald, L. (Ed.). (2002). *Florence Nightingale's theology: Essays, letters and journal notes.* Waterloo, Canada: Wilfrid Laurier University Press. ISBN: 0-88920-371-7.

McDonald, L. (Ed.). (2003). *Florence Nightingale on society and politics, philosophy, science, education, and literature.* Waterloo, Canada: Wilfrid Laurier University Press. ISBN: 0-88920-429-2

McDonald, L. (Ed.). (2004). *Florence Nightingale on public health care.* Waterloo, Canada: Wilfrid Laurier University Press. ISBN: 0-88920-446-2.

McDonald, L. (Ed.). (2005). *Florence Nightingale on women, medicine, midwifery and prostitution.* Waterloo, Canada: Wilfrid Laurier University Press. ISBN: 0-88920-466-7.

McDonald, L. (Ed.). (2009). *Florence Nightingale: Extending nursing.* Waterloo, Canada: Wilfrid Laurier University Press. ISBN: 978-1-55458-170-2.

McDonald, L. (Ed.). (2010). *Florence Nightingale and the Crimean War.* Waterloo, Canada: Wilfrid Laurier University Press. ISBN: 978-1-55458-245-7.

McDonald, L. (Ed.). (2011). *Florence Nightingale on wars and the War Office.* Waterloo, Canada: Wilfrid Laurier University Press. ISBN: 978-1-55458-382-9.

McDonald, L. (Ed.). (2012). *Florence Nightingale and hospital reform*. Waterloo, Canada: Wilfrid Laurier University Press. ISBN: 978-0-88920-471-3.

Nightingale, F. (1858a). *Answers to written questions addressed to Miss Nightingale by the commissioners. Report of the commissioners appointed to inquire into the regulations affecting the sanitary condition of the army and the treatment of the sick and wounded* (pp. 361–394). London, UK: Her Majesty's Stationery Office.

Nightingale, F. (1858b). *Notes on matters affecting the health, efficiency, and hospital administration of the British Army*. London, UK: Harrison.

Nightingale, F. (1859). *A contribution to the sanitary history of the British Army during the late War with Russia*. London, UK: Harrison.

Nightingale, F. (1860a). Hospital statistics. Paper submitted to the Second Section of the congress.

Nightingale, F. (1860b). *Notes on nursing: What it is and what it is not*. (New ed., rev., enlarged). London, UK: Harrison (library standard version).

Nightingale, F. (1862). Note on the supposed protection afforded against venereal disease, by recognizing prostitution and putting it under police regulation. Private and Confidential paper.

Nightingale, F. (1863a). *Notes on hospitals* (3rd ed.). London, UK: Longmans, Green.

Nightingale, F. (1863b). Sanitary statistics of native colonial schools and hospitals. *Transactions of the National Association for the Promotion of Social Science, 475–488.*

Nightingale, F. (1869, November). *Memorandum regarding sanitary progress at home and foreign military stations and in India in conformity with the principles and recommendations of the Army Sanitary Commission*. Printed paper.

Nightingale, F. (1870, November 19). Letter to the editor. *The Lancet, 96*(2464), 725.

Nightingale, F. (1871). *Introductory notes on lying-in institutions*. London, UK: Longmans, Green.

Nightingale, F. (1873, July). A sub "note of interrogation." what will be our religion in 1999? *Fraser's Magazine* (new series), *8*(43), 25–36.

Nightingale, F. (1879, May 31). Irrigation and water transit in India. *Illustrated London News, 10*(35), 495.

Registered Nurses Association of Ontario. (2015). *Cap and trade program design options. Submission to the Ministry of Environment and Climate Change*. Retrieved from http://rnao.ca/sites/rrnao-ca/files/Cap_and_Trade_Program.pdf

Sattler, B., & Lipscomb, J. (Eds.). (2003). *Environmental health and nursing practice*. New York, NY: Springer Publishing. ISBN: 0826142826.

Statistics of the general hospitals of London. (1862, September). *Journal of the Statistical Society of London, 25,* 3384–3385.

Treiber, L., & Jones, J. H. (2015). The care/cure dichotomy: Nursing's struggle with dualism. *Health Sociology Review, 24*(2), 152–162. doi:10.1080/14461242.2014.999404

Vallée, G. (Ed.). (2006*). Florence Nightingale on health in India*. Waterloo, Canada: Wilfrid Laurier University Press. ISBN: 10-0-88920-468-3.

Watts, N., Stott, R., & Rafferty, A. M. (2015, November). Combating climate change. *British Medical Journal, 18,* 351. doi:10.1136/bmj.h6178

Webb, B. (1906). *Methods of investigation*. London Sociological Society.

Part II: In Nightingale's Own Words

In Part II, we trace Nightingale's ideas as they evolved over the years. In Part I, numerous instances are given of the errors people—even academicians!—make about Nightingale by consulting only her *Notes on Nursing*. That book is the key for her statements on healing as a restorative process and her environmental theory, but it does not reflect Nightingale's social justice goal of quality health care for all. For that, one *must* turn to her later works, especially her brief to the Parliamentary committee on workhouse infirmary nursing and her work on district nursing, presented in Chapter 11. *Notes on Nursing* reflects her ideas before the opening of her school. Over the years, the quality of care nurses could give and the complexity of tasks they could perform increased enormously. Physicians were pleased with their work and wanted them to do more. The last papers, published between 1883 and 1893, show the much greater demands made on nurses than the very limited expectations at the start in 1860. *Notes on Nursing* represents only the rock-bottom minimum.

We begin, in Chapter 10, with Nightingale's work of 1858 to 1859, her first papers on hospital reform after finishing her mammoth analysis of Crimean War mortality (she returned from the war in 1856). This first version of what became *Notes on Hospitals*, in turn, shaped her best-known book, *Notes on Nursing*. It can be seen as the positive response to the lessons learned from the defective army hospitals of the war. It is grounded on the belief that high death rates can be prevented by careful, sturdy measures of hygiene.

Chapter 11 relates Nightingale's work directed to providing care for the most disadvantaged sick, getting quality nursing into the workhouse infirmaries, and avoiding workhouse infirmaries entirely by providing care at home by visiting or district nurses. Chapter 12, the final chapter, excerpts her last papers, by 1893 after 35 years of experience. For this late writing, she could draw on advances in medicine, nursing, and health care generally, from an ever-widening network of friends and colleagues.

Part II enables readers to look at Nightingale's work from the perspective of today. The selections are all her writing, selected because of their ongoing significance. Part I reports the views of many experts on her contributions to nursing and public health care more generally. Too often, there was reason to complain that even leading experts missed what she had written. That so few nurses, or doctors, or health scientists, read history is all too obvious. Many simply missed the fact that Nightingale paid great attention to updating her own knowledge.

In Part II, the reader can trace the evolution of her ideas, on the significant components of nursing and public health care. All three chapters contain little-known material: in Chapter 10, her papers from before her famous *Notes on Nursing*; in Chapter 11, papers on extending quality health care to those who could not pay for it (a concern no less in public policy debates of the 21st century); and in Chapter 12, her late papers, which show how much her ideas took into account new work. In all these respects, she outdoes expectations, and thus again is a model for us today.

Chapter 10: Nightingale's Early Writing on Hospitals and Nursing

Sick people are more susceptible than healthy people, and if such people be shut up together without sufficient space and sufficient fresh air, there will be produced, not only fever, but erysipelas, pyemia, and the usual tribe of hospital-generated epidemic diseases.

—Nightingale (1858c)

FIRST EDITION OF *NOTES ON HOSPITALS*, 1858

This, the original version of what became a full book in 1863, *Notes on Hospitals*, consists of the two papers Nightingale wrote for the National Association for the Promotion of Social Science, which met in Liverpool in October 1858. They draw on her earlier work on the Crimean War hospitals (Nightingale, 1858a, 1858b).

The papers were read on two consecutive days by the secretary of the association, Dr. Holland. The chair was Lord Shaftesbury, Nightingale's ally on so many issues. The sessions were well attended and the discussion exceptionally well informed. There were papers also in that section by sanitary expert Edwin Chadwick and Robert Rawlinson, the civil engineer on the Sanitary Commission who had gone to the Crimean War. Newspaper coverage of the sessions was sympathetic and detailed, especially for the second paper (*The Times*, 1858).

In the papers, Nightingale held that good nursing depended greatly on the hospital itself, its design and materials. The influence of the war hospital experience is obvious, although both papers included much material on civil hospitals, as did her war analyses. Hospitals—all hospitals—had and still have much in common; sociologists call them "total institutions" and include prisons and barracks in the category.

The papers were first published in the association's *Transactions* (Nightingale, 1859a) then republished by Nightingale herself, with additional material (Nightingale, 1859b), in both cases with slight changes in the text and titles from the original handwritten papers (Nightingale). In the papers, we see her advancing her ideas on adequate space, air, and light that would be featured in *Notes on Nursing*. The first paper specifies four defects in the hospital construction, the second no fewer than 16 defects.

There are two important connections between this hospital material and nursing. One is that Nightingale considered it to be the nurse's task to ensure fresh air, light, and so on for the patient. The second is that nurses themselves were vulnerable to sickness and death from defects in hospital construction. Nightingale wanted to build a new profession, without losing its valuable recruits to sickness and death from hospital-acquired infections.

She used Dr. William Farr's term "zymotic disease," derived from the Greek word for fermentation, for such epidemic diseases as typhus and typhoid fever, cholera, smallpox, scarlet fever, and measles, before the bacilli causing them had been identified. It can be seen as a step in the direction of germ theory, for it presupposes a living entity, as opposed to a chemical poison, although the terms "poison" and "noxious" continue to appear in her writing and other sources.

Nightingale considered that good hospital construction was crucial to efficient nursing as well as to the safety of patients and staff. Hospital design should ensure adequate space for bedside care and minimize the distance nurses had to walk to provide it. In her brief to the Parliamentary committee on cubic space, she argued that "the efficiency of nursing is to a considerable extent dependent on hospital construction" (Nightingale, 1867, in Chapter 11). The large number of deaths from hospital-acquired infections that continue to occur shows that safety continues to be a major concern.

The titles given to the papers here are the original ones, as read to the Liverpool meetings. The source lines give a cross-reference to the volume and page numbers of the work in the *Collected Works of Florence Nightingale*, where the full work is available, with much more context.

* * * * *

Source: Florence Nightingale, Notes on the Sanitary Condition of Hospitals, and on Defects in the Construction of Hospital Wards (McDonald, 2012, pp. 47–60)

No stronger condemnation of any hospital or ward could be pronounced than the simple fact that any zymotic disease has originated in it, or that such diseases have attacked other patients than those brought in with them (Nightingale, 1858c).

Feeling very desirous of contributing whatever I can to aid to improvement in hospital construction and administration—especially at this time, when several new hospitals are being built—it has occurred to me to transmit a few notes on defects which have come under my own observation in an extended experience of these institutions.

No one, I think, who brings ordinary powers of observation to bear on the sick and maimed can fail to observe a remarkable difference in the aspect of cases, in their duration, and in their termination, in different hospitals. To the superficial observer, there are two things only apparent—the disease and the remedial treatment, medical or surgical. It requires a considerable amount of experience, in hospitals of various constructions and varied administrations, to go beyond this....

The facts flow almost of necessity from ascertained sanitary experience. But it is not often, excepting perhaps in the case of intelligent house surgeons, that the whole process whereby the sick, who ought to have had rapid recoveries, are retained week after week, or perhaps month after month, in hospital....I have known a case of slight fever received into hospital, the fever passed off in less than a week, and yet the patient, from the foul state of the wards, not restored to health at the end of eight weeks.

The defects to which such occurrences are mainly to be attributed are four:

1. The agglomeration of a large number of sick under the same roof.
2. Deficiency of space.
3. Deficiency of ventilation.
4. Deficiency of light.

These are the four radical defects in hospital construction....

It is an all-important question to decide whether the propagation of such diseases is inevitable or preventable. If the former, then the whole question must be considered as to whether hospitals, necessarily attended with results so fatal, should exist at all. If the latter, then it is our duty to prevent their propagation....

Sick people are more susceptible than healthy people, and if such people be shut up together without sufficient space and sufficient fresh air, there will be produced, not only fever, but erysipelas, pyemia, and the usual tribe of hospital-generated epidemic diseases.

Again, if we have a fever hospital with overcrowded, badly ventilated, wards, we are quite certain to have the air become so infected as to poison the blood, not only of the sick, so as to increase their mortality, but also of the medical attendants and nurses, so that they also shall become subjects of fever. It will be seen at a glance that, in every such case and in every such

example, the "infection" is not inevitable, but simply the result of carelessness and ignorance....

No stronger condemnation of any hospital or ward could be pronounced
than the simple fact that any zymotic disease has originated in it, or that
such diseases have attacked other patients than those brought in with them.
And there can be no stronger condemnation of any town than the outbreak
of fatal epidemics in it....

It is a vulgar error to suppose that epidemics are occasioned by the
spread of disease from person to person, either by infection or contagion.
Epidemics do not *spread*—they develop themselves in constitutions already
made ripe for them by neglect of natural laws. Unless these laws be ignored,
epidemics, as experience seems to show, will not occur, the epidemic being,
in fact, the last or, so to speak, retributive stage of a succession of antecedent
phenomena extending over months or years, and all traceable to the neglect
of natural laws....

It was necessary to say thus much to show to what hospital diseases are
not due. To defects in site and construction and to defective management
they are mainly to be attributed.

1. *The Agglomeration of a Large Number of Sick Under One Roof:* It is a well-
    established fact that, other things being equal, the amount of sickness
    and mortality on different areas bears a ratio to the degree of density of
    the population. Why should undue agglomeration of sick be any excep-
    tion to this law? Is it not rather to be expected that, the constitutions of
    sick people being more susceptible than those of healthy people, they
    should suffer more from this cause?

But, if anything were wanting in confirmation of this fact, it would
be the enormous mortality in the hospitals which contained perhaps the
largest number of sick ever at one time under the same roof, viz., those at
Scutari. The largest of these two famous hospitals had at one time 2500 sick
and wounded under its roof, and it has happened that, out of these, two out
of every five have died. In the hospital tents of the Crimea, although the
sick were almost without shelter, without blankets, without proper food or
medicines, the mortality was not above one half what it was at Scutari. Nor
was it even so high as this in the small Balaclava General Hospital, while
in the huts of the Castle Hospital, on the heights above Balaclava, at a subsequent period, the mortality among the wounded did not reach 3 percent.

But it is not to this, however, that we appeal as the only proof of the
danger of surface overcrowding so much as it is to the fact of 80 cases of
hospital gangrene having been recorded during one month at Scutari (and
many, many, more passed unrecorded), to the fact that, out of 44 secondary

amputations of the lower extremities consecutively performed, 36 died, and to the cases of fever which broke out in the hospital, not by tens but by hundreds.

All experience tells the same tale, both among sick and well. Men will have a high rate of mortality in large barracks, a low one in separate huts, even with a much less amount of cubic space. (It must never be forgotten that, during the last six months of our occupation in the Crimea, the death rate among our men barracked in huts was actually less than it is among the men in barracks at home.)...

2. *Deficiency of Cubic Space:* The master of some large works in London lately mentioned the following fact: he was in the habit of sending those of his workmen who met with accidents to two different metropolitan hospitals. In one, they recovered quickly; in the other, they were frequently attacked with erysipelas, and some cases were fatal. On inquiry, it appeared that, in the former hospital, a larger amount of cubic space was allowed than in the latter, which is also so deficient in external ventilation and in construction that nothing but artificial ventilation could effectively change its atmosphere.

It is no less important to have a sufficient surface area between the adjoining and the opposite beds. Piling cubic space above the patient is not at all that is wanted. In the lofty corridors of Scutari, I have seen two long rows of opposite beds with scarcely three feet from foot to foot. Certainly it cannot be thought too much, under any circumstances, to give to each bed a territory to itself of at least eight feet wide by twelve feet long.

3. *Deficiency of Ventilation:* The want of fresh air may be detected in the appearance of patients sooner than any other want. No care or luxury will compensate indeed for its absence. Unless the air *within* the ward can be kept as fresh as it is *without*, the patients had better be away. Except in a few cases well known to physicians, the danger of admitting fresh air directly is very much exaggerated. Patients in bed do not catch cold....Although in badly constructed hospitals, or in countries where fuel is dear and the winter very cold, artificial ventilation may be necessary, it never can compensate for the want of the open window. The ward is never fresh....

If this be so for the well, how much more will it be so for the sick? for the sick, the exhalations from whom are always highly morbid and dangerous, as they are one of Nature's methods of eliminating noxious matter from the body, in order that it may recover health.

One would think that the first and last idea in constructing hospitals would be to contrive such means of ventilation as would be perpetually and instantly carrying off these morbid emanations. One would think that it would be the first thing taught to the attendants to manage such means of ventilation. Often, however, it is *not even* the *last* thing taught to them....

4. *Deficiency of Light:* What is the proportionate influence of the four defects enumerated in delaying recovery I am not competent to determine.

Second only to fresh air, however, I should be inclined to rank light in importance for the sick. Direct sunlight, not only daylight, is necessary for speedy recovery, except, perhaps, in ophthalmic and a small number of other cases. Instances could be given, almost endless, where, in dark wards or in wards with a northern aspect, even when thoroughly warmed, or in wards with borrowed light, even when thoroughly ventilated, the sick could not by any means be made speedily to recover....

Among kindred effects of light I may mention, from experience, as quite perceptible in promoting recovery, the being able to see out of a window, instead of looking against a dead wall, the bright colours of flowers, the being able to read in bed by the light of a window close to the bedhead. It is generally said that the effect is upon the mind. Perhaps so, but it is no less so upon the body on that account.

All hospital buildings in this climate should be erected so that as great a surface as possible should receive direct sunlight—a rule which has been observed in several of our best hospitals but, I am sorry to say, passed over in some of those most recently constructed. Window blinds can always moderate the light of a light ward, but the gloom of a dark ward is irremediable.

The axis of a ward should be as nearly as possible north and south, the windows on both sides so that the sun shall shine in (from the time he rises till the time he sets) at one side or the other. There should be a window to at least every two beds, as is the case now in our best hospitals.... But, while we *can* generate warmth, we cannot generate daylight, or the purifying and curative effect of the sun's rays.

* * * * *

SIXTEEN SANITARY DEFECTS IN THE CONSTRUCTION
OF HOSPITAL WARDS

In this second paper, given only the following day at the same conference (paper given at the National Association for the Promotion of Social

Science, Liverpool. Manuscript, Liverpool Record Office, in McDonald, 2012, pp. 60–72), Nightingale went into much more detail on what was wrong with the hospital design. There are points on the necessary cubic space for safety and much on sewers and drains, favorite Nightingale themes. Here we see her focus not only on ventilation but also on the importance of sunlight, for which she had no hard evidence but only her suspicions. She would pursue evidence on the value of sunlight in *Notes on Nursing*.

Today's reader feels some relief that so many of the urgent defects she portrayed have been dealt with, thanks to improved technology.

Nightingale used this second paper also to raise her philosophical/religious objections to utility theory—the greatest good for the greatest number. She noted the appearance of the idea in a government report, calling for "what is best for the *majority* of the sick in a hospital." Her opposition was faith based, for God's love was for all, not only the majority. She countered, if we cannot do the best possible for *all* the sick, by all means let us leave the rest at home" (Nightingale, 1858c, Part II, section 13). She wanted no less than that hospitals be built and administered so as to be of benefit to *all* their patients, not only a portion of them.

This second paper ended with a political crack at France, which was ahead of Britain in hospital design at that time. She regretted that great advances were being made by a "despotic government," meaning that of Emperor Napoleon III, when (democratic) England "ought to take the lead in everything good" (Nightingale, 1858c, Part II, section 16).

* * * * *

Sewers may become cesspools of the most dangerous description, if improperly made and placed. At Scutari, if the wind changed so as to blow up the open mouths of the sewers, such change was frequently marked by outbreaks of fever among the patients, and by relapses among the convalescents from fever.

—Nightingale (1858c, Part II, Section 15.)

Considering, then, that the conditions essential to the health of hospitals are principally these (a) fresh air, (b) light, (c) ample space, and (d) subdivision of sick into separate buildings or pavilions, let us examine the causes in the usual ward construction that prevent us from obtaining these conditions. The principal causes are as follows:

1. Defective means of natural ventilation and warming;
2. Defective height of wards;

3. Excessive width of wards between the windows;
4. Arranging the beds along the dead walls;
5. Having more than two rows of beds between the opposite windows;
6. Having windows only on one side or having a closed corridor connecting the wards;
7. Using absorbent materials for walls and ceilings;
8. Defective condition of water closets;
9. Defective ward furniture;
10. Defective accommodation for nursing and discipline;
11. Defective hospital kitchens;
12. Defective hospital laundries;
13. Selection of bad sites and bad local climates for hospitals;
14. Erecting hospitals in towns;
15. Defects of drainage;
16. Construction of hospitals without free circulation of external air.

1. *Defective means of ventilation and warming.* When the question of ventilation first assumed a practical shape in this country, it was supposed that 600 cubic feet of air per hour were sufficient for a healthy adult, in a room where a number of people are congregated together. Subsequent experience, however, has shown that this is by no means enough. As much as 1,000 cubic feet have been found insufficient to keep the air free from closeness and smell, and it is highly probable that the actual quantity required will ultimately be found to be at least 1500 cubic feet per hour per man.

   In sick wards, we have more positive experience as to the quantity of air required to keep them sweet and healthy. It has been found in certain Parisian hospitals in which the ventilating arrangements were deficient that pyemia and hospital gangrene had appeared among the patients. These diseases disappeared on the introduction of ventilating arrangements whereby 2,500 cubic feet of air per bed per hour was supplied to the wards....

2. *Defective height of wards.* It is not possible to ventilate sufficiently a ward of 10 or 12 feet high. And, again, it is not possible to ventilate a ward where there is a great height above the windows. A ward of 30 beds can be well ventilated with a height of about 17 feet, provided the windows reach to within one foot of the ceiling. Otherwise, the top of the ward becomes a reservoir for foul air.

3. *Too great width of wards between the opposite windows.* It does not appear as if the air could be thoroughly changed if a distance of more than 30 feet intervenes among the opposite windows....If you make your length too great in proportion to the width, your ward becomes a tunnel—a

form fatal to good ventilation. This was the case with the great corridor wards at Scutari.

If, on the other hand, you make your wards too short in proportion to this width, you multiply corners in a greater ratio than you multiply sick. And direct experiment has shown that the movement of the air in the centre of a ward is three or four times as great as it is at the corners....

4. *Arranging the beds along the dead walls.* This deprives the patient of the amount of light and air necessary to his recovery and has, besides, the disadvantage that, when the windows are opened, the effluvia must blow over all the intervening beds before escaping....

5. *Having more than two rows of beds between the windows....* These double wards are nearly 20 feet wider than they ought to be between the opposite windows for a thorough ventilation. The partition down the middle, with apertures, makes matters rather worse....

6. *Having windows only on one side, or having a closed corridor connecting the wards.* These corridors are the certain means of engendering a hospital atmosphere. If anyone had wished to see the corridor plan in all its horrors, Scutari would have shown them on a colossal scale. But they may be seen on a smaller scale in almost every hospital in London....

7. *Absorbent materials for floors, walls, and ceilings of hospitals....* The amount of organic matter given off by respiration and in other ways from the sick is such that the floors, walls, and ceilings of hospital wards—if not of impervious materials—become the most dangerous absorbents. The boards are in a time saturated with organic matter and only require moisture to give off noxious effluvia....

In Scutari, where the wards were overcrowded, the cases offensive and the floors ill-laid, rotten, and dirty, the accumulated saturations of weeks and months were such that the floors could not be scoured without literally poisoning the patients....

As to the walls and ceilings of wards, plaster or brick white-washed are equally objectionable. Pure, white, polished nonabsorbent cement is the only material fit for hospital walls....

8. *Defective condition of water closets.* It is hardly necessary to say more than this. There can be no safety for the sick if any but water closets of the best construction are used, as also, if they are not built *externally* to the main building, and cut off by a lobby, separately lighted and ventilated, from the ward....

9. *Defective ward furniture.* Hospital bedsteads should always be of iron, the rest of the furniture of oak....For all eating, drinking, and washing vessels, and for other utensils, the use of glass or earthenware is

superior to that of tin or any other metal, on account of its greater cleanliness.

10. *Defective accommodation for nursing and discipline.* The simplicity of construction in hospitals is essential to discipline. Effectual and easy supervision is essential to proper care and nursing.

Every unneeded closet, scullery, sink, lobby, and staircase represents both a place that must be cleaned, which must take hands and time to clean, and a hiding or skulking place for patients or servants disposed to do wrong. And no hospital will ever be free. Every 5 minutes is wasted upon cleaning what had better not have been there to be cleaned is something taken from and lost by the sick....

Distribution of sick in convenient numbers for attendance and position of nurses' rooms.... To return to large general hospitals, these "casualty" wards, as they are called, for noisy or offensive cases, are much better placed apart, with a completely appointed staff of their own, than attached one small ward to each larger one. Patients requiring much attention, whose condition fits them the most for the small wards, cannot be put there because either they are more or less neglected or they unduly monopolize the service of the ward attendants....

11. *Defective hospital kitchens.* Two facts every careful, experienced observer of the sick can establish from experience:

(1) The necessity of variety in food as an essential element of health, owing to the number of materials required to preserve the human frame. In sickness, it is still more important because, the frame being in a morbid state, it is scarcely possible to prescribe beforehand with certainty what it will be able to digest and assimilate. The so-called fancies of disease are in many cases valuable indications.

(2) The importance of cooking to secure the greatest digestibility and the greatest economy in nutritive value of food....

I have often been surprised by the primitive kitchens of some of our civil hospitals with which little variety of cooking is possible. These things show how little diet and cooking are even thought of as sanitary and curative agents....

12. *Defective hospital laundries.* It is hardly necessary to go back to the time of the Crimean War when, in a Scutari hospital, six shirts were washed in a month for a number of 2,000 patients, which was constantly changing, when the number per man per month of all articles of all descriptions washed was less than three. The pestilential filth of that time is known now to all....

Let laundries be constructed with sufficient area and cubic space for each washer, with an abundance of water, with proper means of drainage and ventilation for removing the vapor, properly constructed drying and ironing rooms, and we shall cease to hear of washerwomen "catching" fever.

13. *Selection of bad sites and bad local climates for hospitals.* As the object to be attained in hospital construction is to have pure, dry, air for the sick, it is evident that this condition cannot be fulfilled if a damp climate is selected.... Self-draining, gravelly, or sandy subsoils are best. River banks, estuary shores, valleys, marshy, or muddy ground ought to be avoided. It might seem superfluous to state that a hospital should not be built over an old dung heap, or over a crowded graveyard, did we not know that such things were being done at the present moment.

Although hospitals are intended for the recovery of health, people are very apt to forget this, and to be guided in the selection of sites by other considerations—such as cheapness, convenience, and the like— whereas, the professed object in view being to secure the recovery of the sick in the shortest time and to obtain the smallest mortality, that object should be distinctly kept in view as one that must take precedence over all others.

A doctrine has recently been promulgated, in a government report, that we are only to consider what is best for the *majority* of the sick in a hospital. If we cannot do the best possible for *all* the sick, by all means, let us leave the rest at home. In practice, a hospital may be found to benefit a majority and to inflict suffering on the remainder. Let us use our intelligence to see whether we cannot have hospitals constructed so as to be of equal benefit to all.

14. *Erecting hospitals in towns.* Nearly all that has been said under the last head, mutatis mutandis (with appropriate changes), may be repeated here. If the recovery of the sick is to be the object of hospitals, they will not be built in towns. If medical schools are the object, surely it is more instructive for students to watch the recovery from, rather than the long duration of, sickness....

According to all analogy, the duration of cases, the chances against complete recovery, the rate of mortality, must be greater in town than in country hospitals....

15. *Defects in drainage.* Sewers may become cesspools of the most dangerous description if improperly made and placed. At Scutari, if the wind changed so as to blow up the open mouths of the sewers, such change was frequently marked by outbreaks of fever among the patients, and by relapses among the convalescents from fever. Where there are no means for externally ventilating the sewers, no means for cleansing or flushing them, and where the bottoms are rough and uneven, such

occurrences cannot fail to take place....Where sewers pass close to or under occupied rooms, the walls or covers being defective, exhalations infallibly escape into those rooms. Such could be distinctly perceived in Scutari hospitals, and cases of cholera distinctly traced to such a cause.

Not very long ago, five fatal cases of fever occurred in rapid succession in one of our best civil hospitals, which were traced to a defective drain....

16. *Construction of hospitals without free circulation of external air.* To build a hospital with one closed court with high walls, or, what is worse, with two closed courts, is to stagnate the air....

Even in the pavilion structure, unless the distance between the pavilions is double the height of the walls, the ventilation and light are seriously interfered with. For this, among other reasons, two stories are better than three, and one is preferable to two....

To build a hospital in the midst of a crowded neighborhood of narrow streets and high houses, as is now being done in the case of a well-known London hospital, is to ensure a stagnation of the air outside, which no ventilation within, no cubic space, however ample, will be able to remedy.

I have here given the defects; few have had so sad or large an experience of their results as I have had. I appeal to those who are wiser and have more practical power than I have for the remedies, architects, hospital committees, civil and royal engineers, medical officers, officers of health, to all the men of science and benevolence, of whom our country is so justly proud. It is hard that, in a country where everything is done by a despotic government [France under Napoleon III], such advances in the sanitary construction of hospitals should have been made, and that our England, which ought to take the lead in everything good, should be left behind.

* * * * *

NOTES ON NURSING, 1860

I use the word nursing. It has been limited to signify little more than the administration of medicines and the application of poultices. It ought to signify the proper use of fresh air, light, warmth, cleanliness, quiet, and the proper selection and administration of diet—all at the least expense of vital power to the patient.

—Nightingale (1860)

Notes on Nursing: What It Is and What It Is Not was the original title of Nightingale's best-known book. The title was shortened to *Notes on Nursing* in the edition published soon after her death. She revised the text significantly twice. The version used here is the second, called by the editor of the first critical edition of the book, the "library standard version" (Skretkowicz, 1996). It was published only months after the first, badly printed edition. Nightingale not only corrected the many typographical errors in it but added much new material, such as quotations from eminent scientists and literary and political figures. It is far more sophisticated in language than the original. For the following edition, *Notes on Nursing for the Labouring Classes*, 1861, she removed all the extraneous material, simplified the language, and added the famous chapter "Minding Baby."

As anyone reading the material now is well educated compared with women during Nightingale's time, this second edition seems the best to use. "Minding Baby" is largely advice to girls looking after their younger siblings at home, not pediatric nursing. Sadly, the edition most available is the first, with all its misprints, and without the merits of either of the subsequent two editions.

Most of the material, in every version of *Notes on Nursing*, is out-of-date, ventilation, heating, water supply, beds, bedding, and so on, have all been improved, and adequate, sanitary toilets greatly reduce the need for bedpans. Thus, the excerpts here give the bare bones of principle, with as little dated material as possible. Anyone reading the full text, however, is struck with its guiding principle of patient care and comfort: patients come first.

It is also obvious, even in the extracts selected here, that Nightingale drew on her experience of being ill. She remarked on the "most acute suffering produced" from not being able "to see out the window," when "the knots in the wood" were her only view, and recalled how "a nosegay of wild flowers" sped her recovery (Nightingale, 1860a, 1860b, Chapter 5). Her disease was probably brucellosis (Young, 1995), one that would be easily treated today with antibiotics but back then had a high mortality rate. For survivors, chronic pain, partial paralysis, and fatigue typically followed.

Nightingale's reference to diarrhea "merging into cholera" reflects thinking before germ theory. Under germ theory, cholera is a specific disease, produced by a distinct bacillus, while diarrhea simply refers to the looseness of stools, which could be caused by any number of bacilli or parasites. In a hospital with a large number of bowel patients, of diarrhea, dysentery, and cholera, it might well seem that diarrhea merged into cholera.

Some of the comments on disease are not of concern to nurses in developed countries, where "consumption," or tuberculosis, is now rare, as is scrofula (a tubercular disease), pyemia, and erysipelas. Moreover, in most places, people do not bring in "organic matter," manure, on their feet into a sickroom, as they did in Nightingale's days when horse-drawn conveyances were in common use. It is also not necessary now to warn against the evils of the four-poster bed. Given that modern hospitals have adjustable mattresses, the advice on arranging pillows for patient comfort is not needed, although one can imagine that the human interaction in such arrangement might be comforting.

Some of Nightingale's advice, in every edition of *Notes on Nursing*, is as useful now as it was when it was written, none more than, "Every nurse ought to be careful to wash her hands very frequently during the day. If her face, too, so much the better." Still in the 21st century, "proper hand hygiene" remains "the primary method for reducing infections" (Gawande, 2004).

Notes on Nursing is also the source of key Nightingale definitions, such as disease being a "reparative process" of nature, the nurse's task being to aid it. Nightingale made the point that the patient might suffer as much from bad conditions in the sick room as from the disease itself.

Advertisements for the sale of the book, and then excerpts from it, began to appear in *The Times* and other British newspapers in January 1860. Small provincial newspapers often reprinted reviews and excerpts from the major London dailies (*Hampshire Advertiser*, 1860; *Liverpool Mercury*, 1860).

Notes on Nursing soon appeared in an American edition, followed by serialization in the *Saturday Evening Post* (1860). *Scientific American* published an excerpt (*Scientific American*, 1860). Notices of the book began to appear in Canadian newspapers in February 1860, and soon after reviews and excerpts followed (*Toronto Globe*, 1860).

The distinguished Boston doctor, Oliver Wendell Holmes, Sr. (father of the Supreme Court justice) was an early reader, pleased with Nightingale's making disease a "reparative process." He praised her in a famous article, "Currents and Counter-Currents," after noting that Hippocrates, "august father of the healing art," had made a case for nature 2000 years earlier, "Miss Florence Nightingale begins her late volume with a paraphrase of his statement. But from a very early time to this there has been a strong party against 'Nature' " (Holmes, 1861). It is noteworthy that the very first sentence of *Notes on Nursing* makes a point of disease as a "reparative process."

The book reached Australia by steamer in April 1860, duly listed among recently arrived "New Publications." Again, it was widely advertised. Newspapers in the Australian colonies, Tasmania, and New Zealand soon produced reviews and excerpts, some of them lengthy (*Bathurst Free Press and Mining Journal*, 1860; *Hawke's Bay Herald,* 1860; *Hobart Town Daily Mercury*, 1860; *Illawarra Mercury*, 1860; *Nelson Examiner and New Zealand Chronicle*, 1860; *Perth Gazette and Independent Journal of Politics and News*, 1860; *South Australian Advertiser*, 1860; *South Australian*

Register, 1860; *Sydney Morning Herald*, 1860). Key points of her message were highlighted and applied to local circumstances:

> Were these Notes of Miss Nightingale's, together with her Notes on Hospitals, taken advantage of, we should not see the corridors of a main part of an hospital ventilated from the passages of a fever ward when, by a slight sacrifice, they could be made to communicate directly with the external air. (*Cornwall Chronicle* [Tasmania], 1860)

On the 1930 sale of the publishing company that had published *Notes on Nursing*, the price paid to Nightingale was noted, a considerable £1,000. The book was reprinted "again and again" and still found large sales (*The Times*, 1930).

Although *Notes on Nursing* won wide praise, there were dissenters from the start. Elizabeth Blackwell, the first woman to qualify as a medical doctor and a friend of Nightingale's, called it, in a private letter, a "capital little book in its way," even useful, practical, and readable, but not a book "in the usual meaning of the word." Nightingale threw together "a mass of hints and experiences," but was "not able to digest them into a book which will remain as a classic" (Blackwell letter, April 25, 1860, cited in Boyd, 2005, p. 185).

A 1992 Commemorative Edition of *Notes on Nursing* (the badly printed first edition) has comments by 12 American nursing leaders on their use, or not, of Nightingale in their work. All but one were highly positive, as would be expected for a commemorative edition. Several provide a good discussion of her environmental theory (Commemorative Edition, 1992). Several presented Nightingale's ideas well and brought in the pertinent material of their own (Roy, Newman, & Rogers). Roy showed how her adaptation theory was "congruent" with Nightingale's (Roy, in Commemorative Edition, 1992, p. 64). Thompson flagged the emphasis on prevention and noted its influence on nursing in the American Civil War (Thompson, Commemorative Edition, 1992, p. 76). Some held that Nightingale's ideas were still needed (Watson, Newman, & Rogers, in Commemorative Edition, 1992). One saw her importance as a "symbol" of nursing (Styles, in Commemorative Edition, 1992, p. 74).

There are odd errors, also, in these introductions, such as that Nightingale "assigned readings in the humanities" to increase nursing students' understanding "of human ethics and morals," which she could not have done, for she never taught a class in her school. A largely instructive chapter misinterprets Nightingale's views of philosophers, turning her negative views of Hegel and Comte into commendation (Schuyler, in Commemorative Edition, 1992, pp. 11, 13). Fitzpatrick read Nightingale as an empiricist, while Schuyler had her integrating idealism with empiricism (Fitzpatrick, in Commemorative Edition, 1992, p. 5). Watson had her repudiate empiricism to root her instead in "ancient feminine wisdom and knowledge, a cosmology of wholeness, connectedness, and harmony." Watson gave no specific reference, nor do any spring to mind, for Nightingale's supposed use of "women's wisdom and knowledge" (Watson, in Commemorative Edition, 1992, p. 81). Nightingale was a thorough and consistent empiricist.

Several commentators castigated Nightingale for failures in theory, even that she never defined "caring" or "other key terms (Leininger, in Commemorative Edition, p. 30). Levine had her accepting "false theory, laden with superstition and error"; she "stubbornly preached 'atmospherics' while scientific evidence of contagion was being gathered around her" (Levine, in Commemorative Edition, 1992, p. 40). Nightingale's detailed advice on avoiding septicemia includes the necessity of nurses knowing the difference between "contagion and infection, and the distinctions between deodorants, disinfectants, and antiseptics" (Nightingale, 1883; see Chapter 12). Several commentators, as other authors noted in Chapter 1 of this book, chided Nightingale for (supposedly) rejecting germ theory, when in fact in time she came to accept it.

Peplau's Critique of Notes on Nursing

A major American nursing theorist, Hildegard E. Peplau, thoroughly derided *Notes on Nursing* in her chapter, calling it at best a "notable marker in Nursing's progress toward becoming a profession." It was a "period piece," a reflection of Nightingale's "commonly held views about women," a "failure to specify processes," although it "skirts discussion of nurse-patient interactions or relationships." She further faulted Nightingale for, when specifying pure air, failure to state "respiratory processes." She complained that Nightingale sometimes spelled Nature with a capital N, sometimes lower case. God or Nature confused her, although for Nightingale there was no contradiction, God ran the world by laws, which were scientific, discoverable laws of natural and social science. She has Nightingale ignoring Darwin and rejecting germ theory (Peplau, in Commemorative Edition, 1992, pp. 49–52).

Peplau was also critical of Nightingale for excluding men from nursing, and not recognizing male nurses of previous centuries in religious orders (Peplau, in Commemorative Edition, 1992, p. 148). These orders, notably the Knights of St. John of Jerusalem, the "Johanniter," existed in Nightingale's time and were prominent in the Franco-Prussian War. The Crown Princess of Prussia judged that all their hospitals were "so bad, not only at first but continuously," inferior "in cleanliness, ventilation, management, in every vital sanitary condition," to the regular military hospitals (Crown

Princess, letter, September 22, 1870, in McDonald, 2011, p. 715). Letters to Nightingale from other sources refer to these male nurses as being, with some exceptions, ignorant, unhygienic, unqualified, incompetent, heartless, and dishonest—and they diverted donations to the Prussian military (letter, November 16, 1870, Wellcome Ms 9004/145, and letters, December 9, 1870, ca. January 1871, February 1, 1871, April 16, 1871, in McDonald, 2011, pp. 711, 770, 772, 790).

Peplau, a pioneer in psychiatric nursing, was also critical of Nightingale for not including the subject in any of her published works, stating that mental illness and asylums existed in her time (Peplau, in Commemorative Edition, 1992, p. 49). Not one asylum in Nightingale's time—and Peplau named not a single one—had anything close to professional nursing. Nightingale, in fact, was well aware of the horrors of most mental asylums of her day and knowledgeable about the early efforts at humane care, such as by Dr. John Conolly.

Peplau did not like Nightingale's definition of nursing as a restorative process. She proposed instead,

> The work of nurses is to support the person's processes of bodily repair until the functional bodily processes are restored and begin to function fully again, or nurses support the person's functional bodily processes in some way until their normal functions are restored. (Peplau, in Commemorative Edition, p. 52)

Is this a "refinement" of Nightingale's too simplistic wording?: "Nursing is putting us in the best possible conditions for Nature to restore or to pre-serve health—to prevent or to cure disease or injury" (Nightingale, 1882, p. 1043; see Chapter 12).

Overall, the great failure in the commemorative commentaries are the authors' apparent ignorance of Nightingale's later writing. *Notes on Nursing* seems to them to be the first, last, and only book she wrote. One commentator acknowledged the production of 147 books, articles, pamphlets, and other publications, over her lifetime (Schuyler, in Commemorative Edition, 1992, p. 8); they are listed in an appendix in the official biography (Cook, 1913, Vol. 2). However, no commentator made any comparisons from *Notes on Nursing* to these later works. Those who pointed out the lack of discussion of germ theory reveal a critical lapse, for a book written in 1859 could hardly have discussed a theory nowhere then in the literature.

For our purposes, these commentaries serve to reflect how Nightingale was seen by major nursing leaders over a good part of the 20th century and in the 21st century. The extent of the misrepresentation of her views, particularly by failure to look at anything she wrote after *Notes on Nursing*, applies to the present also.

* * * * *

Source: Florence Nightingale. (1860b). *Notes on Nursing: What It Is and What It Is Not* (2nd ed.).

Preface

The following notes are by no means intended as a rule of thought by which nurses can teach themselves to nurse, still less as a manual to teach nurses to nurse. They are meant simply to give hints for thought to women who have personal charge of the health of others....Everyday sanitary knowledge, or the knowledge of nursing, or in other words of how to put the constitution in such a state as that it has no disease, or that it can recover from disease, takes a higher place. It is recognized as the knowledge which everyone ought to have—distinct from medical knowledge—which only a profession can have.

Introductory

Shall we begin by taking it as a general principle that all disease, at some period or other of its course, is more or less a reparative process, not necessarily accompanied with suffering, an effort of Nature to remedy a process of poisoning or of decay which has taken place weeks, months, sometimes years beforehand, unnoticed, the termination of the disease being then, while the antecedent process was going on, determined? ...

In watching disease, both in private houses and in public hospitals, the thing which strikes the experienced observer most forcibly is that the symptoms or the sufferings generally considered to be inevitable and incident to the disease are very often not symptoms of the disease at all, but of something quite different—the want of fresh air, or of light, or of warmth, or of quiet, or of cleanliness, or of punctuality and care in the administration of diet, of each or of all of these....The reparative process which Nature has instituted, and which we call disease, has been hindered by some want of knowledge or attention in one or in all of these things, and pain, suffering, or interruption of the whole process sets in....

I use the word nursing for want of a better. It has been limited to signify little more than the administration of medicines and the application of poultices. It ought to signify the proper use of fresh air, light, warmth, cleanliness, quiet, and the proper selection and administration of diet—all at the least expense of vital power to the patient.

Chapter 1. Ventilation and Warming

The very first canon of nursing, the first and the last thing upon which a nurse's attention must be fixed, the first essential to the patient, without which all the rest you can do for him is as nothing...is this: TO KEEP THE AIR HE BREATHES AS PURE AS THE EXTERNAL AIR, WITHOUT CHILLING HIM....

To have the air within as pure as the air without, it is not necessary, as often appears to be thought, to make it as cold....It is very desirable that the windows in a sick room should be such as that the patient shall if he can move about, be able to open and shut them easily himself (*Note*: Delirious fever cases, where there is any danger of the patient jumping out of window, are, of course, exceptions. ...).

In laying down the principle that the first object of the nurse must be to keep the air breathed by her patient as pure as the air without, it must not be forgotten that everything in the room which can give off effluvia, besides the patient, evaporates itself into his air. And it follows that there ought to be nothing in the room, excepting him, which can give off effluvia or moisture. Out of all damp towels, etc., which become dry in the room, the damp, of course, goes into the patient's air....

Of the fatal effects of the effluvia from the excreta it would seem unnecessary to speak, were they not so constantly neglected....The use of any chamber utensil [bedpan] *without a lid* should be utterly abolished....But never, never, should the possession of this indispensable lid confirm you in the abominable practice of letting the chamber utensil remain in a patient's room unemptied, except once in the twenty four hours....

Let no one ever depend upon fumigations, "disinfectants," and the like for purifying the air. The offensive thing, not its smell, must be removed.

Chapter 2. Health of Houses

There are five essential points in securing the health of houses:

1. Pure air
2. Pure water
3. Efficient drainage
4. Cleanliness
5. Light

Without these, no house can be healthy. And it will be unhealthy just in proportion as they are deficient....Without cleanliness within and without your house, ventilation is comparatively useless....

A dark house is always an unhealthy house, always an ill-aired house, always a dirty house. Want of light stops growth and promotes scrofula, rickets, etc., among the children. People lose their health in a dark house, and if they get ill, they cannot get well again in it.

Chapter 3. Petty Management

All the results of good nursing, as detailed in these notes, may be spoiled or utterly negatived by one defect, viz., in petty management, or in other words, by not knowing how to manage that what you do when you are there shall be done when you are not there....

Apprehension, uncertainty, waiting, expectation, fear of surprise, do a patient more harm than any exertion. Remember, he is face to face with his enemy all the time, internally wrestling with him, having long conversations with him. You are thinking of something else. "Rid him of his adversary quickly" is a first rule with the sick....

To be "in charge" is certainly not only to carry out the proper measures yourself but to see that everyone does so too.

Chapter 4. Noise

Unnecessary noise, or noise that creates an expectation in the mind, is that which hurts a patient. It is rarely the loudness of the noise, the effect upon the organ of the ear itself, which appears to affect the sick. How well a patient will generally bear, e.g., the putting up of a scaffolding close to the house, when he cannot bear the talking, still less whispering, and especially if it be of a familiar voice, outside his door....

I need hardly say that the other common course, namely, for a doctor or friend to leave the patient and communicate his opinion on the result of his visit to the friends just outside the patient's door...is, if possible, worst of all....

All hurry or bustle is peculiarly painful to the sick....

The friend who remains standing and fidgeting about while a patient is talking business to him, or the friend who sits and proses, the one from an idea of not letting the patient talk, the other from an idea of amusing him, such is equally inconsiderate.

Always sit down when a sick person is talking business to you; show no signs of hurry, give complete attention and full consideration if your advice is wanted, and go away the moment the subject is ended.

How to visit the sick and not hurt them: always sit within the patient's view, so that when you speak to him he has not painfully to turn his head round in order to look at you....If you make this act a wearisome one on the part of the patient, you are doing him harm. So also, if by continuing to stand, you make him continuously raise his eyes to see you.... This brings us to another caution. Never speak to an invalid from behind, nor from the door, nor from any distance from him, nor when he is doing anything....

Conciseness and decision are, above all things, necessary with the sick. Let your thought expressed to them be concisely and decidedly expressed. What doubt and hesitation there may be in your own mind must never be communicated to them.

Chapter 5. Variety

The effect in sickness of beautiful objects, of variety of objects, and especially of brilliancy of colour, is hardly at all appreciated. Such cravings are usually called the "fancies" of patients. And often doubtless patients have "fancies," as, e.g., when they desire two contradictions. But, much more often, their (so-called) "fancies" are the most valuable indications of what is necessary for their recovery. And it would be well if nurses would watch these (so-called) "fancies" closely....

People say the effect is only on the mind. It is no such thing. The effect is on the body, too. Little as we know about the way in which we are affected by form, by colour and light, we do know this, that they have an actual physical effect. A variety of form and brilliancy of colour in the objects presented to patients are actual means of recovery....

Flowers. The folly and ignorance which reign too often supreme over the sick room cannot be better exemplified than by this: while the nurse will leave the patient stewing in a corrupting atmosphere, the best ingredient of which is carbonic acid [carbon dioxide], she will deny him, on the plea of unhealthiness, a glass of cut flowers or a growing plant. Now, no one ever saw "overcrowding" by plants in a room or ward. And the carbonic acid they give off at nights would not poison a fly. Nay, in overcrowded rooms, they actually absorb carbonic acid and give off oxygen. Cut flowers also decompose water and produce oxygen gas. It is true there are certain flowers, e.g., lilies, the smell of which is said to depress the nervous system. These are easily known by the smell and can be avoided.

Volumes are now written and spoken upon the effect of the mind on the body. Much of it is true. But I wish a little more thought of the effect of the body on the mind....

Sick suffer to excess from mental as well as bodily pain. It is a matter of painful wonder to the sick themselves how much painful ideas predominate over pleasurable ones in their impressions; they think themselves ungrateful; it is all of no use.... A patient can just as much move his leg when it is fractured as change his thoughts when no external help from variety is given him. This is, indeed, one of the main sufferings of sickness, just as the fixed posture is one of the main sufferings of the broken limb....

We will suppose the diet of the sick is to be cared for. Then, this state of nerves is most frequently to be relieved by care in affording them a pleasant view, a judicious variety as to flowers, and pretty things. Light by itself will often relieve it. (No one who has watched the sick can doubt the fact.)

Chapter 6. Taking Food

Every careful observer of the sick will agree in this, that thousands of patients are annually starved, in the midst of plenty, from want of attention to the ways which alone make it possible for them to take food. This want of attention is as remarkable in those who urge upon the sick to do what is quite impossible to them, as in the sick themselves, who will not make the effort to do what is perfectly possible to them.

For instance, to the large majority of very weak patients, it is quite impossible to take any solid food before 11 A.M., nor then, if their strength is still further exhausted by fasting till that hour....A spoonful of beef-tea, of arrowroot, and wine, of egg flip, every hour, give them the requisite nourishment, and prevent them from being too much exhausted to take, at a later hour, the solid food which is necessary for their recovery....

To leave the patient's untasted food by his side from meal to meal, in hopes that he will eat it in the interval, is simply to prevent him from taking any food at all....A patient should, if possible, not see or smell either the food of others, or a greater amount of food than he himself can consume at one time, or ever hear food talked about or see it in the raw state....

That the more alone an invalid can be when taking food the better is unquestionable, and, even if he must be fed, the nurse should not allow him to talk, or talk to him, especially about food, while eating....

You cannot be too careful as to quality in sick diet: a nurse should never put before a patient milk that is sour, meat or soup that is turned, an egg that is bad, or vegetables underdone.

Chapter 7. What Food

Common errors in diet....One is the belief that beef-tea is the most nutritive of all food articles. Now, just try and boil down a pound of beef into beef-tea, evaporate your beef-tea and see what is left of your beef....Eggs, again, it is an ever ready saw that an egg is equivalent to a lb. of meat, whereas it is not at all so. Also, it is seldom noticed with how many patients, particularly of nervous or bilious temperament, eggs disagree....

Milk and the preparations from milk are a most important article of food for the sick. Butter is the lightest kind of animal fat, and though it wants the sugar and some of the other elements which are there in milk, yet it is most valuable both in itself and enabling the patient to eat more bread. Flour, oats, groats, barley, and their kind are, as we have already said, preferable in all their preparations to all the preparations of arrowroot, sago, tapioca, and their kind. Cream, in many long chronic diseases, is quite irreplaceable by any other article whatever. It seems to act in the same manner as beef-tea, and to most it is much easier of digestion than milk. In fact, it seldom disagrees. Cheese is not usually digestible by the sick, but it is pure nourishment for repairing waste, and I have seen sick, and not a few either, whose craving for cheese showed how much it was needed for them.

In the diseases produced by bad food, such as scorbutic dysentery and diarrhea, the patient's stomach often craves for and digests things, some of which certainly would be laid down in no dietary that ever was invented for sick, and especially not for such sick. These are fruit, pickles, jams, gingerbread, fat of ham or of bacon, suet, cheese, butter, milk. These cases I have seen, not by ones nor by tens, but by hundreds. And the patient's stomach was right, and the book was wrong....

There is often a marked difference between men and women in this matter of sick feeding. Women's digestion is generally slower...

But, if fresh milk is so valuable food for the sick, the least change or sourness in it makes it, of all articles perhaps, the most injurious; diarrhea is a common result of fresh milk allowed to become at all sour....

In laying down rules of diet by the amounts of "solid nutriment" in different kinds of food, it is constantly lost sight of what the patient requires to repair his waste, what he can take, and what he can't. You cannot diet a patient from a book; you cannot make up the human body as you would make up a prescription—so many parts "carboniferous," so many parts "nitrogenous," will constitute a perfect diet for the patient. The nurse's observation here will materially assist the doctor—the patient's "fancies" will materially assist the nurse.

For instance, sugar is one of the most nutritive of all articles, being pure carbon, and is particularly recommended in some books. But the vast majority of patients in England, young and old, male and female, rich and poor, hospital and private, dislike sweet things, and, while I have never known a person take to sweets when he was ill, who disliked them when he was well, I have known many fond of them when in health, who in sickness would leave off anything sweet, even to sugar in tea—sweet puddings, sweet drinks, are their aversion—the furred tongue almost always likes what is sharp or pungent. Scorbutic patients are an exception; they often crave for sweetmeats and jams.

Jelly is another article of diet in great favor with nurses and friends of the sick; even if it could be eaten solid, it would not nourish, but it is simply the height of folly to take 1/8 oz. of gelatine and make it into a certain bulk by dissolving it in water, and then to give it to the sick as if the mere bulk represented nourishment....

Chemistry has as yet afforded little insight into the dieting of the sick. All that chemistry can tell us is the amount of "carboniferous" or "nitrogenous" elements discoverable in different dietetic articles. It has given us lists of dietetic substances, arranged in order of their richness in one or other of these principles, but that is all. In the great majority of cases, the stomach of the patient is guided by other principles....No doubt, in this as in other things, Nature has very definite rules for her guidance, but these rules can only be ascertained by the most careful observation at the bedside. She teaches us that living chemistry, the chemistry of reparation, is something different from the chemistry of the laboratory. Organic chemistry is useful, as all knowledge is when we come face to face with Nature, but it by no means follows that we should learn in the laboratory any one of the reparative processes going on in disease.

Again, the nutritive power of milk and of the preparations of milk, is very much undervalued; there is nearly as much nourishment in half a pint of milk as there is in a quarter of a lb. of meat. But this is not the whole question or nearly the whole. The main question is what the patient's stomach can assimilate or derive nourishment from, and of this the patient's stomach is the sole judge. Chemistry cannot tell this. The diet which will keep the healthy man healthy will kill the sick one....

Home-made bread or brown bread is a most important article of diet for many patients. The use of aperients [laxatives] may be entirely superseded by it. Oat cake is another.

To watch for the opinions, then, which the patient's stomach gives, rather than to read "analyses of foods," is the business of all those who have to settle what the patient is to eat—perhaps the most important thing to be provided for him after the air he is to breathe....

A great deal too much against tea is said by wise people, and a great deal too much of tea is given to the sick by foolish people. When you see the natural and almost universal craving in English sick for their "tea," you cannot but feel that nature knows what she is about. But a little tea or coffee restores them quite as much as a great deal, and a great deal of tea and especially of coffee impairs the little power of digestion they have....

Cocoa is often recommended to the sick in lieu of tea or coffee. But, independently of the fact that English sick very generally dislike cocoa, it has quite a different effect from tea or coffee. It is an oily starchy nut, having no restorative power at all, but simply increasing fat. It is pure mockery of the sick, therefore, to call it a substitute for tea.

Chapter 8. Bed and Bedding

A few words upon bedsteads and bedding, and principally as regards patients who are entirely, or almost entirely, confined to bed. Feverishness is generally supposed to be a symptom of fever—in nine cases out of ten it is a symptom of bedding. The patient has had reintroduced into the body the emanations from himself, which, day after day and week after week, saturate his unaired bedding...

If you consider that an adult in health exhales by the lungs and skin in the twenty four hours three pints at least of moisture, loaded with organic matter ready to enter into putrefaction, that in sickness the quantity is often greatly increased, the quality is always more noxious—just ask yourself next where does all this moisture go? Chiefly into the bedding, because it cannot go anywhere else. And it stays there because, except perhaps a weekly change of sheets, scarcely any other airing is attempted....

The only way of really nursing a real patient is to have an *iron* bedstead, with rheocline springs, which are permeable by the air up to the very mattress (no vallance, of course), the mattress to be a thin hair one, the bed to be not above 3½ feet wide.

If the patient be entirely confined to his bed, there should be *two* such bedsteads, each bed to be "made" with mattress, sheets, blankets, etc., complete—the patient to pass twelve hours in each bed, on no account to carry his sheets with him. The whole of the bedding to be hung up to air for each intermediate twelve hours. Of course, there are many cases where this cannot be done at all–many more where only an approach to it can be made. I am indicating the ideal of nursing, and what has actually been done....

A patient's bed should always be in the lightest spot in the room, and he should be able to see out of window....

It may be worthwhile to remark that, where there is any danger of bedsores, a blanket should never be placed *under* the patient. It retains damp and acts like a poultice.

Chapter 9. Light

It is the unqualified result of all my experience with the sick that, second only to their need of fresh air, is their need of light, that, after a close room, what hurts them most is a dark room, and that it is not only light, but direct sunlight, they want.... People think the effect is upon the spirits only. This is by no means the case....Without going into any scientific exposition, we must admit that light has quite real and tangible effects upon the human body....

A very high authority in hospital construction has said that people do not enough consider the difference between wards and dormitories in planning their buildings. But I go further and say that healthy people never remember the difference between *bed*rooms and *sick* rooms in making arrangements for the sick. To a sleeper in health, it does not signify what the view is from his bed....

But the case is exactly reversed with the sick, even should they be as many hours out of their beds as you are in yours, which probably they are not. Therefore, that they should be able, without raising themselves or turning in bed, to see out of a window from their beds, to see sky and sunlight at least, if you can show them nothing else, I assert to be, if not of the very first importance for recovery, at least something very near it....

Again, the morning sun and the midday sun—the hours when they are quite certain not to be up—are of more importance to them, if a choice must be made, than the afternoon sun....

It is hardly necessary to add that there are acute cases (particularly a few ophthalmic cases and diseases where the eye is morbidly sensitive), where a subdued light is necessary. But a dark north room is inadmissible even for these....

Heavy, thick, dark window or bed curtains should, however, hardly ever be used for any kind of sick in this country. A light white curtain at the head of the bed is, in general, all that is necessary, and a green blind to the window, to be drawn down only when necessary....

Without sunlight, we degenerate body and mind. One of the greatest observers of human things (not physiological) [statistician L.A.J. Quetelet], says, in another language [French], "Where there is sun, there is thought." All physiology goes to confirm this. Where is the shady side of deep valleys, there is cretinism. Where are cellars and unsunned sides of narrow streets, there is the degeneracy and weakness of the human race—mind and body equally degenerating. Put the pale withering plant and human being into the sun, and, if not too far gone, each will recover health and spirit.

It is a curious thing to observe how almost all patients lie with their faces turned to the light, exactly as plants always make their way toward the light.

Chapter 10. Cleanliness of Rooms and Walls

It cannot be necessary to tell a nurse that she should be clean or should keep her patient clean—seeing that the greater part of nursing consists in preserving cleanliness. No ventilation can freshen a room or ward where the most scrupulous cleanliness is not observed....

Without cleanliness, you cannot have all the effect of ventilation; without ventilation, you can have no thorough cleanliness.

Very few people, be they of what class they may, have any idea of the exquisite cleanliness required in the sickroom. For much of what is here said applies less to the hospital than to the private sickroom....

"What can't be cured must be endured," is the very worst and most dangerous maxim for a nurse which ever was made. Patience and resignation in her are, but, other words for carelessness or indifference—contemptible if in regard to herself, culpable if in regard to her sick.

Chapter 11. Personal Cleanliness

Ventilation and skin cleanliness equally essential. The amount of relief and comfort experienced by sick after the skin has been carefully washed and dried is one of the commonest observations made at a sickbed. But it must not be forgotten that the comfort and relief so obtained are not all. They are, in fact, nothing more than a sign that the vital power have been relieved by removing something that was oppressing them....

Just as it is necessary to renew the air round a sick person frequently, to carry off morbid effluvia from the lungs and skin, by maintaining free ventilation, so it is necessary to keep the pores of the skin free from all obstructing excretions. The object both of ventilation and of skin cleanliness is pretty much the same, to wit, removing noxious matter from the system as rapidly as possible.

Care should be taken in all these operations of sponging, washing, and cleansing the skin not to expose too great a surface at once, so as to check the perspiration, which would renew the evil in another form....

In several forms of diarrhea, dysentery, etc., where the skin is hard and harsh, the relief afforded by washing with a great deal of soft soap is incalculable. In other cases, sponging with tepid soap and water, then with tepid water and drying with a hot towel, will be ordered.

Every nurse ought to be careful to wash her hands very frequently during the day. If her face too, so much the better....

Compare the dirtiness of the water in which you have washed when it is cold without soap, cold with soap, hot with soap. You will find the first has hardly removed any dirt at all, the second—a little more, the third a great deal more....

Washing, however, with a large quantity of water, has quite other effects than those of mere cleanliness. The skin absorbs the water and becomes softer and more perspirable. To wash with soap and soft water is, therefore, desirable from other points of view than that of cleanliness. But the water must be soft.

Chapter 12. Chattering Hopes and Advices

Wonderful is the face with which many friends, lay and medical, will come in and worry the patient with recommendations to do something or other, having just as little knowledge as to its being feasible or even safe for him, as if they were to recommend a man to take exercise, not knowing he had broken his leg....

No mockery in the world is so hollow as the advice showered upon the sick....How little the real sufferings of illness are known or understood. How little does anyone in good health fancy him or even herself into the life of a sick person.

Do you who are about the sick or who visit the sick try and give them pleasure, remember to tell them what will do so....A sick person does so enjoy hearing good news, for instance, of a love and courtship while in progress to a good ending. If you tell him only when the marriage takes place, he loses half the pleasure, which God knows he has little enough of, and ten to one, but you have told him of some lovemaking with a bad ending....

Tell him one benevolent act which has really succeeded practically—it is like a day's health to him.

A small pet animal is often an excellent companion for the sick, for long chronic cases especially. A bird in a cage is sometimes the only pleasure of an invalid confined for years to the same room. If he can feed and clean the animal himself, he ought always to be encouraged and assisted to do so. An invalid, in giving an account of his nursing by a nurse and a dog, infinitely preferred that of the dog; "above all, it did not *talk*." ...

Do observe these things, especially with invalids. Do remember how their life is is to them disappointed and incomplete. You see them lying there with miserable disappointments from which they can have no escape but death, and you can't remember to tell them of what would give them so much pleasure, or at least an hour's variety. They don't want you to be lachrymose and whining with them—they like you to be fresh and active and interested, but they cannot bear absence of mind, and are so tired of the advice and preaching they receive from everybody.

Chapter 13. Observation of the Sick

The most important practical lesson that can be given to nurses is to teach them what to observe—how to observe—what symptoms indicate improvement—what is the reverse—which are of importance—which are of none—which are the evidence of neglect—and of what kind of neglect.

All this is what ought to make part, and an essential part, of the training of every nurse. At present how few there are, either professional or unprofessional, who know at all whether any sick person they may be with is better or worse....

Leading questions useless or misleading....The question is generally a leading question, and it is singular that people never think what must be the answer to this question before they ask it, for instance, "Has he had a good night?" Now, one patient will think he has a bad night if he has not slept ten hours without waking. Another does not think he has a bad night if he has had intervals of dosing occasionally....

Why cannot the question be asked, How many hours' sleep has __ had? and at what hours of the night? This is important because on this depends what the remedy will be. If a patient sleeps two or three hours early in the night, and then does not sleep again at all, ten to one it is not a narcotic he wants, but food or stimulus, or perhaps only warmth. If on the other hand, he is restless and awake all night, and is drowsy in the morning, he probably wants sedatives, either quiet, coolness or medicine, a lighter diet, or all four....

It is useless to go through all the particulars, besides sleep, in which people have a peculiar talent for gleaning inaccurate information. As to food, for instance, I often think that most common question, How is your appetite? can only be put because the questioner believes the questioned has really nothing the matter with him....Again, the question, How is your appetite? is often put when How is your digestion? is the question meant. No doubt the two things often depend on one another. But they are quite different....

There may be four different causes, any one of which will produce the same result, viz., the patient slowly starving to death from want of nutrition.

1. Defect in cooking;
2. Defect in choice of diet;
3. Defect in choice of hours for taking diet;
4. Defect of appetite in patient

Yet all these are generally comprehended in the one sweeping assertion that the patient has "no appetite."

Surely many lives might be saved by drawing a closer distinction, for the remedies are as diverse as the causes. The remedy for the first is to cook better; for the second to choose other articles of diet; for the third to watch for the hours when the patient is in want of food; for the fourth to show him what he likes, and sometimes unexpectedly. But no one of these remedies will do for any other of the defects not corresponding with it....

Again, the question is sometimes put, Is there diarrhea? and the answer will be the same whether it is just merging into cholera, whether it is a trifling degree brought on by some trifling indiscretion, which will cease the moment the cause is removed, or whether there is no diarrhea at all, but simply relaxed bowels....

In the case of infants, *everything* must depend upon the accurate observation of the nurse or mother who has to report. And how seldom is this condition of accuracy fulfilled. It is the real test of a nurse whether she can nurse a sick infant....

Almost all superstitions are owing to defective knowledge, to bad observation, the *post hoc, ergo propter hoc* [after this, therefore because of this], and bad observers are almost all superstitious. Farmers used to attribute disease among cattle to witchcraft....

The nurse's attention should be directed to the extreme variation there is not unfrequently in the pulse of such patients during the day. A very common case is this: between 3 and 4 A.M. the pulse becomes quick, perhaps 130, and so thready it is not like a pulse at all, but like a string vibrating just underneath the skin. After this, the patient gets no more sleep. About midday the pulse has come down to 80, and, though feeble and compressible, is a very respectable pulse. At night, if the patient has had a day of excitement, it is almost imperceptible. But, if the patient has had a good day, it is stronger and steadier and not quicker than at midday....

A nurse ought to be able to understand what the variations of the pulse imply, what its character indicates. It is not the absolute rate of the pulse, which it signifies so much, for you to know. At least, you ought to be able to form an accurate enough guess at its rate without counting. It is the character of the pulse which signifies. There is the "splashing" pulse, which implies aneurysm. There is the pulse without an edge, which feels not like a ribbon, but a thread running along a space which it does not fill. There is the intermittent pulse of heart disease, the pulse of acute pleurisy, the pulse of peritonitis, the throbbing pulse which indicates acute inflammation or risk of hemorrhage. There is the rapid pulse of exhaustion in fever, which is the sign that the time has come for wine and stimulants....

In dwelling upon the vital importance of *sound* observation, it must never lose sight of what observation is for. It is not for the sake of piling up miscellaneous information or curious facts, but for the sake of saving life and increasing health and comfort....

And remember every nurse should be one who is to be depended upon, in other words, capable of being a "confidential" nurse. She does not know how soon she may find herself placed in such a situation; she must be no gossip, no vain talker; she should never answer questions about her sick, except to those who have a right to ask them; she must, I need not say, be strictly sober and honest, but more than this, she must be a religious and devoted woman; she must have a respect for her own calling, because God's precious gift of life is often literally placed in her hands; she must be a sound and close and quick observer, and she must be a woman of delicate and decent feeling.

Conclusion

The whole of the preceding remarks apply even more to children and puerperal [birthing] women than to patients in general. They also apply to the nursing of surgical, quite as much as to that of medical, cases. Indeed, if it be possible, cases of external injury require such care even more than sick. In surgical wards, one duty of every nurse certainly is *prevention*. Fever, or hospital gangrene, or pyemia, or purulent discharge of some kind may else supervene. Has she a case of compound fracture, of amputation, or of erysipelas, it may depend very much on how she looks upon the things enumerated in these notes, whether one or other of these hospital diseases attacks her patient or not. If she allows her ward to become filled with the peculiar close fetid smell, so apt to be produced among surgical cases, especially where there is great suppuration and discharge, she may see a vigorous patient in the prime of life gradually sink and die, where, according to all human probability, he ought to have recovered. The surgical nurse must be ever on the watch, ever on her guard, against want of cleanliness, foul air, want of light, and of warmth.

Nevertheless, let no one think that, because *sanitary* nursing is the subject of these notes, therefore what may be called the handicraft of nursing is to be undervalued. A patient may be left to bleed to death in a sanitary palace. Another who cannot move himself may die of bedsores, because the nurse does not know how to change and clean him, while he has every requisite of air, light, and quiet....

To revert to children. They are much more susceptible than grown people to all noxious influences. They are affected by the same things, but much more quickly and seriously, viz., by want of fresh air, of proper warmth, want of cleanliness in house, clothes, bedding, or body, by startling noises, improper food, or want of punctuality, by dullness, and by want of light, by too much or too little covering in bed or when up, by want of the spirit of management generally in those in charge of them. One can, therefore, only press the importance as being yet greater in the case of children, greatest in the case of sick children, of attending to these things.

That which, however, above all, is known to injure children seriously is foul air, and most seriously at night. Keeping the rooms where they sleep tight shut up is destruction to them. And, if the child's breathing be disordered by disease, a few hours only of such foul air may endanger its life, even where no inconvenience is left by grown-up person in the same room....

Pathology teaches the harm that disease has done. But it teaches nothing more. We know nothing of the principle of health, the positive of which pathology is the negative, except from observation and experience. And nothing but observation and experience will teach us the ways to maintain or to bring back the state of health. It is often thought that medicine is the curative process. It is no such thing: medicine is the surgery of functions, as surgery proper is that of limbs and organs. Neither can do anything but remove obstructions: neither can cure; nature alone cures. Surgery removes the bullet out of the limb, which is an obstruction to cure, but nature heals the wound. So it is with medicine; the function of an organ becomes obstructed; medicine, so far as we know, assists nature to remove the obstruction, but does nothing more. And what nursing has to do in either case is to put the patient in the best condition for nature to act upon him.

Supplementary Chapter: What Is a Nurse?

This book takes away all the poetry of nursing, it will be said, and makes it the most prosaic of human things....

What is it to feel a *calling* for anything? Is it not to do your work in it to satisfy your own high idea of what is the *right*, the *best*, and not because you will be "found out" if you don't do it? This is the "enthusiasm" which everyone from a shoemaker to a sculptor must have in order to follow his "calling" properly. Now the nurse has to do, not with shoes or with chisel and marble, but with human beings, and if she, for her own satisfaction, does not look after her patients, no *telling* will make her capable of doing so.

* * * * *

REFERENCES

Bathurst Free Press and Mining Journal [New South Wales]. (1860, June 13). Ventilation of the sick room, 3.

Boyd, J. (2005). *The excellent doctor Blackwell: The life of the first woman physician*. Stroud, Australia: Sutton. ISBN: 9780750941402.

Cook, E. T. (1913). *The life of Florence Nightingale* (Vol. 2, pp. 437–458). London, UK: Macmillan.

Cornwall Chronicle [Tasmania] (1860, May 23). Review, 2.

Empire [Sydney]. (1860, May 9). Victoria, 5.

Florence Nightingale's notes on nursing. (1860, July 16). *The Mercury* [Hobart, Tas.]. 3.

Gawande, A. (2004). Notes of a surgeon: On washing hands. *New England Journal of Medicine, 350*, 1283–1286. doi:10.1056/NEJMp048025

Hampshire Advertiser & Salisbury Guardian. (1860, January 21). Notes on nursing: What it is and what it is not, 6.

Hawke's Bay Herald. (1860, July 14). Review, 1.

Hobart Town Daily Mercury [Tasmania]. (1860, May 25). Latest from Europe, Florence Nightingale's notes on nursing, 3.

Holmes, O. W. (1861). *Currents and counter-currents in medical science: Other addresses and essays.* Boston, MA: Ticknor & Fields.

Illawarra Mercury. (1860, July 27). A sensible word on disease.

Launceston Examiner [Tasmania]. (1860, May 19). Children's diseases, 2.

Liverpool Mercury. (1860, January 29). Miss Florence Nightingale on nursing the sick.

McDonald, L. (Ed.). (2001–2012). *Collected works of Florence Nightingale*, 16V. Waterloo, ON, Canada: Wilfred Laurier University Press.

McDonald, L. (Ed.). (2011). *Florence Nightingale on wars and the war office.* Waterloo, ON, Canada: Wilfrid Laurier University Press. ISBN: 978-1-55458-382-9.

McDonald, L. (Ed.). (2012). *Florence Nightingale and hospital reform.* Waterloo, ON, Canada: Wilfrid Laurier University Press. ISBN: 978-0-88920-471-3.

Nelson Examiner and New Zealand Chronicle. (1860, June 13), 4.

Nightingale, F. (1858a). *Answers to written questions addressed to Miss Nightingale by the Commissioners. Report of the Commissioners appointed to inquire into the regulations affecting the sanitary condition of the Army and the treatment of the sick and wounded* (pp. 361–394) London, UK: Her Majesty's Stationery Office.

Nightingale, F. (1858b). *Notes on matters affecting the health, efficiency, and hospital administration of the British Army.* London, UK: Harrison.

Nightingale, F. (1858c, September 22). *Part I: Notes on the Health of Hospitals, and Part II: Sixteen sanitary defects in the construction of hospital wards.* Papers given at the National Association for the Promotion of Social Science. Liverpool, UK: Manuscript, Liverpool Record Office.

Nightingale, F. (1859a). Notes on the sanitary condition of hospitals, and on the defects in the construction of hospital wards. In *Transactions of the National Association for the Promotion of Social Science 1858* (pp. 462–482). London, UK: John W. Parker & Son.

Nightingale, F. (1859b). *Nightingale, notes on hospitals, being two papers read before the National Association for the Promotion of Social Science, at Liverpool, in October 1858, with evidence given to the Royal Commissioners on the State of the Army in 1857* (2nd ed.) London, UK: John W. Parker.

Nightingale, F. (1860a). *Notes on nursing: What it is, and what it is not.* London, UK: Harrison.

Nightingale, F. (1860b). *Notes on nursing: What it is, and what it is not.* Rev., enlarged. London, UK: Harrison.

Nightingale, F. (1861). *Notes on nursing for the labouring classes.* London, UK: Harrison.

Nightingale, F. (1863). *Notes on hospitals.* (3rd ed.). London, UK: Longmans, Green.

Nightingale, F. (1867). *Suggestions on the subject of providing training and organizing nurses for the sick poor in workhouse infirmaries* (pp. 64–76). London, UK: Her Majesty's Stationery Office.

Nightingale, F. (1883). Nurses, training of and nursing the sick. In R. Quain (Ed.), *A dictionary of medicine* (pp. 1038–1049). London, UK: Longman, Green.

Nightingale, F. (1992). *Notes on nursing: What it is and what it is not* (Commemorative edition). Philadelphia, PA: J.B. Lippincott. ISBN: 0397550073.

Perth Gazette and Independent Journal of Politics and News [Western Australia]. (1860, July 27). *Miss Nightingale's Notes on Nursing.*

Saturday Evening Post. (1860, March 10 to May 26).

Scientific American. (1860, July 2). Tea, coffee, and cocoa for the sick. *Scientific American, 3.* Retrieved from https://app2.scientificamerican.com/magazine/sa/1860/07-02/

Skretkowicz, V. (Ed.)., (1996). *Florence Nightingale's notes on nursing.* London, UK: Baillière Tindall. ISBN: 1-871364-63-9.

South Australian Advertiser. (1860, April 20). Miss Nightingale's notes, 3.

South Australian Register. (1860, July 30). Miss Nightingale's *Notes on Nursing, 3.*

Sydney Morning Herald. (1860, May 25). Bed fever, 8.

The Times. (1858, October 15 & 16). National Association of Social Science, 6EF and 7F.

The Times. (1930, February 8). St. Martin's Lane, 21C.

Toronto Globe. (1860, February 13 and 21). *Notes on Nursing,* 4 and 2.

Young, D. A. B. (1995, December 23–30). Florence Nightingale's fever. *British Medical Journal, 311,* 1697–1700.

Chapter 11: Nightingale's Writing on Nursing for the Poorest

Years ago, when I visited in one of the great London workhouses, I felt that visiting had no other effect but to break the visitor's heart. To nurse efficiently is what is wanted.

—Nightingale (letter, October 13, 1864,
Cambridge University Library and Archives, Add 8546/1/170)

Reforming the workhouse infirmaries had long been on Nightingale's heart when she started her nursing school in 1860. She had the chance in 1865, thanks to the offer of philanthropist William Rathbone to fund trained nursing in one workhouse, Liverpool—qualified nurses had to be paid a decent salary, while the old "pauper nurses" got only a token pay, typically spent on alcohol. Thanks to Rathbone's "munificence," Nightingale could now finally act. The experiment brought good results; the workhouse authorities found that more patients got better and could leave. This saved them money, and they agreed to take over the funding for the nursing staff.

When a scandal arose in 1865 owing to a lack of nursing care in a London workhouse infirmary, which caused a man's death, Nightingale used the ensuing press coverage to argue for a wider reform (McDonald, 2010, pp. 141–151). The bad publicity led to the doctors and medical journals taking up the issue.

BRIEF TO A PARLIAMENTARY COMMITTEE, 1867

That there has been hitherto nothing of nursing but the name in workhouse infirmaries in general, I believe the committee and I shall be agreed.

—Nightingale (1867, p. 64)

The British government's response to revelations of lack of care was to establish a Parliamentary committee in 1867 on workhouse infirmaries, preliminary to bringing in new legislation. Nightingale's brief to it, however, had little to do with its ostensible subject, the necessary minimum cubic space needed in workhouse infirmaries. She was no expert on such technicalities, although her brief shows that she mastered the key points. Rather, she argued that, for the care of the patient, the superficial area was more important than cubic space. Nightingale then bootlegged her concerns about good nursing care, which required that scarce commodity, the trained nurse, into her remarks.

The Times gave her good coverage, publishing a lengthy, detailed, article on the brief, focusing on her core concern of training rather than cubic space (*The Times*, 1867).

At the time she wrote the brief, very few workhouses, the hospitals used by the vast majority of patients, had any trained nurses on their staff giving patient care. Some just had one trained nurse who acted as the manager. Otherwise, the people called "nurses" were pauper inmates.

Nightingale offered to arrange for trained nurses in one of the London workhouse infirmaries, doubtless an attractive offer, and one consistent with her belief in the need to see the first results before extending any new reform. It turned out to be Highgate, the new location of the old St. Pancras Workhouse.

It is also clear that her aim was the establishment of a regular, professional, nursing service at workhouse infirmaries, with possibilities of promotion based on merit. She asserted the necessity of nurses controlling the nursing, not a male manager or doctor. Nightingale throughout her life strenuously insisted that nurses control the hiring, promotion, discipline, and dismissal of nurses. Doctors would give medical orders on their cases, but they would have to take any complaints they had about the nursing care to the director of nursing.

The brief is noteworthy also for stating a core belief of Nightingale's that the sick poor deserve to be well cared for. She accepted harsh treatment for those who would later be called the "willfully unemployed," although she did not believe that there were many. When a poor man or woman became sick, however, "he [or she] ceases, by the fact, from being the legitimate object of any such repressive measure." Indeed, it was good economy "to cure him [or her] as quickly as possible," so that the patient could return to work and cease causing expense to the taxpayer. Her high principle, in short, was also sound economics for the whole society.

Nightingale recognized that the stigma of the workhouse would affect the reputation of any infirmary as a hospital. Thus, she urged a strict separation in administration between the two buildings, which were no better related, she quipped, than an infirmary with a railway. This, in fact, was gradually done, and indeed workhouse infirmaries were renamed to give them a new identity. Many were, in time, amalgamated with regular hospitals, so great were the improvements in the care they gave and the training they provided. The (model) Chorlton Union Workhouse Infirmary, near Manchester, became Withington Hospital, later to be incorporated into the University Hospitals of South Manchester. The Shoreditch Workhouse Infirmary was renamed St. Leonard's Hospital in 1920; the St. Marylebone Workhouse Infirmary became St. Charles Hospital in 1930.

* * * * *

Source: Florence Nightingale. (1867). Brief to the Committee Appointed to consider Cubic Space of Metropolitan Workhouses.

In order to reply in detail to the request I have had the honor to receive through you, from the committee appointed by the president of the Poor Law Board, for suggestions on the subject of providing training and organizing nurses for the sick poor in workhouse infirmaries, I begin by taking it for granted that we understand the same thing as to what is meant by the word "nursing." The word "nursing" has very much improved in its meaning during the last ten years, and is improving its meaning every year more and more.

That there has been hitherto nothing of nursing but the name in workhouse infirmaries *in general*, I believe the committee and I shall be agreed. But, as a great experiment has been now for eighteen months in operation to nurse the Liverpool Workhouse Infirmary by trained nurses, as there are few or none of the London workhouses which have not now one or two or more paid head nurses, and as I read the terms of the question which the committee have done me the honor of putting to me, I will take for granted that the intention is now really to inquire into the best system of nursing (best as conducing to the cure of the sick), and how to obtain it, and that there is no difference of opinion as to what nursing *is*.

Latterly there has been all over England a great movement to substitute for "paid nursing" paid TRAINED nursing. And, as it is not the payment but the training which makes the high efficiency of the medical officer, so and still more in the case of the nurse, it is not the payment but the training of the nurse which makes her efficiency (though high efficiency will always be highly paid).

Method of Improving the Supply of Trained Nurses

Supposing that an efficient staff was obtained to undertake the nursing of one large workhouse infirmary and that the superintendent were to proceed to train nurses, the next question is, how to train? A reply to this question is furnished by our experience and, resting on this, the following system, or something like, might be adopted.

It has answered sufficiently for all practical purposes, and would probably answer in a workhouse infirmary where the required number of patients and the means of training were to be found. I would add what I think is important, that there is this advantage in organizing a special infirmary nursing service, an advantage which attaches to any regular service, namely, that a prospect of promotion may be held out, not, of course, by seniority, but by selection for superior merit and distinguished service, in which the length of service would be considered. . . .

Supposing, then, for the sake of argument, that you have the means of training, namely, a capable matron, medical officers willing to help, and suitable material, probably you could not do better than frame your procedure on the Rules for Admission and Training Nurses at St. Thomas' and King's College Hospitals under the "Nightingale Fund." The probationer [student] nurses at St. Thomas' are trained in general nursing duties, those at King's College Hospital especially in midwifery and midwifery nursing. The following are the steps in the process of training.

Every woman applying for admission is required to fill up the Form of Application, which is supplied to her by the matron of St. Thomas' Hospital on the application. . . . After being received on a month's trial and trained for a month, if the woman shows sufficient aptitude and character, and is herself desirous to complete her training, she is required to come under the obligation, . . . binding her to enter into hospital service for at least four years. This is the only recompense the committee exact for the costs and advantages of training.

The List of Duties . . . is put into the hands of every probationer on entering the service as a general instruction for her guidance, and she is checked off by the matron and "sister" (head nurses) in these same duties.

Relation of Hospital Management to Efficient Nursing

The nature of the hospital authority is as important as the provision of trained nurses, as these nurses have to perform their duties under this authority itself. Unless an understanding is arrived on this point, the very existence of good nursing is an impossibility. In dealing with this question, I may state at once that to turn any number of trained nurses into a workhouse infirmary to act under the superintendence or instructions of any workhouse master, or workhouse matron or medical officer would be a sheer waste of good money. This is not matter of opinion, but of fact and experience. The "original sin" of this part of the workhouse infirmary system, or no system, has been (a) the nature of the authority; and (b) the nature of the nursing material on which the authority has been exercised.

There has never been any express provision made for the care of the sick in workhouses. The reception of sick is, in them, an accident, an excrescence. The law is perfectly right in limiting the comforts of able-bodied poor in workhouses to those required simply for preserving life in health. There must be some check on the constant tendency for a certain class to descend into pauperism.... However, the very opposite conditions are required to cure the sick, and the very opposite is the object.

By curing the sick you prevent pauperism, both for themselves and their families, and you do not cure the sick by the measures which repress pauperism. From the instant the poor man becomes sick, he ceases, by the fact, from being the legitimate object of any such repressive measure. On the contrary, the best policy and economy (leaving motives of humanity out of the question) are to cure him as quickly as possible, so that he may return to his work and cease to be a cause of expense to the rates [taxes].

The principle is so obvious a one that it is scarcely necessary to enunciate it were it not that it must be prominently recognized if we are to improve the administration. To make improvement possible in the nursing of workhouse infirmaries, the very best workhouse master and mistress would, from their very efficiency against the spread of pauperism, be the very worst to place over any efficient nursing staff (There is, besides, absolutely no more real connection between an infirmary and a workhouse than between an infirmary and a railway establishment.).

I have made special inquiry as to the superficial area found to be required for efficient nursing in those hospitals where nurses are trained under the "Nightingale Fund." At King's College Hospital, it is found that 105 square feet is sufficient for good nursing and ward administration, except in the lying-in [maternity] wards, where the superficial area is much more. I have already given the space in old St. Thomas' at 101 square feet. When the plans of the new St. Thomas' were under consideration, it was at one time proposed to give as much as 120 sq. ft. per bed, but the exigencies of the site rendered it necessary to reduce this amount to 112 sq. ft., which, I am informed, is sufficient.

All these superficial areas are intended for general hospitals, but it is in the highest degree doubtful whether any of them would be enough for a lying-in or special hospital.

In fever hospitals, there is a great and constant sacrifice of life in the establishment itself. Scarcely a year passes in which some most valuable lives, both among medical and nursing attendants, are not lost in consequence of defective structural arrangements and bad sanitary conditions, under which they have to do their work.

It may be said that you must fit your nursing arrangements to your sick and not your sick to your nursing arrangements and that nurses must take their chance of fevers. Perfectly true as far as the sick are concerned, but most untrue as far as the hospital arrangements are concerned.

Every employer of labor is bound to provide for the health of the workers. And any society which professes to provide for sick, and so provides for them that the lives of nurses and medical officers have to be sacrificed in the discharge of their duty, gives sufficient proof that providing for the care of the sick is not its calling. For, as it happens, the arrangements required for the welfare of sick are the very same which is required for the health of nurses. However, in dealing with the question of superficial area required for nursing, it is said that the special class of cases to be nursed must be considered. We must also take into consideration the fact that many hospitals have large medical schools attached to them, wherein a ward where all the cases are of a severe character, a larger nursing staff and, in consequence, more area, is required than where all the cases are of a comparatively slight character.

Whatever apparent truth there may be in such a statement, we must not lose sight of the fact that nurses are there because patients are there, and not because case A is severe and case B is not severe. The previous question is whether there should be an infirmary with patients in it at all, and if this is decided in the affirmative, then a nursing staff, with the required conditions for good nursing, must be provided. If severe cases occur, a good superintendent or a good head nurse always economize her staff so as to provide attendance for them, except, for example, in a severe epidemic outbreak, such as cholera, when temporary assistance may be required.

It has been said that, a considerable proportion of the workhouse sick being infirm and aged, they cannot require such a good nursing as hospital sick require, but this is a mistake. Many of these are "helpless cases," "dirty cases." As such, they require more careful nursing than any, and must receive it in all good establishments for infirm and invalids, both in England and abroad. I cannot suppose that in any improved nursing arrangements, it can be contemplated to neglect this class of patients. However, as such distinctions have been made, it is necessary to refer to them. Again, it may not always be possible to define what cases are "acute" and what cases are "infirm," but this cannot alter the relation of nursing.

Summary

I have entered into considerable detail in the preceding remarks because it is absolutely indispensable that the relation of efficient infirmary nursing to training, organization, management, and construction should be thoroughly understood before a trustworthy decision can be arrived at on the question of your committee. Moreover, I shall conclude with a recapitulation of those requirements, without which any attempt, not at ostensibly improving (for that is to "keep the word of promise to our ear and break it to our hope"), but at really improving the nursing of the sick poor at present admitted into workhouses would be attended with results not worth the trouble and outlay.

1. Hired nurses, unless they are also *trained* nurses, are not worth their hire, unless by accident. There must be trained matrons (superintendents) to superintend trained nurses.
2. At the present time, it is impossible to obtain either trained matrons or trained nurses for the London workhouse infirmaries.
3. An attempt should be made (in which I should be glad to render any assistance in my power) to obtain, by training, a sufficient staff to undertake the work in one of the largest metropolitan workhouse infirmaries.
4. Every trained and organized nursing staff should, as one of its duties, undertake the training of nurses for infirmary work on some such plan as that, the details of which have been given earlier.
5. The government of the infirmary should in future be separated from the government of the workhouse as an indispensable condition for success.
6. The matron (superintendent) should be responsible to the government of the infirmary alone for the efficient discharge of her duties, and the nurses should be responsible to the matron alone for the discharge of their duties.
7. The larger the number of sick (up to 800 or 1000) under one hospital government and under one matron the better, both for economy and efficiency. Without consolidation of workhouse hospitals, a great and quite needless expenditure must be incurred in attempting to secure the conditions under which efficient nursing can be carried out.
8. It has been proved by experience that the efficiency of nursing is to a considerable extent dependent on hospital construction, and on the kind of accommodation provided for the nursing service.

TRIBUTE TO AGNES JONES, "UNA AND THE LION," 1868

The happiest people, the fondest of their occupation, the most thankful for their lives, are, in my opinion, those engaged in sick nursing.

—Nightingale (1868, p. 364)

Nightingale's article "Una and the Lion" was a tribute to Agnes Jones, the heroic director of nursing at the Liverpool Workhouse Infirmary, the first trained nurse to take on that kind of post. Jones died of typhus fever in her third year on the job. Like Nightingale, she came from a well-off family in which daughters were not expected to work. She also had a partial deafness to overcome. She trained at the Nightingale School at St. Thomas' Hospital, got some experience at another London hospital, and then took on this daunting job. Nightingale mentored her throughout.

Jones, like Nightingale, was deeply religious, and had, like her, spent time at the (Lutheran) Deaconess Institution at Kaiserswerth, Germany. An evangelical Christian, she seemed at first, to Nightingale and others, to be intolerant—Liverpool had a substantial Roman Catholic population, and the philanthropist behind the project was Unitarian. However, she became an effective nursing leader, liked and respected by people of every faith, or, in Nightingale's more colorful words, "Roman Catholic and Unitarian, high church and low church, all literally rose up and called her 'blessed.'" The tribute dwells much on her faith, and anyone interested in it should read the whole article (Nightingale, 1868, in McDonald, 2004, pp. 290–301).

Nightingale took the occasion to put in some practical material, on what was required to become a workhouse nurse—she hoped Jones's example would inspire applications, at a time when the school had difficulty attracting educated candidates. She noted usual salaries and gave the address where to apply. The article had the intended effect, several women who became leaders in British nursing were moved by reading "Una" to enroll in training.

Nightingale explained the need for *teams* of nurses to take on the nursing, not isolated nurses. This, she believed was necessary for any hospital starting professional nursing, but especially so in a workhouse, where the differences between the new professionals and the "pauper nurses" were even greater than with the "Sairey Gamps" of the unreformed, regular, hospitals. The risk was that the trained nurse would sink to the level of the old-style hospital nurse or, worse still, the "pauper nurse."

In the article, Nightingale also addressed the issue of sacrifice and martyrdom—Agnes Jones, after all, died young from a disease acquired at the infirmary. However, Jones's (deeply religious) family understood that she had died doing what she wanted to do, that her 3 years at Liverpool had been the most meaningful of her life. Nightingale in "Una" gave perhaps her most enthusiastic endorsement of nursing as a career, in the epigraph for this section, that the "happiest people" she knew were those who did "sick nursing."

Her expression was vigorous throughout. She remarked facetiously that to rely on "testimonials" for job applicants was hardly better than the Romans seeking advice from "a flight of crows." She evoked the witches of Macbeth: "They keep the word of promise to our ear, but break it to our hope" (Act 5, scene 8).

Harriet Beecher Stowe, the author of *Uncle Tom's Cabin*, was another person touched by "Una." She wrote a long letter to Nightingale with her comments on it, to which Nightingale sent a lengthy reply (Stowe letter, March 20, 1872, British Library Add Mss[1] 45803 f3, in McDonald, 2005, pp. 802–803; Nightingale letter, August 14, 1872, Radcliffe College Beecher Stowe Collection, folder 253, in McDonald, 2005, p. 804).

Nightingale recounted, in her address to nurses of 1872, that Harriet Beecher Stowe had "fallen in love with the character of our Agnes Jones," and asked about the progress of their work, "They wish to 'organize a similar movement' in America, a 'movement' of 'Una's,' what a great thing that would be!" (Nightingale, 1872a, May, in McDonald, 2005, p. 801).

Stowe's brother, the Rev. Henry Ward Beecher, had "Una" reprinted in the United States with a new introduction (Nightingale, 1872b).

* * * * *

Source: Florence Nightingale, Una and the lion. Good Words, 1868 (McDonald, 2004, pp. 296–298)

We require that a woman be sober, honest, truthful, without which there is no foundation on which to build. We train then in habits of punctuality, quietness, trustworthiness, personal neatness. We teach her how to manage the concerns of a large ward or establishment. We train her in dressing wounds and other injuries, and in performing all those minor operations which nurses are called upon day and night to undertake. We teach her how to manage helpless patients in regard to moving, changing, feeding, temperature, and the prevention of bedsores.

She has to make and apply bandages, line splints for fractures, and the like. She must know how to make beds with as little disturbance as possible

---

[1] Further references to Add Mss (Additional Manuscripts) are also to the British Library.

to their inmates. She is instructed how to wait at operations, and as to the kind of aid the surgeon requires at her hands. She is taught cooking for sick, the principles on which sick wards ought to be cleansed, aired, and warmed, the management of convalescents, and how to observe sick and maimed patients so as to give an intelligent and truthful account to the physician or surgeon in regard to the progress of cases in the intervals between visits, a much more difficult thing than is generally supposed.

We do not seek to make "medical women" [doctors] but simply nurses acquainted with the *principles* which they are required constantly to apply at the bedside. For the future superintendent is added a course of instruction in the administration of a hospital....

Hitherto we have been compelled to confine ourselves to sending out staffs of nurses to hospitals or workhouses, with a view to their becoming, in their turn, centers of training, because the applications we receive for trained nurses are far more numerous and urgent than we have power to answer. But, did a greater number of probationers [nursing students] suitable for superior situations offer themselves, we could provide additional means for training and answer applications for district nurses and many others. These probationers receive board, lodging, training, entirely free, a certain amount of uniform dress, and a small amount of pay during their year of training.

For the efficiency, comfort, and success of a nursing staff thus sent out it is, of course, essential that the trained nurses should not go without the trained superintendent, nor the trained superintendent without the trained nurses.

There are two requisites in a superintendent: (1) character and business capacity, (2) training and knowledge. Without the second, the first is of little avail. Without the first, the second is only partially useful, for we can't bring out of a person what is not in her. *We* can only become responsible for the training; the other qualifications can only be known by trial. Now to take superintendents or head nurses, as is done every day, by receiving and comparing of testimonials...this is hardly more to the purpose than to do as the Romans did, when they determined the course of conduct they should take by seeing whether there were a flight of crows.

The future superintendent would be a great deal the better for two years of training for so difficult and responsible a post. But such are the calls upon us that we can often give her scarcely one. If the lady in training for a superintendent can pay for her own board, it is, of course, right that she should do so (everything else is, in all cases, given free). At the present time, we are able to admit a few gentlewomen free of all expense, and with the small salary above mentioned during the year of training. We have applications from institutions in want of trained superintendents (or matrons), and trained head nurses for hospitals in India and in England and for a large workhouse infirmary....

I give a quarter of a century's European experience when I say that the happiest people, the fondest of their occupation, the most thankful for their lives, are, in my opinion, those engaged in sick nursing. In my opinion, it is a mere abuse of words to represent the life, as is done by some, as a sacrifice and a martyrdom. But there *have* been martyrs in it. The founders and pioneers of almost everything that is best must be martyrs. But these are the last ever to think themselves so. And, for all, there must be constant self-sacrifice for the good of all. But the distinction is this—the life is not a sacrifice—it is the engaging in an occupation the happiest of any. But the strong, the healthy, wills in any life must determine to pursue the common good at any personal cost, at daily sacrifice. And we must not think that any fit of enthusiasm will carry us through such a life as this. Nothing but the feeling that it is God's work more than ours, that we are seeking, His success and not our success, and that we have trained and fitted ourselves by every means which He has granted us to carry out His work, will enable us to go on.

* * * * *

FUND-RAISING FOR DISTRICT NURSING, 1876

Nursing requires the most undivided attention of anything I know, and all the health and strength, both of mind and body.

—Nightingale (1876)

Nightingale's (substantial) letter to the editor that follows was a plea for donations to support a residence for district nurses, trained nurses who provided care for the poor at home, so that they could avoid entering a workhouse infirmary. "Nursing the room," often in a tenement building, typically crowded, small, dark, and often dirty, was a requirement, but, teaching the mother or another family member how to give care and keep the room clean was another.

A nurses' residence was essential in Nightingale's time, for the nurses then would almost all be single women, the hours long, and such conveniences as takeout food, pizza deliveries, and microwave dinners simply did not exist. Nightingale accepted the long working day for nurses and students, but she always insisted on efficient working conditions, comfortable quarters, and a decent, cooked, meal at the end of the day, with a glass of wine.

Nightingale's environmental theory claimed that the physical environment of the home, be it a hovel or small, cramped, room, influenced, for better or worse, the course of the patient's healing. Nightingale also made the much-quoted statement that hospitals were "only an intermediate stage of civilization." She looked forward to their not being needed.

Nightingale's letter to *The Times* attracted a response by an anonymous critic in *The Lancet*. Her "noble example" during the Crimean War was superior to "the somewhat rambling and incoherent precepts" of this later, "wonderfully vague," project. The writer thought that the sick poor would be better removed "to a cheerful hospital, where they may receive not only the best of nursing, but many a hygienic lesson as well, which they may carry home with them" ("Letter to the editor", 1876, p. 611). This is a wildly optimistic assessment of the real hospital options the sick poor had at the time.

* * * * *

Source: Florence Nightingale, Trained nurses for the sick poor, *The Times*, April 14 1876, p. 6CD

The beginning has been made, the first crusade has been fought and won, to bring a truly *national* undertaking—real nursing, trained nursing—to the bedsides of cases wanting real nursing among the London sick poor, in the only way in which real nurses can be so brought to the sick poor, and this by providing a real home within reach of their work for the nurses to live in, a home which gives what real family homes are supposed to give: materially, a bedroom for each, dining, and sitting rooms in common, all meals prepared and eaten in the home; morally, direction, support, sympathy, in a common work, further training and instruction in it, proper rest and recreation and a head of the home who is also and preeminently trained and skilled head of the nursing—in short, a home where any good mother, of whatever class, would be willing to let her daughter, however attractive or highly educated, live. But all this costs money.

Allow an old nurse to say her word on what a district nurse is to be. This system, which twenty years ago was a paradox, twenty years hence will be a commonplace. If a nurse has to…cook for herself when she comes home "dog tired" from her patients, to do everything for herself, she cannot do real nursing, for nursing requires the most undivided attention of anything I know, and all the health and strength, both of mind and body. If, then, she has to provide for herself, she can only be half a nurse, and one of two things happens. Either she is of the level of her patients, or she sinks to the level of her patients and actually makes apologies for their dirt and disorderliness, instead of remedying these…. Nay, as the old hospital nurse did thirty years ago, she may even come to prey upon what is provided for her patients. There is a third alternative: that she breaks her heart….

What is a district nurse to do? A nurse is, first, a nurse. Secondly, to nurse the room as well as the patient, to put the room into nursing order, that is, to make the room such as a patient can recover in, to bring care and cleanliness into it, and to teach the inmates to keep up that care and cleanliness. Thirdly, to bring such sanitary defects as produce sickness and death, and, which can only be remedied by the public, to the notice of the public officer whom it concerns.

A nurse cannot be a cook (though sweet Jack Falstaff says she is), a relieving officer, district visitor, letter writer, general storekeeper, upholsterer, almoner [social worker], purveyor, lady bountiful, head dispenser, and medical comforts shop. A district nurse can, rather less than a hospital nurse, be all this, though, where things are wanting and wanted for recovery, she or her head know how and where to apply for them. There are agencies for all these things....

1.   A district nurse must first nurse. She must be of a yet higher class and of a yet fuller training than a hospital nurse, because she has not the doctor always at hand, because she has no hospital appliances at hand at all, and because she has to take notes of the case, for the doctor, who has no one but her to report to him. She is his staff of clinical clerks, dressers, and nurses. These district nurses—and it is the first time that it has even been done—keep records of the patient's state, including pulse, temperature, etc., for the doctor. One doctor stated that he knew when an operation ought to be performed by reading the nurse's report on the case. Another, that by hearing the nurse's history of the case, he found patients to be suffering from typhoid fever who had been reported as consumptive. A hospital doctor, who had admitted patients into hospital with the nurse's written history of the case "doubted if many of our medical students could have sent a better report." Further, if the hospital must "first of all be a place which shall do the sick no harm," this was even more important for the sick person's room.

2.   If a hospital must first of all be a place which shall do the sick no harm, how much more must the sick poor's room be made a place not to render impossible recovery from the sickness which it has probably bred? This is what the London district nurses do; they nurse the room as well as the patient, and teach the family to nurse the room. It requires a far higher stamp of woman to do this....

3.   A district nurse must bring to the notice of the officer of health, or proper authority, sanitary defects which he alone can remedy. Thus, dustbins [garbage cans] are emptied, waterbutts [tanks] cleaned, water supply and drainage examined and remedied which look as if this had not been done for 100 years.

Hospitals are but an intermediate stage of civilization. At present hospitals are the only place where the sick poor can be nursed or, indeed, often the sick rich. But the ultimate object is to nurse all sick at home. Where can the sick poor in general be sick? At home; it is there that the bulk of sick cases are. Where can nurses be trained for them? In hospitals; it is there only that skilled nurses can be trained. All this makes real nursing of the sick at home the most expensive kind of nursing at present. Yet no one would wish to convey the whole sick population into hospital, even were it possible, and even if it did not often break up the poor man's home....

All this costs money. The district nurses cost money and the district home costs money. Each district nurse must have, before she is qualified (1) a month's trial in district work, (2) a year's training in hospital nursing, (3) three months' training in district nursing under the superintendent-general....

I ask the public not to add one more charity or relief agency to the many that are already, but to support a charity truly *metropolitan* in its scope, and truly *national* if carried out, which never has been before. Subscriptions may be sent to the Secretary of the Metropolitan and National Nursing Association, 23 Bloomsbury Square, W.C.

* * * * *

REFERENCES

McDonald, L. (Ed.). (2004). *Florence Nightingale on public health care*. Waterloo, Canada: Wilfrid Laurier University Press. ISBN: 0-88920-446-2.

McDonald, L. (Ed.). (2005). *Florence Nightingale on women: Medicine, midwifery and pros-titution*. Waterloo, Canada: Wilfrid Laurier University Press. ISBN: 0-88920-466-7.

McDonald, L. (2010). *Florence Nightingale at first hand*. London, UK: Bloomsbury.

Nightingale, F. (1867, January 19). Brief to the committee appointed to consider cubic space of Metropolitan workhouses. *Paper No. 16. HMSO*, 64–76.

Nightingale, F. (1868, June). Una and the lion. *Good words* (pp. 360–366). London, UK: Strahan and Co.

Nightingale, F. (1872a). Address. *Claydon House Bundle*, 386.

Nightingale, F. (1872b). *"Una and her paupers," Memorials of Agnes Elizabeth Jones, by her sister*. Introductory preface by the Rev H.W. Beecher. New York, NY: G. Routledge.

Nightingale, F. (1876, April 14). Trained nurses for the sick poor. *The Times*, 6CD.

The Lancet (1876, April 22), *Letter to the editor*, 610.

The Times (1867, March 6). *Miss Nightingale on training of nurses*, 12C.

Chapter 12: Nightingale's Late Writing on Nursing, Hospitals, and Disease Prevention

In these later works, we see Nightingale's writing at its polished best, ideas that she first expressed in *Notes on Nursing* in 1860 now finely honed. To some extent, her new wordings reflect lessons learned from having to make the case for her point so many times. In other respects, she added material from new developments in medicine, nursing, and public health.

Her much-quoted definition of health dates from this late period, the second item, of 1883, not her far better known *Notes on Nursing*: "Health is not only to be well, but to be able to use well every power we have to use."

The impetus for the first article is not known, but the three following contributions were all solicited by others, a leading British doctor for his medical dictionary, an American newspaper for advice on an expected cholera epidemic, and lastly a paper for a world congress on women's charities meeting in Chicago.

HOSPITALS AND PATIENTS, 1880

> *Do we care for the patients in hospital? Hospitals were made for patients—not patients for hospitals.*
>
> —Nightingale (1880, p. 1)

Nightingale wrote this next paper in 1880 for publication in a progressive journal, *The Nineteenth Century*. It was set in print, but in fact not published there or anywhere else at the time. Now 20 years after the opening of her school, she could suggest that hospitals would come to consider that nursing schools were as necessary to them as medical schools. She also argued that training schools for nurses could only be at their best "where there *is* a medical school."

Nightingale highlighted the need for "the free outer air of public opinion" in hospitals as a means of preventing abuse, although her words were more positive, "to keep up the highest standard of care, including nursing care." As scandals of shoddy care hit the media today, the need for public opinion continues.

"Intelligent obedience" gets a mention, as it did in so many places, here with a negative reference to the "military discipline" of the Prussian Army for comparison. Nurses were not to be automatons.

* * * * *

Source: Florence Nightingale, Hospitals and patients, 1880, in McDonald, 2012, p. 829–833

Do we care for the patients in hospitals? Hospitals were made for patients—not patients for hospitals. Yet sometimes it would seem as though the patients were the only things left out of the consideration: the play of *Hamlet* with the part of Hamlet left out.

What is the "new system" of hospital nursing for?... Is it that we are to learn how to do the best for the sick, how to advance the methods for doing this best, how to educate men and women, the physicians and nurses, for the sick, how to advance science and practice for curing and preventing disease and smoothing the path of the dying and the incurable?...

What is true nurse craft? What is true nurse training? The essence, the object, of all training is *intelligent* obedience to medical orders, to teach the nurse how to obey intelligently, so that the orders which are for the good of the patients shall be carried out so as to be for the patients' good.

What possible meaning can be attached to military discipline or training, to the Prussian, for example, of which we have heard so much as being the highest standard—but to obey orders with the utmost intelligence and perfection of detail, which details must have been taught beforehand—but now they must be carried out not by an automaton, but by an intelligent human being who has to do with matters of life and death....

If "trained nurses" are less obedient to the medical authorities than charwomen nurses, it is not from training but from *want* of training—from defect in (so-called) training.... As well might we say that an educated physician knows less than the old village crone or bone setter. What possible meaning can be attached to the word "training" if it were otherwise?...

Ought not the nursing staff to hold much the same relation to the medical officers that the building staff does to the architect? That the nurse should know her business, that each individual employed by the builder should know his business, is of the first, the most essential, importance to the physician or surgeon as it is to the architect. It is indeed the *sine qua non* [without which there is nothing]. And how can either know his or her business if he or she is not trained to it?...

The training school for nurses can only be at its best where there *is* a medical school. This is almost a truism, most truly felt to be so by the best nurse.

It is not a cricket match that we are playing, with patients as balls, and [medical] students as one eleven against nurses as the other. The object is far other than this, it is that the whole building, civil administration, medical staff, and school, nursing staff and training school, matron and all, shall be one great and organized whole to be worked and harmonized for one purpose—that purpose the good of the patients—that which doctors and nurses alike are there for.

It is again a truism that the more the free outer air of public opinion is brought into the hospital the better, in order to keep up the highest standard of care, including nursing care, of the patients. The [medical] students are thus an advantage to the nursing, as a highly educated element among the trained nurses undoubtedly is to the [medical] students.... The time will soon come when the public, including especially "the doctors," will consider a great hospital incomplete without its training school for nurses as without its medical school for students....

We cannot enter here into technical points of what constitutes a good training school for nurses, what constitutes a failure. But there are two or three common sense points, and common sense applies, or ought to apply, to all things.... One is nothing can be more wholesome (for the patients) than a friendly rivalry between one ward head nurse (sister) and another, as to the respective merits of the visiting physicians and surgeons. If every head nurse thinks her physician or surgeon greater than any other, so much the better....

The convenience of the matron is a misnomer. The good of the patients *is* the convenience of the matron, of course, and of every official there.

It follows that the whole regulation of the nurse's life, including her hours of recreation, is to preserve a human being (who is not a piece of furniture) in such health of body and mind, as will enable her to do her duty best for the patients....

Do we care for the patients first and foremost? That is the last and the first keynote. The alpha and omega is, do we wisely care for the patients?

> *Do we care for the patients first and foremost? That is the last and the first keynote.*

—Nightingale (1880, p. 4)

* * * * *

DICTIONARY OF MEDICINE ARTICLES ON NURSE
TRAINING AND HOSPITAL NURSING, 1883

Health is not only to be well, but to be able to use well every power we have to use.
—Nightingale (1883, p. 1043 in McDonald, 2009, pp. 735–736, p. 1043)

Nightingale wrote two articles on nursing for Richard Quain's *Dictionary of Medicine*, in dictionary language, "Nurses, training of" and "Nursing the sick." The second meant hospital nursing only, thus excluding health promotion, community health, midwifery nursing, and military nursing. She even advised on the two articles Douglas Galton wrote for the *Dictionary*, on hospital construction and hospital administration. He read and advised on her two—Galton was an expert on hospital construction but deferred absolutely to her on all matters of nursing.

Nightingale's articles reflect the state of nursing in the late 1870s—the volume did not appear until 1883, but correspondence shows that she had written them earlier. Her school by then had been in operation for nearly 20 years. She had sent out nurses to many hospitals in several countries, and they reported back to her. She was well versed, in other words, with the best of nursing from many places. Later editions of the *Dictionary* show that she had updated the articles (Nightingale, 1894).

For nurses acquainted only with her *Notes on Nursing*, these dictionary articles are an excellent corrective. They notably demonstrate the higher technical proficiency required of nurses, both as medical technology improved, and as nurses were trusted to do more. From the simple admonition in *Notes on Nursing* for frequent handwashing—still a good idea—there are specifications for using "carbolic soap," "chlorinated soda," separate towels for different uses, and a list of rules for avoiding finger poisoning (septicemia). Precautions after treating certain cases were added, such as nose blowing, expectoration, and mouth and throat rinsing with a disinfectant. "The nurse must be taught the nature of contagion and infection, and the distinctions between deodorants, disinfectants, and antiseptics" (Nightingale, 1883, p. 1047). There were explicit warnings, similar to Semmelweis's on maternity cases in Vienna, on not conveying "contagious matter" from one patient to another. The specific points are similar to those in Exhibit 5.1 in Chapter 5. Nightingale drew on the expertise and advice developed at St. Thomas' Hospital for a more general readership.

It must be remembered that in those days, no hospital nurse or trainee had any university experience, few even had anything equivalent to secondary school; nor did the tutor or heads of wards, who did much of the training. The academic material was taught by the resident medical officer, a qualified doctor

Nightingale gave 10 qualities of character required in a nurse in "Nursing the sick." They overlap somewhat with the initial qualities stipulated at her school in 1860 but go further.

She repeated some of the best ideas of her earlier works, "The physician prescribes for supplying the vital force—but the nurse supplies it" and nursing "is to help the patient to live." However, her much-quoted definition of health appears here first, "Health is not only to be well but to be able to use well every power we have to use." She repeated this in her 1893 paper for the Chicago congress.

Most of the material in the article is obsolete, especially that on nurses residences, and accordingly is omitted here. Even the core points repeated from *Notes on Nursing*, on ventilation, light, and cleanliness, are omitted as already covered.

By the last revision of the *Dictionary of Medicine*, for the 1894 edition, Nightingale argued the need for updating nurse training "every five or ten years," what would now be called "continuing education." Although, earlier she had referred to medicine, surgery, and hygiene all making progress, here she added pathology but specified that hygiene, or public health, had made the greatest strides (Nightingale, 1894, p. 236, in McDonald, 2009, p. 734).

* * * * *

Source: Florence Nightingale. (1883). Nurses, training of. (in McDonald, 2009, pp. 723–734)

> *The physician prescribes for supplying the vital force—but the nurse supplies it.*
> —Nightingale (1883, p. 1043)

Training is to teach not only what is to be done, but how to do it. The physician or surgeon orders what is to be done. Training has to teach the nurse how to do it to his order and to teach not only how to do it, but *why* such and such a thing is done, and not such and such another, as also to teach symptoms. And what symptoms indicate what of disease or change, and the "reason why" of such symptoms.

Nearly all physicians' orders are conditional. Telling the nurse what to do is not enough and cannot be enough to perfect her—whatever her surroundings. The trained power of attending to one's own impressions, made by one's senses, so that these should *tell* the nurse how the patient is, is the *sine qua non* [without which there is nothing] of being a nurse at all. The nurse's eye and ear must be trained—smell and touch are her two right hands, and her taste is sometimes as necessary to the nurse as her head. Observation may always be improved by training—will indeed seldom be found without training—for otherwise, the nurse does not know what to look for....

The nurse is told by the medical attendant, "If such or such a change occur, or if such or such symptoms appear, you are to do so and so, or to vary my treatment in such or such a manner." In no case is the physician or surgeon always there. The woman must have trained powers of observation and reflection, or she cannot obey. The patient's life is lost by her blunder, or "sequelae" of incurable infirmity make afterlife a long disease.

A conscientious nurse is not necessarily an observing nurse, and life or death may lie with the good observer. Without a trained power of observation, no nurse can be of any use in reporting to the medical attendant....

Medicine, surgery, pathology, and above all hygiene, have made immense strides, partly in consequence of improved tools, improved instruments of observation. Nursing, their agent, has to be trained up to them. A good nurse 20 years ago had not to do the twentieth part of what she is required by her physician or surgeon to do now.

Nursing needs its instruments nearly as much as surgery, and yet more than medicine. The physician prescribes for supplying the vital force—but the nurse supplies it. Training is to teach the nurse how God makes health and how He makes disease. Training is to teach a nurse to know her business, that is, to observe exactly, to understand, to know exactly, to do, to tell exactly, in such stupendous issues as life and death, health and disease. Training is to enable the nurse to act for the best in carrying out her orders, not as a machine but as a nurse....

Training has to make her, not servile, but loyal to medical orders and authorities. True loyalty to orders cannot be without the independent sense or energy of responsibility, which alone secures real trustworthiness.... Training must show her how the effects on life of nursing may be calculated with nice precision—such care or carelessness, such a sick rate, such a duration of case, such a death rate.

* * * * *

Source: Florence Nightingale. (1883). Nursing the Sick (in McDonald, 2009, pp. 735-752)

Nursing is putting us in the best possible conditions for Nature to restore or to preserve health—to prevent or to cure disease or injury.

—Nightingale (1883, p. 1043)

Nursing proper, that is, nursing the sick and injured, will be here treated of, and not preventive or sanitary nursing, or nursing healthy children....

Nursing is putting us in the best possible conditions for Nature to restore or to preserve health—to prevent or to cure disease or injury. The physician or surgeon prescribes these conditions—the nurse carries them out. Health is not only to be well but to be able to use well every power we have to use. Sickness or disease is Nature's way of getting rid of the effects of conditions which have interfered with health. It is Nature's attempt to cure—we have to help her. Partly, perhaps mainly, upon nursing must depend whether Nature succeeds or fails in her attempt to cure by sickness. Nursing is therefore to help the patient to live. *Training* is to teach the nurse to help the patient to live. Nursing is an art, and an art requiring an organized, practical, and scientific training. For nursing is the skilled servant of medicine, surgery, and hygiene.

Nursing may be divided under four heads: *(a) hospital* nursing; *(b) private* nursing, that is, nursing one sick or injured person at a time, at home, ... generally of the richer classes; *(c) district* nursing, that is, nursing the sick or injured poor at home, taking as many cases as can be well attended to by one nurse...; (d) *midwifery* nursing, including the nursing of the healthy mother and infant after natural childbirth....

No disinfection will enable dirty linen to be kept with safety a single day in the same building with the sick. It is cruel to allow dirty linen from "infectious" patients to be taken home by the relatives to be washed in the crowded rooms of the poor. Dirty linen should be removed immediately from the sick room and sent to the laundry, at least every day....

It must not be supposed that even a good sprinkling of carbolic powder (which, besides, injures the sheets) over the dirty linen lying in a basket, will at all obviate the necessity of instant removal. Steeping in boiling water with an antiseptic solution (carbolic acid 1 in 100) is the only safe method of disinfection. All washing of dirty linen and bandages should be done outside of the sick room and, if possible, of the house. In a hospital, the laundry should be in a separate building. *Bandages* with pus on them are always to be burnt at once—to be carried straight to the ward fire, or to a furnace. The best economy is to burn them, but one must make up the fire so that the burning shall not smell. Bandages used for fractures, etc., are the only bandages that may be washed. Soak these with chlorinated soda, a diluted pint, then boil them all night with soft soap, soda, and chlorinated soda—a quart bottle for the two....

Absolute cleanliness is the true disinfectant, but chlorinated soda, if disinfectants are to be used, is about the best. Always have chlorinated soda for nurses to wash their hands, especially after dressing or handling a suspicious case. "It may destroy germs at the expense of the cuticle," but, "if it takes off the cuticle it must be bad for the germs," said the same surgeon. Fire is the right way, if a thing is so bad that it wants a disinfectant....

There should always be water and a tap in every water closet for rinsing.

Towels in a hospital should be kept separate for three separate uses, changed for clean ones as often as possible, and marked "Hands," "Bedpans," and "Basins." A bottle of chlorinated soda and a bottle of glycerine should always be by, to wash the hands....

Precautions against finger poisoning, etc. One of the most important points nurses have to be taught on beginning surgical ward work (and, indeed, surgeons also), is how not to poison their fingers. No good nurse will poison her own fingers any more than her patient's....

The fear of dirt is the beginning of good nursing. With all internal cases, keep the nails short, fill the same with carbolic soap, and carefully anoint the fingers you are about to use, especially the first and second fingers in attending on vaginal cases, with carbolic oil (1 in 20). Oil the tube or nozzle, etc., to be used for any internal application, with carbolic oil (1 in 20). Otherwise, the appliance used might convey contagious matter from one patient to another. Always use two basins in washing wounds, so as not to dip the fingers in dirty water. Catheters must be cleansed and disinfected, first with a stream of warm water, and then with a stream of watery solution of carbolic acid (1 in 40). Catheters of other material than silver should *not be soaked* in carbolic acid solutions, as the acid injures varnish and gum. Never "blow down" towards the eye *first* instead of last, for so some lodgement will always be effected at the bottom.

Never fail to take your own carbolic soap, with which you will be provided, in your own soap tin, into the ward each morning and evening in your pocket. But take it out before beginning "dressings," as otherwise you put a dirty hand into your pocket. Always dry your cleaned fingers and hands on towels *not* used for any other purpose. After offensive cases, blow the nose and expectorate, and rinse mouth and throat with Condy [a disinfectant] and water, or with permanganate of potassium—a few grains in water.

Cuffs and sleeves and stuff dresses are possible carriers of contagious matter. Always change the apron and oversleeves, which you have worn about the sick before eating or drinking....

The nurse must be taught the nature of contagion and infection, and the distinction between deodorants, disinfectants, and antiseptics. Mischief done by students and dressers might have been saved, and valuable lives spared, even among surgeons, if such precautions had been always scrupulously observed by them....

Application of remedies. The physician or surgeon requires the nurse: To be able to dress blisters, burns, sores. To administer stimulants and medicines as ordered, enemas and injections to men and women, and suppositories. To manage trusses, appliances in uterine complaints; to pass the catheter—at least for women....

To use the best methods of friction to the body and extremities; to make and apply fomentations, poultices, and minor dressings, wet and dry or greasy; syringe wounds; to syringe the vagina.

To manage helpless patients—fever, operation, and surgical cases—that is to move, to change them, to keep them personally clean, warm, or cool.... To give food and stimulants to helpless patients—fever, operation, and surgical cases; manage the position of such cases; to prevent or to dress bed sores....

To prepare the bed for fever, for accidents, for ovariotomy [removal of ovarian cysts], and various kinds of operations; to undress, handle, and put to bed accident cases.

To attend at and prepare for operations including ovariotomy, lithotomy, hernia; to prepare patients for and manage them after operations and anesthetics, and all this with the least call on their small strength. To be able to do the first thing in case of hemorrhage, namely, compression by hand or finger, by extemporary tourniquet and plugging.

To bandage all the various parts of the body, arm, leg, and chest.... To make bandages of the various kinds used.... The nurse should be able to give subcutaneous injections, to use the galvanic battery, to dry and wet cup, and to apply leeches externally and internally....

Observation of patients. The physician and surgeon require every nurse to be able to observe correctly, and to report correctly on the state or character of secretions, expectoration, pulse, skin, appetite; effect of diet, of stimulants and of medicines; eruptions; the formation of matter; as to intelligence, with regard to delirium, stupor, etc.; as to breathing, whether quick or slow, regular or irregular, difficult, etc.; as to sleep, whether sound, starting, heavy, etc.; and as to the state of wounds. The physician also requires the nurse to be able to "take" and to record the temperature—sometimes every quarter of an hour in critical cases, the pulse, the respiration; to measure, and sometimes to test, the urine for him. She will be required to make these observations—if possible still more accurately—for child patients, who cannot tell what is the matter with them; to understand the management of sick children and children's wards, which need a yet more exquisite cleanliness....

A really good nurse must needs be of the highest class of character. It need hardly be said that she must be: (1) chaste, in the sense of the Sermon on the Mount, (2) sober, in spirit as well as in drink, and temperate in all things, (3) honest, not accepting the most trifling fee or bribe from patients or friends, (4) truthful—and to be able to tell the truth includes attention and observation, to observe truly—memory, to remember truly—power of expression, to tell truly what one has observed truly—as well as intention to speak the truth; (5) trustworthy, to carry out directions intelligently and perfectly;... (6) punctual to a second and orderly to a hair—having everything ready and in order before she begins her dressings or her work about the patient, nothing forgotten; (7) quiet, yet quick, quick without hurry, gentle without slowness, discreet without self-importance; no gossip, (8) cheerful, hopeful, not allowing herself to be discouraged by unfavorable symptoms... (9) cleanly to the point of exquisiteness, both for the patient's sake and her own, neat and ready, (10) thinking of her patients and not of herself....

A patient wants according to his wants and not according to any nurse's theory of his wants or "occasions." "Tender over his occasions" [a quotation from *Romeo and Juliet*] she must be, but she must have a rule of thought and this the physician or surgeon has to give her in his directions, which her training must have fitted her to obey intelligently, using discretion. The nurse must have simplicity and a single eye to the patient's good. She must make no demand upon the patient for reciprocation.... The nurse must always be kind and sympathetic, but never emotional.

* * * * *

SCAVENGE, SCAVENGE, SCAVENGE, *THE NEW YORK HERALD*, 1884

Since the Crimean War of 1854 to 1856, Nightingale was well known in the United States, thanks to the considerable attention American newspapers gave to her and her writing. That her *Notes on Nursing* was serialized in the *Saturday Evening Post* (copyright be damned!) is an example. American doctors began writing her and visiting her in London on their projects of starting nurse training and/or building a new hospital. She met many and corresponded with more.

The approach made to her in 1883, however, was different, a request, by C. Harry Meltzer, a correspondent for *The New York Herald*, for advice on confronting an impending cholera epidemic. Meltzer, then in London, missed a meeting Nightingale tried to arrange for him with Douglas Galton. She urged him to make some alternative arrangement to see him, but to no avail. Meltzer was "quite innocent," Nightingale told Galton, of "the terrible cholera failure" in Egypt, then under the British control. "Out of thirty-seven attacks of cholera among our officers and men, twenty-five have died!!!! and nine more since!! out of how many attacks?" She could report a telegram she had received that the nursing sisters were safe. Next, "the *New York Herald* man asks me to let him publish *my letter* to him not only in the *N.Y. Herald* but in a '*London paper.*' What do you say? I have told him to send my letter back to me to see." She asked Galton, "Is it possible now to stir up anything about sending out a scavenging staff? to Cairo?" (letter, July 29, 1883, British Library Add Mss[1] 45765 ff215-216).

A letter the next day to her closest collaborator, Dr. John Sutherland, told of meeting the correspondent on his request for "*practical* advice about prophylactic measures," and that he believed in "quarantine!!!" She sent Meltzer to meet Dr. Sutherland, urging her colleague: "Please keep him straight about cholera. It is of such terrible importance that America and England should be put right on such subjects." She wrote the letter Meltzer wanted for his newspaper and also sent him an epidemiological lecture, by a cholera expert Dr. Cunningham, which she had quoted. Again, she flagged the need for practical action: "the Foreign Office should send out a scavenging staff to Cairo," and if it had earlier, "cholera would never have been." She called for "inspectors and men for a scavenging staff to undertake the cleansing of Cairo under Dr. Hunter," another cholera expert with vast Indian experience (letter, July 30, 1883, British Library Add Mss 45758 f171). This was, in fact, done, although whether her advice prompted it or not is not evident.

As was her practice, Nightingale asked Dr. Sutherland to review her draft for *The New York Herald*, which he presumably did. By the time she got the finished statement ready, however, Meltzer had left London. It was not published until the following year. "Scavenge, scavenge, scavenge!" would be much quoted and excerpted. It was reprinted both in an American public health journal, the main source used here (Nightingale, 1884a) and a British one (Nightingale, 1884b, August), although there were excerpts in the popular magazine *Scientific American* (*Scientific American*, 1884). The (British) Ladies Sanitary Association printed up her instructions for use in the U.K. (*The Times*, 1884).

However, a *New York Times* story was critical of Nightingale soon after her letter in *The New York Herald* appeared, insisting that quarantine was the means of prevention. The story (no author named) allowed that the bacteriologist who had only recently identified the disease may have mistaken about the "microbe," but judged Nightingale's view, which it took to be a spontaneous generation from filth, as being "at variance with the facts" (*The New York Times*, 1884). The discovery of the cholera bacillus by Robert Koch

---

[1]Further references to Add Mss (Additional Manuscripts) are also to the British Library.

was, in fact, a great scientific breakthrough, but identification of the bacillus does not prevent outbreaks of the disease.

Nightingale's practical advice on prevention was sound. She insisted that quarantine, or preventing people from getting off a ship from an affected area, did nothing to stop the disease. The cholera bacillus thrives in the bowel and is communicated by fecal-laden water. Contact with a patient with cholera does not spread the disease; a person would have to ingest food or water with cholera bacilli in it. As was her custom, Nightingale cited examples of quarantines that achieved nothing, and cited examples where cholera had started in places in Egypt where no ship stopped.

Her advice was reprinted again in Britain during the cholera epidemic of 1892. There it was noted that the National Health Society was supplying the material, "in quantity, cheap handbills and directions" for use in prevention. This 1892 version added a few more particulars, points that also appeared in a pamphlet issued that same year by the medical officer of health for Buckinghamshire, again with substantial quotations from Nightingale (De'Ath, 1892, p. 3):

> Boil your water or drink a pure natural table water. Boil your milk (and here the lecturer gave an example of a well-defined cholera outbreak spread by contaminated milk). Inspect your fruit, fish, and meat markets. Avoid unsound food and excesses of diet. Feed wholesomely the needy and destitute; help the poor to be as careful in their homes and habits as you will be in yours. (*The Times*, 1892)

* * * * *

Source: Practical advice in view of the rapid spread of cholera: "Scavenge, scavenge, scavenge," (Nightingale, 1884a)

In reply to an inquiry, Miss Florence Nightingale, the Crimean heroine, kindly sent the following to the *New York Herald*:

Sir, I beg to reply to your note asking for "practical advice in view of the rapid spread of cholera." That our whole experience in India, where cholera is never wholly absent, tends to prove—nay, actually does prove—that cholera is not communicable from person to person.

That the disease cannot be ascribed to "somebody else," that is, that the sick do not manufacture a "special poison" which causes the disease.

That cholera is a local disease—an epidemic affecting localities, and there depending on pollution of earth, air, and water, and buildings.

That the isolation of the sick cannot stop the disease, nor quarantine, nor cordons, nor the like. These, indeed, may tend fatally to aggravate the disease, directly and indirectly, by turning away our attention from the only measures which can stop it.

That the only preventive is to put the earth, air, and water and buildings into a healthy state by scavenging, limewashing, and every kind of sanitary work, and, if cholera does come, to move the people from the places where the disease has broken out and then to cleanse.

Persons about cholera patients do not "catch" the disease from the sick any more than cases of poisoning "infect" others. If a number of persons have been poisoned, say by arsenic put by mistake into food, it is because they have each swallowed the arsenic. It is not because they have taken "it," the "mysterious influence" of one another.

In looking sadly at Egypt—Egypt where cholera did not begin anywhere along the route from India to Europe—but at Dametta, where no ship and no passenger ever stops, and where the dreadful unsanitary condition of the place fully accounts for any outbreak of cholera—in sorrowfully looking at Egypt and at Europe now, one might almost say that it is this doctrine of a special poison emanating from the sick man which it is thought can be carried in a package, that has (mentally) "poisoned" us. People will soon believe that you can take cholera by taking railway ticket. They speak as if the only reason against enforcing quarantine were, not that it is an impossibility and an absurdity to stop disease in this way, but that it is impossible to enforce quarantine. "If only we could," they say, "all would be well."

Vigorously enforce sanitary measures, but with judgment, e.g., scavenge, scavenge, scavenge; wash, cleanse, and limewash; remove all putrid human refuse from privies and cesspits and cesspools and dust bins; look to stables and cow sheds and pigsties; look to common lodging houses and crowded places, dirty houses and yards. "Set your house in order" in all ways sanitary and hygienic, according to the conditions of the place, and "all will be well."

I beg to send you the best thing that has been written upon the subject—where also what can be said about quarantine is fully stated in the best manner—the lecture by Dr Cunningham, sanitary commissioner with the Government of India, on the "Sanitary Lessons of Indian Epidemics," at the beginning of the *Medical Times*, which I enclose.

The real danger to be feared is in blaming somebody else and not our own selves for such an epidemic visitation. As a matter of fact, if the disease attacks our neighbors, we ourselves are already liable to it. To trust for protection to stopping intercourse would be just as rational as to try to sweep back an incoming flood instead of getting out of its way.

With the most earnest wish that America, as well as England, may "set her house in order," and so defy cholera and turn its appearance elsewhere into a blessing, pray, believe me
    ever her and your faithful servant
    Florence Nightingale

* * * * *

SICK NURSING AND HEALTH NURSING, WORLD CONGRESS, CHICAGO, 1893

Hospitals are only an intermediate stage of civilization, never intended, at all events, to take in the whole sick population.
                                            —Nightingale (1893, p. 198)

This last major paper that Nightingale wrote, for a world congress in Chicago, is a gem. It was solicited by the nursing director of Johns Hopkins University Hospital, Isabel Hampton, in January 1893, to lead off the section. Hampton read the paper as well as her own, which was itself an important paper calling for higher standards of nursing education. As noted in Chapter 10, Hampton Robb (as she soon became) would herself become the major link between Nightingale and American nursing in the 20th century.

In this paper, Nightingale took the opportunity of revisiting key, central, themes, her thoughts now polished by years of reflection. By 1893, she had had more than 30 years of experience guiding the new profession and had a large network of colleagues who kept her informed of developments. She was well aware of what worked and what did not. Nurses by then were much better educated than when her school opened, but still not a single one had any university experience. Few would have had much secondary schooling. The doctor or surgeon, as before, had sole responsibility to diagnose and direct treatment, although again the nurse's obligation to obedience was "intelligent obedience," meaning with discretion. As before, doctors were not to have administrative control over the nurses or hospitals. Nightingale argued for the *lay* administration of hospitals. Nurses, as always, must be relied on to run the nursing itself.

Nightingale went back to her words on "calling" from *Notes on Nursing*, as doing our work "to satisfy the high idea of what is the *right*, the *best*, and not because we shall be found out if we don't do it" (Nightingale, 1860). Her calling was religious, specifically Christian, but this broader definition suits people of any faith or none. She repeated her definition of health from Quain's *Dictionary of Medicine* as "not only to be well but to be able to use well every

power we have." She went back to the special vulnerability of babies: "The li
duration of babies is the most 'delicate test' of health conditions." She used tl
language also from Quain of sickness being nature's way of curing some co
dition, "we have to help her." She repeated a point from her 1876 letter on di
trict nursing that hospitals were "only an intermediate stage of civilization.'

Nightingale's paper began confidently and boldly on the creation of tl
"new art" and "new science" in the past 40 years. The tone throughout w.
confident and forthright.

* * * * *

Source: Florence Nightingale (1893). Sick Nursing and Health Nursing (
McDonald, 2004, pp. 205-219)

A new art and a new science has been created since and within the last for
years. With it is a new profession, so they say: we say *calling*. One wou!
think this had been created or discovered for some new want or local war
Not so. The want is nearly as old as the world, nearly as large as the worl
as pressing as life or death. It is that of sickness. And the art is that of *nursir
the sick*. Please mark: nursing *the sick*, *not* nursing sickness.

We will call the art nursing proper.... This is one of the distinctior
between nursing proper and medicine, though a very famous and succes
ful physician did say, when asked how he treated pneumonia: "I do n
treat pneumonia, I treat the person who has pneumonia." This is the reaso
why nursing proper can only be taught by the patient's bedside and in tl
sick room or ward. Neither can it be taught by lectures or by books, thoug
these are valuable accessories, if used as such; otherwise what is in the boc
stays in the book....

It is the want of the art of health, then, of the cultivation of health, whic
has only lately been discovered, and great organizations have been made t
meet it, and a whole literature created. We have medical officers of healtl
immense sanitary works. We have not nurses, *missioners* of health-at-hom

How to bring these great medical officers to bear on the families, tr
homes, and households, and habits of the people, rich as well as poor, ha
not been discovered, although family comes before acts of Parliament. On
would think *family* had not health to look after. And woman, the great mis
tress of family life, by whom everybody is born, has not been practicall
instructed at all. Everything has come before health. We are not to look aft
health, but after sickness. Well, we are to be convinced of *error* before we ai
convinced of *right*....

Though everybody *must* be born, there is probably no knowledge mor
neglected than this, nor more important for the great mass of women

namely how to feed, wash, and clothe the baby, how to secure the utmost cleanliness for mother and infant. Midwives certainly neither practise nor teach it. And I have even been informed that many lady doctors consider that they have "nothing to do with the baby," and that they should "lose caste with the men doctors" if they attempted it. One would have thought that the *ladies* "lost caste" with themselves for *not* doing it, and that it was the very reason why we wished for the lady doctors for them to assume these cares which touch the very health of everybody from the beginning. But I have known the most admirable exceptions to this most cruel rule.

I know of no systematic teaching for the ordinary midwife or the ordinary mother, how to keep the baby in health, certainly the most important function to make a healthy nation. The human baby is not an invalid, but it is the most tender form of animal life. This is only one, but a supremely important instance of the want of health nursing....

What is sickness? Sickness or disease is Nature's way of getting rid of the effects of conditions which have interfered with health. It is Nature's attempt to cure. We have to help her.... What is health? Health is not only to be well, but to be able to use well every power we have.

What is nursing? Both kinds of nursing are to put us in the best possible conditions for Nature to restore or to preserve health—to prevent or to cure disease or injury. Upon nursing proper, under scientific heads, physicians or surgeons, must depend partly, perhaps mainly, whether Nature succeeds or fails in her attempt to cure by sickness. Nursing proper is therefore to help the patient suffering from disease to live, just as health nursing is to keep or put the constitution of the healthy child or human being in such a state as to have no disease.

What is training? Training is to teach the nurse to help the patient to live. Nursing the sick is an art, and an art requiring an organized, practical, and scientific training, for nursing is the skilled servant of medicine, surgery, and hygiene. A good nurse of twenty years ago had not to do the twentieth part of what she is required by her physician or surgeon to do now, and so, after the year's training, she must be still training under instruction in her first and even second year's hospital service.

The physician prescribes for supplying the vital force, but the nurse supplies it. Training is to teach the nurse how God makes health, and how He makes disease. Training is to teach a nurse to know her business, that is, to observe exactly, to understand, to know exactly to do, to tell exactly, in such stupendous issues as life and death, health and disease. Training has to make her not servile, but loyal to medical orders and authorities. True loyalty to orders cannot be without the independent sense or energy of responsibility, which alone secures real trustworthiness. Training is to teach the nurse how to handle the agencies within our control which restore health and life, in strict, intelligent obedience to the physician's or surgeon's power and knowledge, how to keep the health mechanism prescribed to her in gear. Training must show her how the effects on life of nursing may be calculated with nice precision, such care or carelessness, such a sick rate, such a duration of case, such a death rate....

What makes a good training school for nurses? The most favorable conditions for the administration of the hospital are:

First, a good lay administration with a chief executive officer, a civilian (be he called treasurer or permanent chairman of committee) with power delegated to him by the committee.... This is the main thing. With a consulting committee, meeting regularly, of businessmen, taking the opinions of the medical officers. The medical officers on the committee must be only consulting medical officers, not executive. If the latter they have often to judge in their own case, which is fatal. Doctors are not necessarily administrators (the executive), any more than the executive are necessarily doctors....

Secondly, a strong body of medical officers, visiting and resident, and a medical school.

Thirdly, the government of hospitals in the point of view of the real responsibility for the conduct and discipline of the nurses being thrown upon the matron (superintendent of nurses), who is herself a trained nurse, and the real head of all the female staff of the hospital. Vest the whole responsibility for nursing, internal management, for discipline, and training of nurses in this one female head of the nursing staff, whatever called. She should be herself responsible directly to the constituted hospital authorities and all her nurses and servants should, in the performance of their duties, be responsible, in matters of conduct and discipline, to her only. No good ever comes of the constituted authorities placing themselves in the office which they have sanctioned her occupying. No good ever comes of anyone interfering between the head of the nursing establishment and her nurses....

Having then, as a basis, a well-organized hospital, we require, as further conditions: (1) a special *organization for the purpose* of training, that is, where systematic technical training is given in the wards to the probationers... (2) a good "home" for the probationers in the hospital, where they learn moral discipline, for technical training is only half the battle... (3) staff of training school: (a) a trained matron over all... (b) a "home" sister (assistant superintendent)... (c) ward sisters (head nurses of wards) who have been trained in the school... for they are the key to the whole situation, matron influencing through them.... For, after all, the hospital is for the good of the patients, not for the good of the nurses....

There should be an *entente cordiale* between matron, assistant matrons, "home" sister [tutor], and whatever other female head there is, with frequent informal meetings, exchanging information, or there can be no unity in training.

Nursing proper means, besides giving the medicines and stimulants prescribed or the surgical appliances, the proper use of fresh air (ventilation), light, warmth, cleanliness, quiet, and the proper choosing and giving of diet, all at the least expense of vital power to the sick. So health-at-home nursing means exactly the same proper use of the same natural elements, with as much life-giving power as possible to the healthy.

We have awakened, though still far from the mark, to the need of training or teaching for nursing proper....

The life duration of babies is the most "delicate test" of health conditions. What is the proportion of the whole population of cities or country which dies before it is five years old? We have tons of printed knowledge on the subject of hygiene and sanitation. The causes of enormous child mortality are perfectly well known: they are chiefly want of cleanliness, want of fresh air, careless dieting, and clothing, want of white washing, dirty feather beds and bedding—in one word, want of *household* care of health. The remedies are just as well known, but how much of this knowledge has been brought into the homes and households and habits of the people, poor or even rich?...

The laws of God—the laws of life—are always conditional, always inexorable. But neither mothers, nor school mistresses, nor nurses of children are *practically* taught how to work within those laws which God has assigned to the relations of our bodies with the world in which He has put them. In other words, we do not study, we do not practise, the laws which make these bodies into which He has put our minds, healthy or unhealthy, organs of those minds; we do not practise how to give our children healthy existences.

It would be utterly unfair to lay all the fault upon us women, none upon the buildings, drains, water supply. There are millions of cottages, more of town dwellings, even of the rich, where it is utterly impossible to have fresh air. As for the workshops, work people should remember that health is their only capital, and they should come to an understanding among themselves not only to have the means, but to use the means, to secure pure air in their places of work, which is one of the prime agents of health....

The crowded national or board school [state-supported], in it how many children's epidemics have their origin! The great school dormitories! [of expensive private schools] Scarlet fever and measles would be no more ascribed to "current contagion" or to "something being much about this year," but to its right cause; nor would "plague and pestilence" be said to be "in God's hands," when, so far as we know, He has put them into our own....

Health in the home can only be learnt from the home and in the home....that as medicine and surgery can, like nursing, only be properly taught and properly learnt in the sick room, and by the patient's side, so sanitation can only be properly taught and properly learned in the home and house....

The work we are speaking of has nothing to do with nursing disease, but maintaining health by removing the things which disturb it, which have been summed up in the population in general as "dirt, drink, diet, damp, draughts, drains."...

4. *Dangers.* After only a generation of nursing arise the dangers: (1) fashion on the one side, and its consequent want of earnestness; (2) mere money getting on the other; woman does not live by wages alone; (3) making nursing a profession and not a calling.

What is it to feel a *calling* for anything? Is it not to do our work in it to satisfy the high idea of what is the *right*, the *best*, and not because we shall be found out if we don't do it? This is the "enthusiasm" which everyone, from a shoemaker to a sculptor, must have in order to follow his "calling" properly. Now the nurse has to do not with shoes or with marble, but with living human beings.

How, then, to keep up the high tone of a calling, to "make your calling and election sure" [2 Peter 1:10]? By fostering that bond of sympathy (*esprit de corps*) which community of aims and of action in good work induces....

(4) There is another danger, perhaps the greatest of all. It is also a danger which grows day by day. It is this: as literary education and colleges for women to teach literary work start and multiply and improve, some, even of the very best women, believe that everything can be taught by book and lecture and tested by examination—that memory is the great step to excellence.

Can you teach horticulture or agriculture by books, for example describing the different manures, artificial and natural, and their purposes?... Could you teach painting by giving, for example, Fuseli's "Lectures"? Fuseli himself said, when asked how he mixed his colours: "With brains, Sir," that is, practice guided by brains. But you have another, a quite other sort of a thing with nursing, for you have to do with living bodies and living minds and feelings of both body and mind....

The physician or surgeon gives his orders, generally his conditional orders, perhaps once or twice a day, perhaps not even that. The nurse has to carry them out, with intelligence, in conditions, every minute of the twenty four hours.

The nurse must have method, self-sacrifice, watchful activity, love of the work, devotion to duty (that is, the service of the good), the courage, coolness of the soldier, the tenderness of the mother, the absence of the prig (that is, never thinking that she has attained perfection or that there is nothing better). She must have a threefold interest in her work: an intellectual interest in the case, a (much higher) hearty interest in the patient, a technical (practical) interest in the patient's care and cure. She must not look upon patients as made for nurses, but upon nurses as made for patients.

There may also now—I only say *may*—with all this dependence on literary lore in nurse training, be a real danger of being satisfied with diagnosis, or with looking too much at the pathology of the case, without cultivating the resource or intelligence for the thousand and one means of mitigation, even where there is no cure. Never, never, let the nurse forget that she must look for the fault of the nursing as much as for the fault of the disease in the symptoms of the patient.

(5) Forty or fifty years ago a hospital was looked upon as a box to hold patients in. The first question never was, will the hospital do them no harm? Enormous strides have had to be made to build and arrange hospitals so as to do the patients no sanitary or insanitary harm. Now there is danger of a hospital being looked upon as a box to train nurses in. Enormous strides must be made not to do them harm, to give them something that can really be called an "all-round" training....

(6) Another danger—that is, stereotyping, not progressing. "No system can endure that does not march." Are we walking to the future or to the past? Are we progressing or are we stereotyping? We remember that we have scarcely crossed the threshold of uncivilized civilization in nursing: there is still so much to do....

The health of the unity is the health of the community. Unless you have the health of the unity, there is no community health.

Competition, or each man for himself and the devil against us all, may be necessary, we are told, but it is the enemy of health. Combination is the antidote, combined interests, recreation, combination to secure the best air, the best food, and all that makes life useful, healthy, and happy. There is no such thing as independence. As far as we are successful, our success lies in combination.

The Chicago Exhibition is a great combination from all parts of the world to prove the dependence of man on man. What a lesson in combination the United States have taught to the whole world, and are teaching!...

May our hopes be that, as every year the technical qualifications constituting a skilful and observing nurse meet with more demands on her from the physicians and surgeons, progress may be made year by year, and that, not only in technical things, but in the qualifications which constitute a good and trustworthy woman, without which she cannot be a good nurse....

We are only on the threshold of nursing. In the future, which I shall not see, for I am old, may a better way be opened! May the methods by which *every* infant, *every* human being, will have the best chance of health—the methods by which *every* sick person will have the best chance of recovery—be learned and practised! Hospitals are only an intermediate stage of civilization, never intended, at all events, to take in the whole sick population.

* * * * *

REFERENCES

De'Ath, G. H. (1892). *Cholera: What can we do?* Buckingham, UK: Walford.

McDonald, L. (Ed.). (2004). *Florence Nightingale on public health care.* Waterloo, Canada: Wilfrid Laurier University Press. ISBN: 0-88920-446-2

McDonald, L. (Ed.). (2009). *Florence Nightingale: The Nightingale School.* Waterloo, Canada: Wilfrid Laurier University Press. ISBN: 978-1-55458-169-6

McDonald, L. (Ed.). (2012). *Florence Nightingale and hospital reform.* Waterloo, Canada: Wilfrid Laurier University Press. ISBN: 978-0-88920-471-3

Nightingale, F. (1860). *Notes on Nursing: What it is and what it is not.* (New ed., rev., enlarged). London, UK: Harrison (library standard).

Nightingale, F. (1880). Hospitals and Patients. Unpublished paper for *The Nineteenth Century.* (September 1880:1–4. British Library Cup.400.i.20(3)

Nightingale, F. (1883). Nurses, training of and nursing the sick. In R. Quain (Ed.), *A dictionary of medicine* (Vol. 2, pp. 1038–1049). London, UK: Longmans, Green.

Nightingale, F. (1884a). Practical advice in view of the rapid spread of cholera: "Scavenge, scavenge, scavenge." In A. N. Bell (Ed.), *The Sanitarian, 13,* 114–115.

Nightingale, F. (1884b, August 15). Miss Florence Nightingale on the cholera. In E. Hart (Ed.), *The Sanitary Record: A Monthly Journal of Public Health and the Progress of Sanitary Science, 6*(73), 66.

Nightingale, F. (1893). Sick nursing and health nursing. In A. Burdett-Coutts (Ed.), *Woman's mission: A series of Congress papers on the philanthropic work of women* (pp. 184–205). London, UK: Sampson, Low, Marston.

Nightingale, F. (1894). Nurses, training of and nursing the sick. In R. Quain (Ed.), *A dictionary of medicine* (Vol. 2, pp. 231–244). London, UK: Longmans, Green.

The New York Times. (1884, July 29). A mischievous letter, 4.

Scientific American. (1884, August 9). Timely advice about the cholera by Florence Nightingale, 89.

The Times. (1884, September 1). Birnam Games, 4A.

The Times. (1892, September 2). The cholera, 9D.

Appendix: Timeline—Nightingale's Nursing and Health Care and Its Influence

This timeline is directed to Nightingale's nursing and health care work, not at all to her personal life. Hence, it begins with her earliest experiences and attempts to gain nursing experience, carrying on through her significant contributions. It includes important nurses she mentored and (highlights only) key publications of theirs that she influenced. It includes work that she inspired, such as starting professional nursing in France and Italy, but in which she was only peripherally involved.

The timeline continues after her death to the present, noting events that she could never have anticipated, such as statements made by the World Health Organization (WHO) and public health care measures brought in by the National Health Act in the United Kingdom in 1948. The listing is far from exhaustive but attempts to include major examples from many countries, both in nursing and health care more broadly.

Note that the term *nurse* here refers to a trained, qualified, person, as opposed to "pauper nurses" in the old workhouses, or the old-style untrained hospital nurses. "Nightingale nurse" refers to one trained at the Nightingale School. References to "Add Mss" are to manuscripts at the British Library.

EVENTS OF THE CRIMEAN WAR

1848–1850   Nightingale travels in Europe, visits hospitals (McDonald, 2004b).
1851–1853   Gets ward experience at the Kaiserswerth Deaconess Institution (McDonald, 2004b, pp. 513–543; 2009b, pp. 49–55) and in Paris hospitals (McDonald, 2009b, pp. 57–60).

1853–October 1854 Superintendent at the Establishment for Gentlewomen during Illness, Upper Harley Street, London (McDonald, 2009b, The Establishment for Gentlewomen During Illness, pp. 60–112).

1854 October Leaves for the Barrack Hospital, Scutari, Turkey, as head of the first nursing team to nurse in war, helps clean up hospitals, establishes kitchens and laundries (McDonald, 2010); in London, improved nursing begins at St. Thomas' Hospital, under nursing director Sarah E. Wardroper.

1855 Establishes nursing at hospitals in the Crimea (McDonald, 2010); Nightingale Fund opened, to honor her for her war work.

1856 Nightingale returns from the Crimean War; meets the Queen, Prince Consort, and the war secretary, Lord Panmure, at Balmoral Castle; war secretary asks her to prepare a "précis" of her analysis (McDonald, 2010); many places join in raising money for the Nightingale Fund throughout the United Kingdom, France, Australia, and New Zealand.

1857 Nightingale begins analysis of Crimean War data, visits army and navy hospitals in England (McDonald, 2010); works on improving plans for the army's Royal Victoria Hospital at Netley, near Southampton.

1858 Nightingale submits Answers to Written Questions to the Royal Commission (Nightingale, 1858a); prints, for private distribution, 853-page *Notes on Matters Affecting the Health, Efficiency and Hospital Administration of the British Army* (McDonald, 2010; Nightingale, 1858b); publishes *Subsidiary Notes on the Introduction of Female Nursing into Military Hospitals in Peace and in War* (Nightingale, 1858c); sends papers on hospital defects to National Association for the Promotion of Social Science meetings in Liverpool (Nightingale, 1858d, in Part II, Chapter 10); publishes three unsigned articles in an architecture journal, on hospital construction, opposing plans for the new army hospital at Netley (Nightingale, 1858, August 28, September 11, and September 25).

1859 Battle of Solférino in Italian War of Independence; Henri Dunant helps on battlefield postbattle, inspired by Nightingale (*The Times*, 1872); Nightingale prepares for the opening of her school; drafts *Notes on Nursing*; her papers on hospitals published by the National Association for the Promotion of Social Science and on her own (Nightingale, 1859a,b).

FROM THE OPENING OF HER SCHOOL

1860 In January, first edition of *Notes on Nursing* published, then library standard version (Nightingale, 1860a,b, in Part II, Chapter 10); American edition appears, soon serialized in the *Saturday Evening Post*; translations into German and Italian published; in June 1860, the Nightingale School opens; Nightingale tries to get questions on health and housing added to the U.K. Census (McDonald, 2003, pp. 95–103); advises on plans for Lisbon Children's Hospital.

1861 to 1864 American Civil War; U.S. Sanitary Commission uses Nightingale's Crimean War analysis and forms; large numbers of women volunteer to nurse, on both sides, inspired by her (Adams, 1952, pp. 150–168); Confederate Army publishes extracts of her material on army cooking (Virginia, 1861) and follows Nightingale principles in hospital hut construction, with cross-ventilation.

1861 Nightingale midwifery ward and training open at King's College Hospital; she publishes *Notes on Nursing for the Labouring Classes* (Nightingale, 1861); begins work on the Royal Commission on India (completed in 1863); her paper "Hospital statistics" read at the International Statistical Congress, London (McDonald, 2003, pp. 83–88); advises on plans for the new St. Thomas' Hospital and for the Leeds General Infirmary; translations of *Notes on Nursing* published in German, Swedish, and Danish.

1862 Nightingale issues paper opposing compulsory inspection of suspected prostitutes, "Note on the Supposed Protection Afforded Against Venereal Diseases" (Nightingale, 1862, in McDonald, 2005, pp. 428–435); submits *Observations by Miss Nightingale on the Evidence contained in Stational Returns sent to her by the Royal Commission on the Sanitary State of the Army in India* (Vallée, 2006, pp. 130–194); War Office issues standard plans for (pavilion) regimental hospitals, on which Nightingale assisted Royal Engineer Douglas Galton; French and Dutch translations of *Notes on Nursing* published.

1863 Publishes third edition of *Notes on Hospitals* (Nightingale, 1863); her first paper on India read, *How people may live and not die in India* given in Edinburgh, and her *Sanitary statistics of native colonial schools and hospitals*, both at meetings of the National Association for the Promotion of Social Science (Nightingale, 1864a,b).

1864 Advises on starting professional nursing in military hospitals; works on getting nurses for Liverpool Workhouse Infirmary, works on getting trained nursing started in Manchester; sends paper on the aboriginal races of Australia to the National Association for the Promotion of Social Science, York (Nightingale, 1864b); advises British delegates to Geneva Convention meetings.

1865 First professional nursing in a workhouse infirmary starts in May, at Liverpool, led by Nightingale nurse Agnes Jones; Nightingale publishes Introduction to William Rathbone's *The Organization of Nursing in a Large Town* (Rathbone, 1865); assists with establishing nursing at the Derby Infirmary; advises on Swansea General Infirmary; issues a proposal for nursing in Indian hospitals (Nightingale, 1865); Herbert Hospital, the model army pavilion hospital, opens.

1866 Nightingale advocates quality care for the poorest, as good as for the rich; proposes abolition of most of the Poor Law (McDonald, 2004a, pp. 337–353); begins correspondence on sending nurses to Australia (McDonald, 2009a, Australian Hospitals, pp. 404–415); begins to assist Crown Princess of Prussia on nursing in Prussia (McDonald, 2009a, pp. 450–453), Princess Alice in Hesse-Darmstadt (McDonald, 2009a, pp. 453–460), and nurse Emmy Rappe for Sweden (Johannson, 1977).

1867 Nightingale submits brief to Parliamentary committee on training and organizing nursing in workhouse infirmaries (Nightingale, 1867, in Part II, Chapter 11); her letter on workhouse nursing published in Rathbone, *Workhouse Nursing: The Story of a Successful Experiment* (Rathbone, 1867).

1868 On death of Agnes Jones (tribute in Part II, Chapter 11). Nightingale seeks replacement for Liverpool; King's College Hospital closes midwifery ward and training program, on account of excessive maternal deaths postchildbirth; Nightingale nurses under Lucy Osburn begin work at the Sydney Infirmary, Australia (McDonald, 2009a, pp. 416–439).

1869 Nightingale starts work on nursing for Highgate Workhouse Infirmary, London; new Leeds General Infirmary, on which she advised, opens; new Nightingale Wing opened at Sydney Infirmary, Australia, a model nursing residence.

1870 Nightingale sends paper on Indian sanitation to Bengal Social Science Association (Nightingale, 1870, in Vallée, 2007, pp. 235–243).

1870–1871 Nightingale assists with relief and nursing, for both sides, of the Franco-Prussian War, decorated by both sides after it (McDonald, 2011, pp. 603–822).

1871 Nightingale publishes pioneering study on maternal mortality, *Introductory Notes on Lying-in Institutions* (McDonald, 2005); Queen opens new St. Thomas' Hospital in London, model civil hospital, with a comfortable nurses' residence.

1872 Nightingale undertakes greater supervision at her school at St. Thomas'; issues first "address" to nurses and student nurses; academic lectures reinstated; "home sister," or tutor, appointed; Nightingale advises Dr. Gill Wylie on nursing for Bellevue Hospital, New York City (McDonald, 2009a, pp. 498–508).

1873 Medical instructor at the Nightingale School publishes his *Notes of Lectures at St. Thomas' Hospital* (Croft, 1873); first three American schools of nursing open using Nightingale methods: Bellevue Hospital, New York City; New England Hospital for Women, Boston; Connecticut Training School, New Haven; Nightingale nurses begin nursing at Edinburgh Royal Infirmary, then take nursing to other Scottish hospitals (McDonald,

2009a, pp. 304–383); first nursing school in Canada with Nightingale principles opens, Mack Training School, St Catherines, Ontario.

1874 Nightingale assists with founding of the Metropolitan and National Nursing Association (McDonald, 2009a, pp. 723–760); advises on children's hospital for Moscow; Florence Lees publishes, with much advice from Nightingale, *Handbook for Hospital Sisters* (Lees, 1874).

1875 Nightingale corresponds with Sir Patrick Dun's Hospital, Dublin, on starting trained nursing; begins work to send nurses to Montreal; issues paper on starting nursing in Belfast; circulates major paper, *The Zemindar, The Sun and the Watering Pot as affecting Life or Death in India* (Nightingale, 1875 in Vallée, 2007, pp. 401–442).

1876 Publishes "Trained Nurses for the Sick Poor" (Nightingale, 1876); advises Dr. John Shaw Billings on plans for Johns Hopkins University Hospital, Baltimore; advises on nursing at St. Mary's, Paddington, London, and at the Belfast Hospital for Sick Children; Nightingale nurses, with Maria Machin as nursing director, start at Montreal General Hospital; Nightingale nurse Jessie Lennox becomes first trained nursing director at Belfast Children's Hospital.

1877 Nightingale advises on nursing for Addenbrooke's Hospital, Cambridge (Alice Fisher, nursing director); Nightingale nurses Rachel Williams and Alice Fisher (1877) publish *Hints for Hospital Nurses*; New York Hospital Training School for Nurses opens, on Nightingale principles.

1878 Nightingale meets with first American trained nurse, Linda Richards; assists with nurses for the Anglo-Zulu War; addresses abuse issues at Buxton Hospital, Derbyshire; Nightingale nurse Elizabeth Vincent starts professional nursing in Lincoln County Hospital; Bellevue Hospital publishes *A Manual of Nursing* for its training school, closely modeled on Nightingale's *Notes on Nursing* (Bellevue Hospital, 1878).

1879 Nightingale publishes "Irrigation and Water Transit in India"; Maria Machin starts as nursing director at St. Bartholomew's Hospital, London.

1880 Nightingale begins work to bring trained nurses into the St. Marylebone Workhouse Infirmary, London.

1881 Nightingale assists with starting nursing at Royal Hospital for Incurables; Elizabeth Vincent starts professional nursing at St. Marylebone workhouse Infirmary, London, with new hospital building, on which Nightingale advised.

1882 Nightingale advises on nursing and relief for the Egyptian campaign; Prince Alfred Hospital, Sydney, opens.

1883 Nightingale publishes articles in Quain's *Dictionary of Medicine* (Nightingale, 1883, in Part II, Chapter 12); Nightingale awarded Royal Red Cross, an award established by Queen Victoria for army nurses.

1884   Nightingale publishes *Practical advice in view of the rapid spread of cholera: "scavenge, scavenge, scavenge"* (Nightingale, 1884, in Part II, Chapter 12); Eva Luckes (1884) publishes *Lectures on General Nursing*; Agnes Snively starts trained nursing at Toronto General Hospital, on Nightingale principles; first Nightingale-type nursing begun in China, in Shanghai (Lin, 1938, p. 3; Yuhong, 2017).

1885   Nightingale assists Nightingale nurse Ella Pirrie in starting nursing at the Belfast Workhouse Infirmary, assists with sending nurses and relief for second Egyptian campaign; Alice Fisher starts professional nursing and nurse training at the Blockley Hospital, Philadelphia.

1886   Nightingale works on medical assistance and health promotion for women in India (Vallée, 2006, Nursing in India, pp. 939–980); assists on nursing and planning for Gordon Boys' Home (Add Mss[1] 45808 & 45809).

1887   Nightingale advises on nursing at the Homerton Fever Hospital; Dr. Joseph Bell, Edinburgh, publishes *Notes on Surgery for Nurses*, dedicated to her (Bell, 1887); her advice on local sanitation quoted at meetings of the Public Health Section of the British Medical Association (*Belfast News-Letter*, 1887).

1888   "Letter from Miss Nightingale" published in *Journal of the Public Health Society* (Nightingale, 1888); advises on plans and helps raise funds for Women's Hospital, Euston Rd., London (McDonald, 2012, pp. 884–891); Nightingale nurse Ella Pirrie starts as nursing director at Union (Workhouse) Infirmary, Belfast, starts first training of workhouse nurses in Ireland (Pirrie letter, July 28, 1888, Add Mss 45808 f177); Nightingale advises army nurses sent to nurse in India (Loch letter, September 18, 1888, Add Mss 45808 f37).

1889   Nightingale begins to mentor Eva Luckes, nursing director, London Hospital; Nightingale nurse Louisa Parsons first trained nursing director at University of Maryland Training School, Baltimore; Florence Lees Craven publishes *A Guide to District Nurses* (Craven, 1889).

1890   Nightingale publishes "Hospitals" in *Chambers's Encyclopaedia* (Nightingale, 1890); does Introduction for *Sketch of the History and Progress of District Nursing* (Rathbone, 1890); publishes revised articles for Quain's *Dictionary of Medicine*.

1891   Trained nursing begins at the Radcliffe Infirmary, Oxford, with Nightingale nurse Flora Masson as nursing director; in the 1890s five nursing schools established in Japan on Nightingale principles (Takahashi, 2004, p. 2).

1892   Nightingale publishes tribute to St. Thomas' nursing director Sarah Wardroper on her death (Nightingale, 1892); her advice on

---

[1] Further references to Add Mss (Additional Manuscripts) are also to the British Library.

cholera prevention quoted by leading doctors at National Health Society meetings (*Dundee Courier & Argus*, 1892 and *Sheffield and Rotherham Independent*, 1892).

1893   Nightingale paper "Sick nursing and health nursing" read at Chicago World Congress (Nightingale, 1893, in Part II, Chapter 12); she accepts honorary degree from the New Jersey Training School for Nurses; meets with Louise Darche, nursing director at the New York Training School for Nurses; sends joint letter, "Royal British Nurses' Association," opposing its proposal for state registration to *The Times* and *The Lancet* (Nightingale et al., 1893, July 3 and July 8); Isabel Hampton Robb publishes *Nursing: Its Principles and Practice for Hospital and Private Use*, using Nightingale principles (Robb, 1893); Lillian Wald establishes "public health nursing" in New York City, similar to U.K. district nursing.

1894   Nightingale publishes on rural health and local government (Nightingale, 1894); meets with Isabel Hampton Robb in London; begins advising on nurse training in Italy (McDonald, 2009a, pp. 480–491).

1895   Corresponds with Dr. Alfred Worcester on nursing at the Waltham Training School, Boston (McDonald, 2009a, pp. 516–519); Nightingale nurse Rebecca Strong gives paper on nurse education, on the new 3-year program, with 3 months of lectures before ward work (Matrons' Council, 1895).

1896   Nightingale publishes Health missioners for rural India (Vallée, 2007, pp. 388–392); mentors Finnish nurse Ellen Ekblom (McDonald, 2009a, pp. 491–495); Nightingale nurse Florence A. Haig Brown publishes *Hints on Elementary Physiology* (Haig Brown, 1896).

1897   Nightingale nurse Amy Hughes publishes *Practical Hints on District Nursing* (Hughes, 1897); Nightingale meets with Elisabeth Robinson Scovil, nursing director at Black Island, New York; advises Georgina Franklin, leaving to do plague nursing in India (Vallée, 2007, pp. 791–796).

1898   Corresponds with Lady Aberdeen on starting district nursing in Canada; Nightingale nurses start nursing in Hong Kong; Louisa Parsons nurses in Spanish-American War; Eva Luckes publishes *General Nursing*.

1899   Nightingale meets with nursing leaders from the United States, Canada, and New Zealand, in London for the International Congress of Women; American nurses with Nightingale training start nursing in Cuba (Hibbard, 1902).

1899–1901   Boer War: Many British and American nurses with Nightingale-type training volunteer to nurse in it, Nightingale only peripherally involved in sending nurses.

1900   Nightingale advises on nursing in Japan; issues last "address" to nurses; stops most active work; International Council of Nurses founded, uses definition of nursing similar to Nightingale's.

1901 A. L. Pringle, long mentored by Nightingale, becomes head of St. Philomena's Training School, Belfast, for the Mater Infirmorum, nursed by the (Irish) Sisters of Mercy; first Nightingale nursing in France, Bordeaux, begun by Dr. Anna Hamilton (Huda, 1979, p. 52); Hamilton publishes first French book on nursing, *Les gardes-malades* (Hamilton & Regnault, 1901).

1902 Nightingale nurse Amy Hughes becomes head of county nursing at Queen Victoria Jubilee Institute of Nursing.

1904 Nightingale sends last, short, letter on district nursing to South Australia.

1905 A. L. Pringle publishes *A Study in Nursing* (Pringle, 1905), becomes nursing director at Waltham, Massachusetts.

1907 Adelaide Nutting becomes first professor of nursing; she and Lavinia Dock publish first two volumes of *History of Nursing* (Waltham, Mass, & Dock, 1907–1912).

1909 Nightingale given a Spanish lace mantilla by Cuban nurse delegates at the International Council of Nurses ("A Sacred Spot," 1909).

1910 Death of Nightingale; University of Minnesota launches first university training of nurses; first nurse training school in Italy opened on "Sistema Florence Nightingale" at Policlinco, Rome (Turton note, Add Mss 47759 f191).

NIGHTINGALE'S INFLUENCE AFTER HER DEATH TO THE END OF THE 20TH CENTURY

1911 Dr. Lauder Brunton publishes Letters from Miss Florence Nightingale on Health Visiting in Rural Districts (Brunton, 1911).

1912 Lavinia Dock publishes last two volumes of History of Nursing (Nutting & Dock, 1907–1912).

1913 Two-volume official biography published (Cook, 1913).

1914 Nightingale cousin Rosalind Nash publishes selection of her addresses to nurses and student nurses (Nash, 1914).

1914–1918 First World War, many Nightingale nurses serve as nursing directors and nurses in war hospitals.

1922 Florence Nightingale School for Nurses opens in Bordeaux on May 12 (her birthday), the first nurse training school in France, with director Dr. Anna Hamilton; Bertha Harmer publishes *Text-Book of the Principles and Practice of Nursing* using Nightingale principles (Harmer, 1922).

1931 Florence Haig Brown publishes *Probationer's Primer: A Guide for the First Year Nurse* (Haig Brown, 1931).

1932 Annie Goodrich publishes *The Social and Ethical Significance of Nursing* using Nightingale principles (Goodrich, 1932).

1939 Bertha Harmer and Virginia Henderson publish *Text-Book of the Principles and Practice of Nursing*, 4th ed., a revision of Harmer, 1922

(Harmer & Henderson, 1939); Nightingale's *Notes on Nursing* published in Finnish and Swahili.

1946 U.K. National Health Service Act adopted; Poor Law abolished.

1948 National Health Service launched in the United Kingdom, establishing quality care for all, regardless of ability to pay, with commitment to health promotion; WHO established, with definition of health similar to Nightingale's.

1950 American Nurses Association adopts Code of Ethics citing her: "Florence Nightingale believed that a nurse's ethical duty was first and foremost to care for the patient."

1953 International Council of Nurses adopts Code of Ethics.

1954 Centennial of Nightingale's arrival at Crimean War celebrated; Florence Nightingale Museum opened at Barrack Hospital, Scutari, Turkey.

1960 Centennial of founding of Nightingale School marked with a publication on it (Seymer, 1960).

1961 Florence Nightingale School of Nursing founded in Istanbul.

1962 Publication of *A Bio-Bibliography of Florence Nightingale* (Bishop & Goldie, 1962).

1976 Sister Callista Roy develops adaptation model of nursing, using Nightingale's environmental principles (Roy & Andrews, 1999).

1978 U.N. Alma Ata Declaration makes health a "human right," its attainment "a most important world-wide social goal," for "access to timely, acceptable and affordable health care" (United Nations, 1978); sixth edition of Harmer's text published, *The Principles and Practice of Nursing* (Henderson & Nite, 1978).

1980s Hospital architects renew interest in Nightingale's principles (Hammond, 2005; Hickman, 2013; Marcus & Barnes, 1999; M. Nightingale [no relation], 1982; Verderber, 2005).

1989 *Notes on Nursing* published in Portuguese.

1992 Commemorative edition of *Notes on Nursing* published by American nursing leaders (Commemorative, 1992).

1996 First critical edition of *Notes on Nursing* published (Skretkowicz, 1996).

NIGHTINGALE'S INFLUENCE IN THE 21ST CENTURY

2001–2012 *Collected Works of Florence Nightingale* makes her work, 16 volumes, published and unpublished, available in print and as ebooks (McDonald, 2001–12): www.uoguelph.ca/~cwfn

2004 Launch of *Collected Works*, Canada House, Trafalgar Sq., London.

2010 U.S. Affordable Care Act adopted, extending health insurance; new critical edition of *Notes on Nursing* published (Skretkowicz, 2010).

2010 Nightingale Chapel dedicated at Westminster Abbey.

2011 Conferences on Nightingale in Tokyo universities.

2012 Nightingale Society formed to promote her work and defend her reputation: nightingalesociety.com. Gottlieb (2012) publishes *Strengths-Based Nursing Care*, drawing on Nightingale principles; Nightingale chairs in nursing practice launched by Florence Nightingale Foundation.

2014 Nightingale's views on fresh air related to microbiome findings (Arnold, 2014); Nightingale named in poll as one of top women "who changed the world," after Marie Curie (twice a Nobel Prize winner), before (former Prime Minister) Margaret Thatcher and Mother Theresa of Calcutta (Winter, 2014)

2016 Commonwealth Nurses and Midwives Federation celebrates Nightingale's work at its congress in London.

REFERENCES

Adams, G. W. (1952). *Doctors in blue: The medical history of the Union army in the civil war*. New York, NY: Henry Schuman.

Arnold, C. (2014, July). Rethinking sterile: The hospital microbiome. *Environmental Health Perspectives, 12*, 7. doi:10.1289/ehp.122-A182

"A sacred spot." (1909, August 7). *British Journal of Nursing, 117.*

Belfast News-Letter. (1887, August 4). British Medical Association.

Bell, J. (1887). *Notes on surgery for nurses.* Edinburgh, UK: Oliver & Boyd.

Bellevue Hospital. (1878). *A manual of nursing prepared for the Training School for Nurses attached to Bellevue Hospital.* New York, NY: G.P. Putnam & Sons.

Bishop, W.J., & Goldie, S. [COMPS.]. (1962). *A bio-bibliography of Florence Nightingale.* London, UK: Dawson.

Brunton, L. (1911). *Letters from Miss Florence Nightingale on health visiting in rural districts.* London, UK: P. S. King.

Commemorative edition. (1992). *Notes on nursing: What it is and what it is not.* (Commemorative edition) Philadelphia, PA: J. B. Lippincott. ISBN: 0397550073.

Cook, E. T. (1913). *The life of Florence Nightingale* (2 vols). London, UK: Macmillan.

Craven, F. L. (1889). *A guide to district nurses.* London, UK: Macmillan.

Croft, J. (1873). *Notes of lectures at St. Thomas' Hospital.* London, UK: St. Thomas/ Blades, East & Blades.

Dundee Courier & Argus. (1892, September 2). A medical authority's warning.

Goodrich, A. W. (1932). *The social and ethical significance of nursing: A series of addresses.* New York, NY: Macmillan.

Gottlieb, L. (2012). *Strengths-based nursing care: Health and healing for person and family.* New York, NY: Springer Publishing. ISBN: 9780826195869.

Haig Brown, F. A. (1896). *Hints on elementary physiology*. London, UK: J. & A. Churchill.

Haig Brown, F. (1931). *Probationer's primer: A guide for the 1st year nurse*. London, UK: H. F. & G. Witherby.

Hamilton, A., & Regnault, F. (1901). *Les gardes-malades: congreganistes, mercenaires, amateurs, professionelles*. Paris, France: Vigot.

Hammond, C. (2005, July). Reforming architecture, defending empire: Florence Nightingale and the pavilion hospital. *Studies in the Social Sciences, 38*, 1–24.

Harmer, B. (1922). *Textbook of the principles and practice of nursing*. New York, NY: Macmillan.

Harmer, B., & Henderson, V. (1939). *Textbook of the principles and practice of nursing* (4th ed.). New York, NY: Macmillan.

Henderson, V., & Nite, G. (1978). *Principles and practice of nursing* (6th ed.). New York, NY: Macmillan.

Hibbard, M. E. (1902, September 1). The establishment of schools for nurses in Cuba. *American Journal of Nursing, 2*(12), 985–991.

Hickman, C. (2013). *Therapeutic landscapes: A history of English Hospital Gardens since 1800*. Manchester: Manchester University Press. ISBN: 978-0-7190-8660-1.

Huda, A.-S. (1979). *Nursing: A world view*. St. Louis, MO: C.V. Mosby. ISBN: 0-8016-6065-0.

Hughes, A. (1897). *Practical hints on district nursing* (3rd. ed.). London, UK: Scientific Press.

Johannson, J. (Ed.). (1977). *"God Bless You, My Dear Miss Nightingale": Letters from Emmy Carolina Rappe to Florence Nightingale 1867–1870*. Stockholm, Sweden: Almqvist & Wiksell.

Lees, F. (Ed.) (1874). *Handbook for hospital sisters*. London, UK: H. W. Acland.

Lin, E. (1938). Nursing in China. *American Journal of Nursing, 38*(1), 1–8.

Luckes, E. (1884). *Lectures on general nursing*. London, UK: Kegan Paul.

Marcus, C. C., & Barnes, M. (Eds.). (1999). *Healing gardens: Therapeutic benefits and design recommendations*. New York, NY: John Wiley. ISBN: 0471192031.

Matrons' Council. (1895). Report. British Library Add Mss 47726 f80

McDonald, L. (Ed.). (2001–2012). *Collected works of Florence Nightingale*. Waterloo, ON, Canada: Wilfrid Laurier University Press.

McDonald, L. (Ed.). (2003). *Florence Nightingale on society and politics, philosophy, science, education, and literature*. Waterloo, ON, Canada: Wilfrid Laurier University Press.

McDonald, L., (Ed.). (2004a). *Florence Nightingale on public health care*. Waterloo, ON, Canada: Wilfrid Laurier University Press. ISBN: 0-88920-446-2.

McDonald, L. (Ed.). (2004b). *Florence Nightingale's European travels*. Waterloo, ON, Canada: Wilfrid Laurier University Press. ISBN: 0-88920-451-9.

McDonald, L. (Ed.). (2005). *Florence Nightingale on women, medicine, midwifery, and prostitution*. Waterloo, ON, Canada: Wilfrid Laurier University Press.

McDonald, L. (Ed.). (2009a). *Florence Nightingale: Extending nursing*. Waterloo, ON, Canada: Wilfrid Laurier University Press. ISBN: 978-1-55458-170-2.

McDonald, L. (Ed.). (2009b). *Florence Nightingale: The Nightingale School* (934 pages). Waterloo, ON, Canada: Wilfrid Laurier University Press. ISBN: 978-1-55458-169-6.

McDonald, L. (Ed.). (2010). *Florence Nightingale and the Crimean war*. Waterloo, ON, Canada: Wilfrid Laurier University Press. ISBN: 978-1-55458-245-7.

McDonald, L. (Ed.). (2011). *Florence Nightingale on wars and the war office*. Waterloo, ON, Canada: Wilfrid Laurier University Press.

McDonald, L. (Ed.). (2012). *Florence Nightingale and hospital reform*. Waterloo, ON, Canada: Wilfrid Laurier University Press. ISBN: 978-0-88920-471-3.

Nash, R. (Ed.). (1914). *Florence Nightingale to her nurses: A selection from Miss Nightingale's addresses to probationers and nurses of the Nightingale School at St. Thomas's Hospital*. London, UK: Macmillan.

Nightingale, F. (1858a). *Answers to written questions addressed to Miss Nightingale by the commissioners. Report of the Commissioners appointed to inquire into the regulations affecting the sanitary condition of the army and the treatment of the sick and wounded* (pp. 361–394). London, UK: Her Majesty's Stationery Office.

Nightingale, F. (1858b). *Notes on matters affecting the health, efficiency, and hospital administration of the British Army*. London, UK: Harrison.

Nightingale, F. (1858c). *Subsidiary notes on the introduction of female nursing into military hospitals in peace and in war*. London, UK: Harrison & Sons.

Nightingale, F. (1858d). *Notes on the sanitary condition of hospitals, and on defects in the construction of hospital wards*. Liverpool, UK: Record Office.

Nightingale, F. (1858, August 28). Sites and construction of hospitals. *The Builder*, *16*, 812.

Nightingale, F. (1858, September 11). Construction of hospitals: The ground plan. *The Builder*, *16*(814), 609–611.

Nightingale, F. (1858, September 25). Hospital construction—Wards. *The Builder*, *16*(816), 641–643.

Nightingale, F. (1859a). Notes on hospitals. *Transactions of the National Association for the Promotion of Social Science*, 462–482.

Nightingale, F. (1859b). *Notes on hospitals, being two papers read before the National Association for the Promotion of Social Science, at Liverpool, in October 1858, With Evidence given to the Royal Commissioners on the State of the Army in 1857*. London, UK: John Parker.

Nightingale, F. (1860a). *Notes on nursing: What it is, and what it is not*. London, UK: Harrison.

Nightingale, F. (1860b). *Notes on nursing: What it is and what it is not* (new ed., rev.). London, UK: Harrison (library standard version).

Nightingale, F. (1861). *Notes on nursing for the labouring classes*. London, UK: Harrison.

Nightingale, F. (1862). Note on the Supposed Protection Afforded Against Venereal Diseases, by recognizing Prostitution and Putting It under Police Regulation. Private and Confidential. Printed paper.

Nightingale, F. (1863). *Notes on hospitals* (3rd ed.). London, UK: Longmans, Green.

Nightingale, F. (1864a). How people may live and not die in India. *Transactions of the National Association for the Promotion of Social Science*.

Nightingale, F. (1864b). *Note on the aboriginal races in Australia* (pp. 552–558). London, UK: *Transactions of the National Association for the Promotion of Social Science*.

Nightingale, F. (1865). *Suggestions on a system of nursing for hospitals in India*. London, UK: Her Majesty's Stationery Office.

Nightingale, F. (1867). *Suggestions on the subject of providing training and organizing nurses for the sick poor in workhouse infirmaries*. London, UK: Her Majesty's Stationery Office.

Nightingale, F. (1870). On Indian sanitation. *Transactions of the Bengal Social Science Association*, 4, 1–9.

Nightingale, F. (1875). *The Zemindar, The Sun and the Watering Pot as affecting Life or Death in India*. Printed paper, British Library Cup 503. p.27.

Nightingale, F. (1876, April 14). Trained nurses for the sick poor. *The Times*, 6CD.

Nightingale, F. (1888, October). Letter from Miss Nightingale. *Journal of the Public Health Society*, 4(2), 62–65.

Nightingale, F. (1883). Nurses, training of, and Nursing the sick. In R. Quain (Ed.), *A dictionary of medicine* (Vol. 2, pp. 1038–1049). London, UK: Longmans, Green.

Nightingale, F. (1884). Practical advice in view of the rapid spread of cholera: "scavenge, scavenge, scavenge." In A. N. Bell (Ed.), *The sanitarian* (Vol. 13, pp. 114–115).

Nightingale, F. (1890). Hospitals. *Chambers's encyclopaedia: A dictionary of universal knowledge* (Vol. 5, pp. 805–807). Edinburgh, UK: W. & R. Chambers.

Nightingale, F. (1892, December 13). The reform of sick nursing and the late Mrs Wardroper: The extinction of Mrs Gamp. *British Medical Journal*, 1448.

Nightingale, F. (1893). Sick nursing and health nursing. In A. Burdett-Coutts (Ed.), *Woman's mission: A series of congress papers on the philanthropic work of women* (pp. 184–205). London, UK: Sampson, Low, Marston.

Nightingale, F., Westminster, J. G., Carter, H. B., Bristowe, J. S., Sharkey, S. J., Gordon, L. M.,...Marsden, A. (1893, July 3). Royal British Nurses' Association. *The Times*, 7C.

Nightingale, F., Westminster (Duke of), J. G., Carter, H. B., Bristowe, J. S., Sharkey, S. J., Gordon, L. M.,...Marsden, A. (1893, July 8). Royal British Nurses' Association. *The Lancet*, 113–114.

Nightingale, F. (1894). *Health teaching in towns and villages: Rural hygiene* (pp. 46–60). Leeds, UK: Official Report of the Central Conference of Women Workers.

Nightingale, M. (1982, July 28). Buildings update: Part 2: Evolving wards. *Architecture Journal*, 47–50.

Nutting, A., & Dock, L.L. (1907–12). *A history of nursing: The evolution of nursing systems from the earliest times to the foundation of the first English and American training schools for nurses* (4 vols). New York, NY: G. P. Putnam's Sons.

Pringle, A.L. (1905). *A study in nursing*. London, UK: Macmillan.

Rathbone, W. (1865). *The organization of nursing in a large town*. Liverpool, UK: Holden.

Rathbone, W. (1867). *Workhouse nursing: The story of a successful experiment*. London, UK: Macmillan.

Rathbone. W. (1890). *Sketch of the history and progress of district nursing from its commencement in the year 1859 to the present date*. London, UK: Macmillan.

Robb, I. H. (1893). *Nursing: Its principles and practice for hospital and private use*. Philadelphia, PA: W. B. Saunders.

Roy, C., & Andrews, H. A. (1999). *The Roy adaptation model* (2nd ed.). Stamford, CT: Appleton & Lange. ISBN: 0838522718.

Seymer, L. (1960). *Florence Nightingale's nurses: The Nightingale Training School 1860– 1960.* London, UK: Pitman Medical.

Sheffield and Rotherham Independent (1892, September 3). More good advice.

Skretkowicz, V. (Ed.) (1996). *Florence Nightingale's notes on nursing.* London, UK: Baillière Tindall. ISBN: 1-871364-63-9.

Skretkowicz, V. (Ed.) 2010. *Florence Nightingale's notes on nursing and notes on nursing for the labouring classes: Commemorative edition with historical commentary.* New York, NY: Springer Publishing. ISBN: 9780826118424.

Takahashi, A. (2004). *The development of the Japanese nursing profession: Adopting and adapting western influences.* London, UK: Routledge Curzon. ISBN: 0-203-32245-2.

The Times (1872, August 7). The treatment of prisoners of war, 3F.

United Nations (1978, September). Declaration of Alma Ata. International Conference on Primary Health Care. Retrieved from http://www.who.int/publications/almaata_declaration_en.pdf?ua=1

Vallée, G. (Ed.) (2006). *Florence Nightingale on health in India.* Waterloo, ON, Canada: Wilfrid Laurier University Press. ISBN: 10-0-88920-468-3.

Vallée, G. (Ed.) (2007). *Florence Nightingale on social change in India.* Waterloo, ON, Canada: Wilfrid Laurier University Press. ISBN: 978-0-88920-495-9.

Verderber, S. (2005). *Compassion in architecture: Evidence-based design for health in Louisiana.* Lafayette: Center for Louisiana Studies. ISBN: 9781887366632.

Virginia, Surgeon General (1861). *Directions for cooking by troops, in camp and hospital, prepared for the army of Virginia.* Richmond, VA: Ritchie & Dunnavant.

Williams, R., & Fisher, A. (1877). *Hints for hospital nurses.* Edinburgh, UK: Maclachlan & Stewart.

Winter, K. (2014). Marie Curie, Florence Nightingale and Margaret Thatcher top list of women who have changed the world. Retrieved from http://www.dailymail.co.uk/femail/article-2847232/Marie-Curie-Florence-Nightingale-Margaret-Thatcher-list-women-changed-world.html

Yuhong, J. (2017, January). Shaping modern nursing development in China before 1949. *International Journal of Nursing Sciences, 4*(1), 19–23. doi:10:1016/j.ijnss.2016.12.009

Index